Prognostic Factors for Pediatric Tumors

Prognostic Factors for Pediatric Tumors

Editors

Maria Kourti
Emmanouel Hatzipantelis

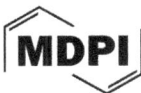

Basel • Beijing • Wuhan • Barcelona • Belgrade • Novi Sad • Cluj • Manchester

Editors
Maria Kourti
Third Department of Pediatrics
Aristotle University
of Thessaloniki
Thessaloniki
Greece

Emmanouel Hatzipantelis
Children & Adolescent
Hematology-Oncology Unit
Aristotle University of Thessaloniki
Thessaloniki
Greece

Editorial Office
MDPI
St. Alban-Anlage 66
4052 Basel, Switzerland

This is a reprint of articles from the Special Issue published online in the open access journal *Diagnostics* (ISSN 2075-4418) (available at: www.mdpi.com/journal/diagnostics/special_issues/prognostic_pediatric_tumors).

For citation purposes, cite each article independently as indicated on the article page online and as indicated below:

Lastname, A.A.; Lastname, B.B. Article Title. *Journal Name* **Year**, *Volume Number*, Page Range.

ISBN 978-3-0365-9703-4 (Hbk)
ISBN 978-3-0365-9702-7 (PDF)
doi.org/10.3390/books978-3-0365-9702-7

© 2023 by the authors. Articles in this book are Open Access and distributed under the Creative Commons Attribution (CC BY) license. The book as a whole is distributed by MDPI under the terms and conditions of the Creative Commons Attribution-NonCommercial-NoDerivs (CC BY-NC-ND) license.

Contents

Preface vii

Maria Kourti and Emmanouel Hatzipantelis
Evolving Aspects of Prognostic Factors for Pediatric Cancer
Reprinted from: *Diagnostics* 2023, 13, 3515, doi:10.3390/diagnostics13233515 1

Maria Kourti, Michalis Aivaliotis and Emmanouel Hatzipantelis
Proteomics in Childhood Acute Lymphoblastic Leukemia: Challenges and Opportunities
Reprinted from: *Diagnostics* 2023, 13, 2748, doi:10.3390/diagnostics13172748 5

Eleni P Kotanidou, Styliani Giza, Vasiliki Rengina Tsinopoulou, Kosmas Margaritis, Anastasia Papadopoulou and Eleni Sakellari et al.
The Prognostic Significance of BRAF Gene Analysis in Children and Adolescents with Papillary Thyroid Carcinoma: A Systematic Review and Meta-Analysis
Reprinted from: *Diagnostics* 2023, 13, 1187, doi:10.3390/diagnostics13061187 23

Chrysoula Margioula-Siarkou, Stamatios Petousis, Aristarchos Almperis, Georgia Margioula-Siarkou, Antonio Simone Laganà and Maria Kourti et al.
Sarcoma Botryoides: Optimal Therapeutic Management and Prognosis of an Unfavorable Malignant Neoplasm of Female Children
Reprinted from: *Diagnostics* 2023, 13, 924, doi:10.3390/diagnostics13050924 41

Anastasios Serbis, Vasiliki Rengina Tsinopoulou, Anastasia Papadopoulou, Savvas Kolanis, Eleni I. Sakellari and Kosmas Margaritis et al.
Predictive Factors for Pediatric Craniopharyngioma Recurrence: An Extensive Narrative Review
Reprinted from: *Diagnostics* 2023, 13, 1588, doi:10.3390/diagnostics13091588 56

Chrysoula Margioula-Siarkou, Stamatios Petousis, Georgia Margioula-Siarkou, George Mavromatidis, Fotios Chatzinikolaou and Emmanouel Hatzipantelis et al.
Therapeutic Management and Prognostic Factors for Ovarian Malignant Tumours in Adolescents: A Comprehensive Review of Current Guidelines
Reprinted from: *Diagnostics* 2023, 13, 1080, doi:10.3390/diagnostics13061080 76

Charikleia Ntenti, Konstantinos Lallas and Georgios Papazisis
Clinical, Histological, and Molecular Prognostic Factors in Childhood Medulloblastoma: Where Do We Stand?
Reprinted from: *Diagnostics* 2023, 13, 1915, doi:10.3390/diagnostics13111915 99

Mirella Ampatzidou, Stefanos I. Papadhimitriou, Anna Paisiou, Georgios Paterakis, Marianna Tzanoudaki and Vassilios Papadakis et al.
The Prognostic Effect of CDKN2A/2B Gene Deletions in Pediatric Acute Lymphoblastic Leukemia (ALL): Independent Prognostic Significance in BFM-Based Protocols
Reprinted from: *Diagnostics* 2023, 13, 1589, doi:10.3390/diagnostics13091589 116

Maria A. Karalexi, Georgios Markozannes, Christos F. Tagkas, Andreas Katsimpris, Xanthippi Tseretopoulou and Konstantinos K. Tsilidis et al.
Nutritional Status at Diagnosis as Predictor of Survival from Childhood Cancer: A Review of the Literature
Reprinted from: *Diagnostics* 2022, 12, 2357, doi:10.3390/diagnostics12102357 132

Kondylia Antoniadi, Nikolaos Thomaidis, Petros Nihoyannopoulos, Konstantinos Toutouzas, Evangelos Gikas and Charikleia Kelaidi et al.
Prognostic Factors for Cardiotoxicity among Children with Cancer: Definition, Causes, and Diagnosis with Omics Technologies
Reprinted from: *Diagnostics* **2023**, *13*, 1864, doi:10.3390/diagnostics13111864 . . . . **145**

Andrada Mara Ardelean, Ioana Cristina Olariu, Raluca Isac, Akhila Nalla, Ruxandra Jurac and Cristiana Stolojanu et al.
Impact of Cancer Type and Treatment Protocol on Cardiac Function in Pediatric Oncology Patients: An Analysis Utilizing Speckle Tracking, Global Longitudinal Strain, and Myocardial Performance Index
Reprinted from: *Diagnostics* **2023**, *13*, 2830, doi:10.3390/diagnostics13172830 . . . . **172**

Preface

Currently, it is estimated that over 80% of children diagnosed with cancer will be cured. This estimate is encouraging and reflects the significant progress made in recent decades, in both supportive care and the risk stratification of patients. Despite these significant advancements in the treatment of childhood cancer, it remains one of the leading causes of death in children and adolescents worldwide. Considerable research efforts have been focused on the biological characterization of the disease in order to refine risk group stratification and facilitate targeted therapies.

Biology has historically played a pivotal role in the prognostic risk assessment of childhood leukemia. The genomic landscape of pediatric leukemia has been mapped and redefined following large-scale sequencing efforts. Pediatric solid tumors are also biologically and morphologically heterogenous, and the interplay between histologic examination and molecular interrogation has a significant role in the prognostication and direction of therapy.

The incorporation of molecularly targeted therapies offers real promise for less toxic and more effective therapy. The identification of novel diagnostic and prognostic markers is required to individualize therapy.

In this Special Issue, recent advancements are discussed, and novel prognostic markers are critically appraised. Greater understanding of the heterogeneity of pediatric cancers will ultimately lead to new therapeutic strategies with the potential to provide new prospects for precision medicine in pediatric oncology.

Maria Kourti and Emmanouel Hatzipantelis
Editors

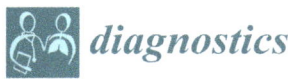

Editorial

Evolving Aspects of Prognostic Factors for Pediatric Cancer

Maria Kourti [1,*] and Emmanouel Hatzipantelis [2]

1. Third Department of Pediatrics, School of Medicine, Aristotle University and Hippokration General Hospital, 54642 Thessaloniki, Greece
2. Children & Adolescent Hematology-Oncology Unit, Second Department of Pediatrics, School of Medicine, Aristotle University of Thessaloniki, 54124 Thessaloniki, Greece; hatzip@auth.gr
* Correspondence: makourti@auth.gr

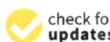

Citation: Kourti, M.; Hatzipantelis, E. Evolving Aspects of Prognostic Factors for Pediatric Cancer. *Diagnostics* **2023**, *13*, 3515. https://doi.org/10.3390/diagnostics13233515

Received: 13 November 2023
Accepted: 20 November 2023
Published: 23 November 2023

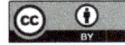

Copyright: © 2023 by the authors. Licensee MDPI, Basel, Switzerland. This article is an open access article distributed under the terms and conditions of the Creative Commons Attribution (CC BY) license (https://creativecommons.org/licenses/by/4.0/).

Advances in risk-directed therapy based on prognostic factors that include clinical, biologic, and genetic features of cancer in children have yielded improved and prolonged responses. This Special Issue of *Diagnostics* consists of ten articles which illuminate different aspects of advances in childhood and adolescent hematology oncology, including original articles and narrative and systematic reviews.

The landmark article of this issue by Kourti et al. provides an extended review of the unanswered challenge of modern omics technology, especially proteomics, in childhood acute lymphoblastic leukemia (ALL) [1]. Proteomic evaluation has impacted the study of solid tumors by increasing the understanding of the underlying tumor biology and, thus, developing promising therapies in the field of oncology by identifying relevant signatures for different cancers [2]. The proteomic profiling of hematologic malignancies creates the opportunity to explore gaps in disease relapse and resistance, as well as to encourage the discovery of novel biomarkers. The identification of proteins and pathways related to the environment and cancer provides an insight into tumor development with the potential to provide new prospects for precision medicine in childhood oncology. Therefore, proteomics may serve as a useful tool for creating innovative and individualized therapy by overcoming increased toxicity from the intensification of treatment in relapsed/refractory childhood ALL.

The genetic landscape of childhood ALL has been broadly studied, yielding novel prognostic markers for risk stratification. Genome-wide technologies and the identification of gene copy-number alterations (CNAs) implicated in leukemogenesis have led to the relentless decoding of the underlying biology of pediatric ALL [3]. One of the most frequent genes affected is the CDKN2A/2B gene, serving as a secondary cooperating event and contributing to cell-cycle regulation chemosensitivity [4]. In the original study by Ampatzidou et al., the CDKN2A/2B deletion was identified as an additive independent prognostic factor for survival in children treated with contemporary BFM-based protocols that can further genetically refine risk stratification based on minimal residual disease [5].

The review by Ntenti et al. summarizes evidence about clinical, histopathological, and molecular factors that have an impact on the prognosis of childhood medulloblastomas (MBs), which are the most common and highly aggressive neoplasms of the central nervous system [6]. New molecular techniques, genomic and transcriptomic analyses, have played an important role in forming novel molecular subgroups of MBs outlined in the recent 2021 WHO molecular classification [7]. Nevertheless, the great heterogeneity within subgroups is challenging. As molecular and genetic pathways in the pathogenesis of MBs are further elucidated, a new risk stratification system will evolve. This landmarks the dawn of a new era in molecular-based MB stratification and prognosis with the optimal goal of developing patient-tailored therapeutic strategies.

Papillary thyroid cancer (PTC) is the most frequent histopathological type in children, with distinct characteristics and prognosis compared to that in adults [8]. This may be attributed to a discrete molecular basis in the activation of the MAPK pathway and its components. Mutated proto-oncogene B-Raf (BRAF) is the most common genetic alteration in adult PTC, and its prognostic significance has been extensively explored in adults [9]. Kotanidou et al. conducted the first systematic review and meta-analysis on the prognostic significance of BRAF gene mutational status in children and adolescents [10]. Since immunomodulation with BRAF inhibitors and molecularly targeted therapy is an appealing contemporary approach, conclusions made from this systematic review may serve as useful tools to establish guidelines in children and adolescent patients with PTC.

Craniopharyngiomas (CPs) are classified as non-malignant neoplasms but their location, growth pattern, and recurrence rate are associated with significant morbidity and mortality. The aim of the extensive narrative review by Serbis et al. is to identify clinical, morphological, and immunohistochemical factors that are associated with the onset and, mainly, the recurrence of CP [11]. Molecular features such as BRAF gene mutations, altered p53 expression, increased Ki-67 expression, higher VEGF and HIF1a expression, and RARs have been extensively studied as potential predictive factors for CP relapse [11]. Moreover, the decision of whether the surgical removal is followed by radiotherapy, age, adherence to surrounding tissues, histology, specific clinical findings, and molecular features remains to be validated through well-designed multicenter prospective studies, with the ultimate goal of developing targeted adjunct therapies [11].

Ovarian cancer in adolescents is challenging not only because of the rarity of the disease but also because of the particularities and substantial differences in incidence, histology, diagnostic work-up, and therapeutic management between adults and the pediatric/adolescent population. Siarkou et al., in their comparative/narrative review, made a great and valuable effort to combine and concisely summarize the existing guidelines from ESMO 2018, ESGO-SIOPE 2020, EXPeRT/PARTNER 2021, and aTRMG 2022 about the diagnosis, prognosis, and management of ovarian malignancies [12]. The reported differences highlight the need for the adoption of an international consensus to further improve the management of adolescent ovarian cancer.

Botryoid rhabdomyosarcoma (RMS), an aggressive subtype of embryonal RMS, is a rare type of tumor mainly affecting very young girls during infancy and early childhood. The narrative review by Siarkou et al. is the first to provide a comprehensive summary of the main outcomes regarding the optimal therapeutic management and prognosis of sarcoma botryoides in female children [13]. It may serve as the initial step towards the globalization of the standards of practice through prospective observational cohorts with the ultimate goal to improve outcomes of this rare but demanding clinical entity.

The impressive increase in survival exceeding 80% for all cancer types and 90% for ALL in many European and North American countries may be attributed not only to the novel multimodal therapies but also to supportive healthcare [14]. Interesting results were achieved in a recent report which showed that mortality among cancer patients is higher than that of the general population, mainly due to increased cardiotoxicity and the development of second neoplasms [15]. Two articles in this Special Issue focus on the risk of cardiotoxicity. The original article by Ardelean et al. explores whether novel echocardiographic measures like speckle-tracking echocardiography (STE), global longitudinal strain (GLS), and the myocardial performance index (MPI) may predict early changes in cardiac function not detected through traditional methods [16]. The promising results that these novel echocardiographic measures contribute to the early detection and long-term prediction of anthracycline-induced cardiotoxicity need to be validated with further longitudinal studies.

The early and preventive diagnosis of cardiotoxicity after chemotherapy treatment in children with cancer using omics technology is extensively reviewed by Antoniadi et al. Conventional biomarkers used for early detection were incorporated into routine diagnosis and monitoring [17]. Their main limitation was that increased levels were detected after the occurrence of significant cardiac damage. On the contrary, omics including genomics, transcriptomics, proteomics, and metabolomics offer new opportunities for biomarker discovery, providing an understanding of cardiotoxicity beyond traditional technologies.

Cardio-specific miRNAs circulating in plasma are promising biomarkers for the detection of subclinical cardiotoxicity, and metabolomics have the potential to revolutionize the ability of individualized cardio-profiles shedding light on the underlying biological processes of cardiotoxicity [17].

Despite the established prognostic factors in childhood malignancies, nutritional status is identified as a crucial factor for optimal clinical outcomes in children with cancer, hence providing a significant modifiable prognostic tool in childhood cancer management. However, scarce studies have examined the impact of nutritional status on the survival of children with cancer, with the majority of them focusing on hematological malignancies [18]. Karalexi et al. summarized published evidence evaluating the association of under-nutrition and over-nutrition with prognosis and treatment-related toxicities (TRT) in children and adolescents treated for cancer [19]. Interestingly, the risk of death and relapse increased by 30–50% in children with leukemia and higher body mass index at diagnosis [19]. Similarly, the risk of TRT was higher in malnourished children with Ewing sarcoma and osteosarcoma. Longitudinal studies utilizing new technologies and assessing the nutritional status in a standardized way are needed in the direction of personalized interventions [19].

In conclusion, in this Special Issue, recent advances are discussed and novel prognostic markers are critically appraised. A greater understanding of the heterogeneity of pediatric cancers will ultimately lead to new therapeutic strategies with the potential to provide new prospects for precision medicine in pediatric oncology.

Conflicts of Interest: The authors declare no conflict of interest.

References

1. Kourti, M.; Aivaliotis, M.; Hatzipantelis, E. Proteomics in Childhood Acute Lymphoblastic Leukemia: Challenges and Opportunities. *Diagnostics* **2023**, *13*, 2748. [CrossRef] [PubMed]
2. Kwon, Y.W.; Jo, H.S.; Bae, S.; Seo, Y.; Song, P.; Song, M.; Yoon, J.H. Application of proteomics in cancer: Recent trends and approaches for biomarkers discovery. *Front. Med.* **2021**, *8*, 747333. [CrossRef]
3. Brady, S.W.; Roberts, K.G.; Gu, Z.; Shi, L.; Pounds, S.; Pei, D.; Cheng, C.; Dai, Y.; Devidas, M.; Qu, C.; et al. The genomic landscape of pediatric acute lymphoblastic leukemia. *Nat. Genet.* **2022**, *54*, 1376–1389. [CrossRef] [PubMed]
4. Feng, J.; Guo, Y.; Yang, W.; Zou, Y.; Zhang, L.; Chen, Y.; Zhang, Y.; Zhu, X.; Chen, X. Childhood Acute B-Lineage Lymphoblastic Leukemia with CDKN2A/B Deletion Is a Distinct Entity with Adverse Genetic Features and Poor Clinical Outcomes. *Front. Oncol.* **2022**, *12*, 878098. [CrossRef] [PubMed]
5. Ampatzidou, M.; Papadhimitriou, S.I.; Paisiou, A.; Paterakis, G.; Tzanoudaki, M.; Papadakis, V.; Florentin, L.; Polychronopoulou, S. The Prognostic Effect of CDKN2A/2B Gene Deletions in Pediatric Acute Lymphoblastic Leukemia (ALL): Independent Prognostic Significance in BFM-Based Protocols. *Diagnostics* **2023**, *13*, 1589. [CrossRef] [PubMed]
6. Ntenti, C.; Lallas, K.; Papazisis, G. Clinical, Histological, and Molecular Prognostic Factors in Childhood Medulloblastoma: Where Do We Stand? *Diagnostics* **2023**, *13*, 1915. [CrossRef] [PubMed]
7. Louis, D.N.; Perry, A.; Wesseling, P.; Brat, D.J.; Cree, I.A.; Figarella-Branger, D.; Hawkins, C.; Ng, H.K.; Pfister, S.M.; Reifenberger, G.; et al. The 2021 WHO Classification of Tumors of the Central Nervous System: A summary. *Neuro Oncol.* **2021**, *23*, 1231–1251. [CrossRef] [PubMed]
8. Bernier, M.O.; Withrow, D.R.; Berrington de Gonzalez, A.; Lam, C.J.K.; Linet, M.S.; Kitahara, C.M.; Shiels, M.S. Trends in Pediatric Thyroid Cancer Incidence in the United States, 1998–2013. *Cancer* **2019**, *125*, 2497–2505. [CrossRef]
9. Rangel-Pozzo, A.; Sisdelli, L.; Cordioli, M.I.V.; Vaisman, F.; Caria, P.; Mai, S.; Cerutti, J.M. Genetic Landscape of Papillary Thyroid Carcinoma and Nuclear Architecture: An Overview Comparing Pediatric and Adult Populations. *Cancers* **2020**, *12*, 3146. [CrossRef] [PubMed]
10. Kotanidou, E.P.; Giza, S.; Tsinopoulou, V.R.; Margaritis, K.; Papadopoulou, A.; Sakellari, E.; Kolanis, S.; Litou, E.; Serbis, A.; Galli-Tsinopoulou, A. The Prognostic Significance of BRAF Gene Analysis in Children and Adolescents with Papillary Thyroid Carcinoma: A Systematic Review and Meta-Analysis. *Diagnostics* **2023**, *13*, 1187. [CrossRef] [PubMed]
11. Serbis, A.; Tsinopoulou, V.R.; Papadopoulou, A.; Kolanis, S.; Sakellari, E.I.; Margaritis, K.; Litou, E.; Ntouma, S.; Giza, S.; Kotanidou, E.P.; et al. Predictive Factors for Pediatric Craniopharyngioma Recurrence: An Extensive Narrative Review. *Diagnostics* **2023**, *13*, 1588. [CrossRef] [PubMed]
12. Margioula-Siarkou, C.; Petousis, S.; Margioula-Siarkou, G.; Mavromatidis, G.; Chatzinikolaou, F.; Hatzipantelis, E.; Guyon, F.; Dinas, K. Therapeutic Management and Prognostic Factors for Ovarian Malignant Tumours in Adolescents: A Comprehensive Review of Current Guidelines. *Diagnostics* **2023**, *13*, 1080. [CrossRef] [PubMed]

13. Margioula-Siarkou, C.; Petousis, S.; Almperis, A.; Margioula-Siarkou, G.; Laganà, A.S.; Kourti, M.; Papanikolaou, A.; Dinas, K. Sarcoma Botryoides: Optimal Therapeutic Management and Prognosis of an Unfavorable Malignant Neoplasm of Female Children. *Diagnostics* **2023**, *13*, 924. [CrossRef] [PubMed]
14. Erdmann, F.; Frederiksen, L.E.; Bonaventure, A.; Mader, L.; Hasle, H.; Robison, L.L.; Winther, J.F. Childhood cancer: Survival, treatment modalities, late effects and improvements over time. *Cancer Epidemiol.* **2020**, *71*, 101733. [CrossRef] [PubMed]
15. World Health Organization. Double Burden of Malnutrition. Available online: https://www.who.int/nutrition/double-burden-malnutrition/en/ (accessed on 15 September 2018).
16. Ardelean, A.M.; Olariu, I.C.; Isac, R.; Nalla, A.; Jurac, R.; Stolojanu, C.; Murariu, M.; Fericean, R.M.; Braescu, L.; Mavrea, A.; et al. Impact of Cancer Type and Treatment Protocol on Cardiac Function in Pediatric Oncology Patients: An Analysis Utilizing Speckle Tracking, Global Longitudinal Strain, and Myocardial Performance Index. *Diagnostics* **2023**, *13*, 2830. [CrossRef] [PubMed]
17. Antoniadi, K.; Thomaidis, N.; Nihoyannopoulos, P.; Toutouzas, K.; Gikas, E.; Kelaidi, C.; Polychronopoulou, S. Prognostic Factors for Cardiotoxicity among Children with Cancer: Definition, Causes, and Diagnosis with Omics Technologies. *Diagnostics* **2023**, *13*, 1864. [CrossRef] [PubMed]
18. Iniesta, R.R.; Paciarotti, I.; Davidson, I.; McKenzie, J.M.; Brougham, M.F.; Wilson, D.C. Nutritional status of children and adolescents with cancer in Scotland: A prospective cohort study. *Clin. Nutr. ESPEN* **2019**, *32*, 96–106. [CrossRef] [PubMed]
19. Karalexi, M.A.; Markozannes, G.; Tagkas, C.F.; Katsimpris, A.; Tseretopoulou, X.; Tsilidis, K.K.; Spector, L.G.; Schüz, J.; Siahanidou, T.; Petridou, E.T.; et al. Nutritional Status at Diagnosis as Predictor of Survival from Childhood Cancer: A Review of the Literature. *Diagnostics* **2022**, *12*, 2357. [CrossRef] [PubMed]

Disclaimer/Publisher's Note: The statements, opinions and data contained in all publications are solely those of the individual author(s) and contributor(s) and not of MDPI and/or the editor(s). MDPI and/or the editor(s) disclaim responsibility for any injury to people or property resulting from any ideas, methods, instructions or products referred to in the content.

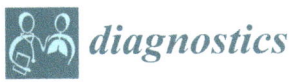

Review

Proteomics in Childhood Acute Lymphoblastic Leukemia: Challenges and Opportunities

Maria Kourti [1,*], Michalis Aivaliotis [2] and Emmanouel Hatzipantelis [3]

1. Third Department of Pediatrics, School of Medicine, Aristotle University and Hippokration General Hospital, 54642 Thessaloniki, Greece
2. Laboratory of Biological Chemistry, School of Medicine, Aristotle University of Thessaloniki, 54124 Thessaloniki, Greece; aivaliotis@auth.gr
3. Children & Adolescent Hematology-Oncology Unit, Second Department of Pediatrics, School of Medicine, Aristotle University of Thessaloniki, 54124 Thessaloniki, Greece; hatzip@auth.gr

* Correspondence: makourti@auth.gr

Abstract: Acute lymphoblastic leukemia (ALL) is the most common cancer in children and one of the success stories in cancer therapeutics. Risk-directed therapy based on clinical, biologic and genetic features has played a significant role in this accomplishment. Despite the observed improvement in survival rates, leukemia remains one of the leading causes of cancer-related deaths. Implementation of next-generation genomic and transcriptomic sequencing tools has illustrated the genomic landscape of ALL. However, the underlying dynamic changes at protein level still remain a challenge. Proteomics is a cutting-edge technology aimed at deciphering the mechanisms, pathways, and the degree to which the proteome impacts leukemia subtypes. Advances in mass spectrometry enable high-throughput collection of global proteomic profiles, representing an opportunity to unveil new biological markers and druggable targets. The purpose of this narrative review article is to provide a comprehensive overview of studies that have utilized applications of proteomics in an attempt to gain insight into the pathogenesis and identification of biomarkers in childhood ALL.

Keywords: acute lymphoblastic leukemia; proteomics; biomarkers

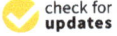

Citation: Kourti, M.; Aivaliotis, M.; Hatzipantelis, E. Proteomics in Childhood Acute Lymphoblastic Leukemia: Challenges and Opportunities. *Diagnostics* **2023**, *13*, 2748. https://doi.org/10.3390/diagnostics13172748

Academic Editor: Eric Deconinck

Received: 30 June 2023
Revised: 20 August 2023
Accepted: 21 August 2023
Published: 24 August 2023

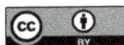

Copyright: © 2023 by the authors. Licensee MDPI, Basel, Switzerland. This article is an open access article distributed under the terms and conditions of the Creative Commons Attribution (CC BY) license (https://creativecommons.org/licenses/by/4.0/).

1. Introduction

Acute lymphoblastic leukemia (ALL) is the most common cancer in children [1]. It is a biologically heterogeneous hematologic malignancy—mainly characterized by chromosomal alterations, and some somatic and genetic mutations—that leads to the dysregulation of cytokine receptors, hematopoietic transcription factors and epigenetic modifiers [2,3]. Contemporary chemotherapy for childhood ALL has resulted in a cure rate of more than 85% in developed countries, representing one of the success stories in treatment of childhood malignancies [4]. This can be attributed to: (i) risk-directed therapy, based on clinical features such as age and initial white blood count, (ii) biologic and genetic features such as karyotype and identification of cryptic translocations, but most importantly (iii) the response to treatment evaluation with minimal/measurable residual disease (MRD) [5,6]. However, despite the observed improvement in survival rates, leukemia remains one of the leading causes of cancer-related deaths [7]. Given the improved cure rates, current research has focused on subgroups of patients with refractory/relapsed disease. Identification of proteins and pathways related to cancer and its environment provides the potential to develop effective individualized treatment, especially in this high-risk group. Proteomics is a cutting-edge technique and a useful tool for creating innovative and customized therapy providing new prospects for precision-medicine strategies [8].

The purpose of this narrative review article is to provide a comprehensive overview of published studies that have utilized applications of proteomics in an attempt to gain insight into the pathogenetic pathway and biomarkers discovery in childhood ALL. A thorough computerized search of the PubMed/Medline database was carried out along with research material from conference proceedings, publications from American Society of Hematology, European Hematology Association, and book chapters. Literature search on PubMed/Medline database was conducted, referring to manuscripts/studies published between 1 January 2010 and 31 January 2023. The last search was carried out on 30 March 2023 with the following keywords: "pediatric" or "children" or "childhood" AND "acute lymphoblastic leukemia" or "ALL" AND "proteomic profile" or "proteomics" or "proteome". Search results were narrowed down to studies published in the English language. Exclusion criteria included studies exclusively conducted in adults, studies involving conditions other than ALL as well as abstracts without full-text articles. Relevance and duplicates were primarily assessed based on the title and abstract screening.

The review comprises three relevant sections: an overview on the molecular basis of childhood ALL, an overview on proteomic analysis and a discussion of the applications of proteomics research in childhood ALL.

2. Molecular Basis of Acute Lymphoblastic Leukemia

Acute lymphoblastic leukemia is a hematologic malignancy of lymphoid origin and the most common childhood cancer representing about 25% of cancer diagnoses [9]. The highest peak age of incidence is between two and five years [10]. It is more frequent in boys than in girls with an approximate ratio of 1.3:1. Children of Hispanic descent are more frequently affected followed by White, and to a lesser percentage, African Americans [11]. Classification, based on immunophenotype, consists of 80–85% B-cell and 15–20% of T-cell, increasing in adolescence. Leukemic cells initiate in the bone marrow (BM) and infiltrate extramedullary sites such as the liver, spleen, mediastinum and lymph nodes and also sanctuary sites, such as the central nervous system (CNS), ovaries in girls and testes in boys.

Although environmental, immunologic, socioeconomic and epidemiologic factors have been evaluated rigorously as contributing factors to leukemogenesis, the exact underlying etiology remains unknown [12]. Before the advent of next-generation sequencing (NGS), only a small number of uncommon constitutional leukemia predisposition syndromes, such as Down syndrome (DS) and Li–Fraumeni syndrome, were associated with the development of ALL [13]. Other genetic syndromes linked to an increased risk of ALL include: Bloom syndrome, ataxia telangiectasia (AT), neurofibromatosis 1 and constitutional mismatch repair deficiency (CMMRD) [13]. The latter, and AT, have a preponderance to T-ALL, while B-ALL occurs almost exclusively in DS-ALL [14,15]. During the last decades, the landscape of germline and somatic mutations in childhood ALL has been unveiled with the aid of a microarray analysis of gene expression and ultra-high throughput sequencing technologies. Based on genomic analysis, childhood ALL is subdivided into genetic subgroups [16–18].

Gross chromosomal alterations in childhood ALL have been associated with outcome. Fluorescence in situ hybridization (FISH) assays and cytogenetics are used to identify structural chromosomal gains or losses in leukemic cells. High-hyperdiploidy (>50 chromosomes: 51–67 chromosomes) with trisomies of chromosomes 4,6,10,14,17,18,21, X occurs in almost 25% of childhood ALL cases and is associated with excellent outcome, even with reduced intensity chemotherapeutic regimens [19,20]. Low-hyperdiploidy with 47–50 chromosomes was traditionally associated with a poor outcome. However, contemporary therapy regimens have significantly improved clinical outcome [21,22]. On the contrary, hypodiploid B-ALL with less than 44 chromosomes is uncommon and associated with a poor outcome, especially in children with positive minimal residual disease at the end of induction. Germline *TP53* mutations consistent with Li–Fraumeni syndrome occur frequently in low-hypodiploid ALL subtype [23,24].

Chromosomal translocations represent a molecular hallmark of childhood ALL and represent a significant prognostic factor. Chimeric fusion genes are created by chromosomal rearrangements and involve epigenetic modifiers, tyrosine kinases and transcription factors [25]. They can be identified with reverse-transcription polymerase chain reaction amplification of the fusion genes created, together with FISH assays. Routine cytogenetic analyses fail to detect some of the cryptic translocations. Almost one fourth of standard-risk B-ALL harbor the cryptic t(12;21)(p13;q22), resulting in ETV6-RUNX1 (TEL-AML1) fusion. It should be noted that this fusion can also be detected in children who do not develop leukemia. It has also been detected in preserved blood spots from children who later develop ALL indicating a potential prenatal origin of leukemogenesis in association with additional necessary co-operating mutations for the development of leukemia [26]. A small group of "ETV6-RUNX1-like" B-ALL has also been reported. These cases lack the classic ETV6-RUNX1 rearrangement and are associated with other ETV6 fusions and with IKZF1 deletions. A unifying and prominent feature of a majority of prognostic studies in pediatric BCP ALL is that the different types of IKZF1 deletions have been constantly linked to an unfavorable clinical outcome of frontline treatment [27]. Most children with ETV6-RUNX1 fusion belong to the standard risk group and exhibit excellent outcome with standard therapy [21].

Other common rearrangements in B-ALL include: t(1;19)(q23;p13.3) resulting in TCF3-PBX1 (E2A-PBX1) fusion, rearrangement of KMT2A (formerly MLL; 11q23), and t(9;22)(q34;q11.2) (the Philadelphia chromosome) resulting in BCR-ABL1 fusion. While TCF3-PBX1 ALL was formerly linked to an intermediate or unfavorable prognosis, modern therapeutic regimens have enhanced outcome; thus, TCF3-PBX1 fusion is no longer considered for risk stratification [28]. Children with TCF3-PBX1 ALL appear to have higher risk of CNS relapse and may warrant intensification of CNS-directed therapy [29]. TCF3-HLF fusion resulting from t(17;19)(q22;p13.3) is very uncommon in patients with B-ALL and, despite its rarity, has been associated with extremely poor outcome [30]. MLL rearrangement involving somatic translocations of the KMT2A gene are common in infant B-ALL. Outcome is generally dismal in infants aged less than 3 months, and clinical prognosis varies according to the specific KMT2 translocation [31]. A trial conducted in KMT2A rearranged infant ALL investigating incorporation of lestaurtinib, an FLT3 inhibitor, with intensive chemotherapy, based on the FLT3 overexpression, revealed that addition of lestaurtinib did not improve outcome [32,33].

An established molecular-targeted therapy paradigm in childhood ALL is Philadelphia positive (Ph+) ALL with the t(9;22)(q34;q11) resulting in BCR-ABL1 oncoprotein. Three BCR-ABL1 protein isoforms are encoded, the p210, the p190, and the p230, which have persistently enhanced tyrosine kinase (TK) activity. The BCR-ABL fusion gene of childhood and adult ALL have a different molecular basis, with the BCR-ABL fusion gene in adult ALL of the "p210" subtype resembling that found in chronic myeloid leukemia (CML), whereas the childhood subtype is mainly "p190" [34]. Historically, the best curative option has been hematopoietic stem cell transplantation (HSCT). The addition of tyrosine kinase inhibitors (TKIs) in the intensive chemotherapy backbone, has significantly improved event-free and overall survival [35,36]. BCR-ABL1-Like or Philadelphia chromosome-like ALL has recently been described as a subset of B-ALL defined by an activated kinase gene expression profile similar to that of Ph+ ALL and is associated with miscellaneous genetic alterations that activate cytokine receptor signaling pathways [37]. In spite of the heterogeneity in Ph-like kinase-activating alterations, JAK-STAT, ABL, Ras/MAPK signaling pathways are activated and can effectively be inhibited by relevant TKIs [38]. The Janus kinase-signal transducer and activator of transcription (JAK-STAT) pathway plays a major role in transmitting signals from cell-membrane receptors to the nucleus leading to important physiological processes such as immune regulation, hematopoiesis, cell proliferation and survival [39]. The mitogen-activated protein kinase (MAPK) pathway, consisting of the Ras-Raf-MEK-ERK signaling cascade, is a crucial cellular network that regulates apoptosis, cellular development, differentiation, and proliferation [40]. Some studies have revealed a functional interaction between the JAK/STAT and RAS/MAPK pathways that promotes leukemogenesis and uncontrolled cell proliferation [41].

In contrast to B-ALL, the identified genetic alterations that occur in T-ALL do not add a substantial prognostic value in the established risk stratification of T-ALL based on CNS and MRD status [42]. Mutation of TAL1 (1p32) is a non-random genetic defect frequently present in childhood T-ALL. The SIL/TAL1 fusion product gives rise to inappropriate expression of TAL1, that may promote T-cell leukemogenesis. The clinical relevance and the prognostic value of this rearrangement remains to be further elucidated [43]. The most common dysregulated signaling pathway is the Notch pathway, either by upregulation with activating mutations of Notch1 or by loss of function of negative regulators such as FBXW7 [44]. Although gamma-secretase inhibitors (GSI) seem promising in the inhibition of the Notch pathway, the gastrointestinal toxicity and lack of efficacy prohibited their use in T-ALL therapy [44]. Interestingly, early T-cell precursor ALL shows JAK-STAT and Ras pathway mutations and is characterized by a distinct gene signature of the JAK-STAT signaling pathway that might explain the chemoresistance of T-ALL. Nevertheless, it can be inhibited by pathway inhibitors in leukemia models [45]. The nucleoside analogue nelarabine has proven to show early activity in patients with relapsed/refractory T-ALL, but it was associated with neurotoxicity [46]. The proteasome inhibitor, bortezomib was examined in the Children's Oncology Group phase III clinical trial AALL123, in which only patients with T-lymphoblastic lymphoma showed a significantly improved survival [47].

The most common translocations in T-ALL involve fusion of T-cell receptor genes. Gene expression signatures define novel oncogenic pathways in T-cell ALL, but their prognostic significance remains unidentified. Although stimulating advances have occurred regarding the genomic characterization of T-ALL, development of precision medicine treatment approaches for T-ALL has proven more challenging [48].

Approximately 20% of pediatric ALL patients experience a relapse with a survival lagging behind newly diagnosed ALL. Major pathways of lymphoid development, kinase signaling, cell cycle regulation and epigenetic modification are involved in the genetic basis of relapsed ALL [49]. Molecular-targeted therapy has shown promising results in early trials, though not translated into improved survival [50,51].

Relapsed and refractory disease pose extreme therapeutic challenges, demonstrating an unmet need for the development of durable therapies. Recent advances in immunotherapy with CD19 inhibitors and CD22 inhibitors (Blinatumomab and Inotuzumab ozogamicin, respectively) and chimeric antigen receptor (CAR)-T cell therapy, have reformed the management of relapsed and refractory ALL with the price of serious adverse events, such as cytokine release syndrome, immune effector neurotoxicity syndrome, prolonged BM suppression and hypogammaglobulinemia [52]. They offer the advantage to act independently of genetic aberrations and overcome drug-resistant mutations enhanced in relapsed ALL [53]. Therefore, these therapies seem ideal for patients who do not express targetable genetic alterations. Whether these immunotherapies could serve as definite therapies rather than bridging therapies to HSCT remains to be elucidated in the near future.

3. The Era of Proteomics

Proteomics studies the structure along with the function of the proteome [54]. The term proteome describes the functional state of the total of proteins, which are responsible for the functional activity of different cells [55]. As a result, study of the proteome correlates the structural and functional multiplicity of proteins during the disease process. The field of proteomics has been developed since genomics is ineffective in unravelling the structure and dynamic state of proteins, which are gene products [56]. In contrast to the steady state of the genome, expression of a protein reflects a dynamic state of processes including RNA transcription, alternative splicing, and/or post-translational modifications (PTM) [57]. PTMs have fundamental regulatory properties, such as converting a protein from its inactive to its active state, or determining a protein's half-life resulting from ubiquitination or acetylation; hence, defining its functional property in a cell and tissue-specific context that ultimately determines the resulting cellular phenotype and its biological significance [58]. Regulation of protein translation, degradation and PTM lead to low association between the cellular proteome and genome/transcriptome [59]. As a result, phenotypical and functional changes are not frequently visible at the genome level but apparent in the proteome.

The general strategy pursued in proteomics is to compare related samples from different disease stages considering that differences in their proteome could reflect a different disease stage. Proteomic studies are carried out mainly in body fluids such as the cerebrospinal fluid (CSF), peripheral blood (PB) and BM. Body fluids exhibit a great emerging potential for biomarker studies, in particular those that can be collected by minimally invasive techniques [60,61]. The high potential of serum/plasma as a source for protein biomarkers is reflective of the overall state of an organism [62–64]. Alternatively, cancer cell lines or patient-derived tumors can also be engrafted into immunocompromised mice to generate the so-called cell line-derived xenografts (CDX) or patient-derived xenografts (PDX), respectively [65–67].

Biomarkers are recognized using mass spectrometry (MS) [68]. Mass spectrometry requires a low-energy ionization source that transfers peptides from solid/liquid to gaseous states (matrix-assisted laser desorption/ionization, MALDI, and electrospray ionization, ESI). The two basic and commonest types of mass analyzers are time of flight (ToF) and ion trap resonance analyzers. Computer algorithms help vastly in the immense task of identifying peptides and ultimately the proteins from which they are derived. Computational methods and statistical algorithms can maximize the mining of proteomic data. Quantification MS-based methods are divided into the label-free and stable isotope label approach. In the label-free approach, individual samples are injected directly in the MS and the relative abundance of peptides is quantified [69]. The major advantage of this technique is minimal sample handling, but problems in reproducibility and accuracy are encountered [69]. Furthermore, the extensive instrument time required is a disadvantage for the large sample sets typical for biological and clinical studies. On the contrary, a stable isotope labeling strategy, such as an isobaric tag, allows for the mixing of multiple samples at different stages [70]. A workflow of proteomics is depicted in Figure 1.

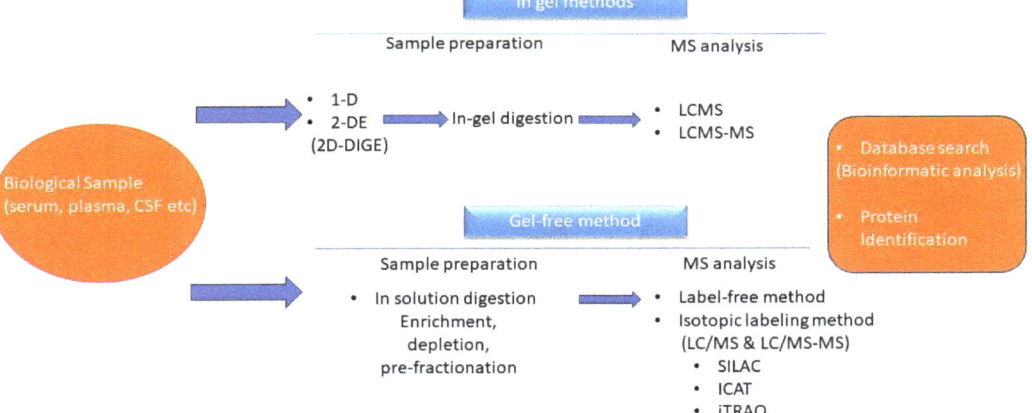

Figure 1. Workflow for proteomic analysis.

There are two different methodological approaches in proteomics. The first, known as top-bottom, is the discovery of a protein through its selective isolation, the characterization of its sequence and structure and the study of function, regulation, interaction and PTM. The second is the bottom-up or the so-called "shotgun" aiming to identify all the proteins present in a sample. In shotgun proteomics, which is a gel-free liquid chromatography (LC)-MS approach, it is essential to know a protein's identity before quantification, as peptides need to be related to each other and to their parent proteins; only then is protein quantification possible. Therefore, gel-based proteomics usually identifies only proteins with different abundances, while LC-MS identifies all detected proteins [71]. Currently, most of proteome analysis is performed with label and label-free shotgun proteomics [72].

4. Discussion—Application of Proteomics in Childhood ALL

Since the hallmark of ALL is the uncontrolled clonal proliferation of poorly differentiated lymphoid progenitor cells inside the bone marrow, interfering with the production of blood cells, serum and plasma may serve as rich sources of blood cancer-associated biomarkers.

In an attempt to determine potential disease markers in childhood B-ALL, a Colombian exploratory study group performed a proteomic study implementing LC-MS/MS and quantification by label-free methods searching for proteins differentially expressed between healthy children and children with B-ALL. They quantified 472 proteins in depleted blood plasma and found that 25 proteins were differentially expressed [73].

Moreover, differential proteins were analyzed by MALDI-TOF-MS and were identified in lymphocytes in patients with childhood ALL and healthy children, by Wang et al. [74]. Among the 25 differential proteins, eight provided a valuable insight into the molecular mechanism of leukemogenesis and could serve as candidate markers or drug targets. Cellular levels of GSTP in c-ALL samples were dramatically up-regulated and may be regarded as a biomarker and drug target together with PHB that was also up-regulated, suggesting that it might be associated with leukemogenesis [74].

Candidate biomarkers for early diagnosis of B-ALL were overexpressed in a proteomic analysis with lectin affinity chromatography LC-MS of serum from pediatric patients with B-ALL performed by Cavalcante et al. [75]. A total of 96 proteins were identified and among them leucine-rich alpha-2-glycoprotein 1 (LRG1), clusterin (CLU), thrombin (F2), heparin cofactor II (SERPIND1), alpha-2-macroglobulin (A2M), alpha-2-antiplasmin (SERPINF2), Alpha-1 antitrypsin (SERPINA1), complement factor B (CFB) and complement C3 (C3) were identified as candidate biomarkers for early diagnosis of B-ALL, as they were up-regulated in the B-ALL group compared to controls after induction therapy [75].

Identification of tumor autoantibodies may be utilized in early cancer diagnosis and immunotherapy. Serological proteome analysis (SERPA) is another proteomic approach and screening autoantibodies as serum biomarkers of B-ALL using SERPA with combination of 2-DE, immunoblotting and MS revealed that α-enolase and VDAC1 autoantibodies were promising biomarkers for children with B-ALL. Evaluation of serum autoantibodies against α-enolase and VDAC1 show promising clinical applications [76].

Braoudaki et al. [77]. evaluated the differential expression detected in the proteomic pro-files of pediatric low- and high-risk ALL patients aiming to characterize candidate biomarkers related to diagnosis, prognosis, and patient-targeted therapy. Proteomic analysis was performed using 2DE and protein identification by MALDI-TOF-MS and revealed that CLUS, CERU, APOE, APOA4, APOA1, GELS, S10A9, AMBP, ACTB, CATA and AFAM proteins play a significant role in leukemia prognosis, potentially serving as distinctive biomarkers for leukemia aggressiveness, or as suppressor proteins in HR-ALL cases. Moreover, bicaudal-D-related protein 1 (BICR1) could probably serve as a significant biomarker for pediatric ALL therapeutics [77].

Xu et al. [78]. performed proteomic analysis comparing the differentially expressed proteins between high-risk and low-risk childhood B-ALL by a label-free quantitative proteomics [78]. In the high-risk childhood B-ALL, 86 differently expressed proteins were depicted, and 35 proteins were predicted to have directive interactions. They found that, in high-risk B-ALL, the aberrant events might happen in pre-mRNA splicing, DNA damage response, and stress response contributing to the high-risk classification [78].

Jiang et al. [79]. using proteomic tools (2DE coupled to MS) in clinically important leukemia cell lines (REH, 697, Sup-B15, RS4.11), together with bone marrow samples from children with ALL, identified potential prognostic protein biomarkers and promising regulators of PRED-induced apoptosis. In patients with a good response to prednisone, down-regulation of PNCA was identified, while in prednisone poor responders (PPRs), proteins remained unchanged [79].

Hu et al. [80]. hypothesized that identification of proteins through proteomic analysis might lead to novel insights into resistance mechanisms in acute leukemia [80]. They applied proteomics tools via DIGE followed by MALDI-TOF, aiming to study the expression difference of cellular proteins between the drug-sensitive HL-60 and adriamycin-resistant HL-60 (HL-60/ADR) cell lines. They found that the up-regulations of nucleophosmin/B23 (NPM B23) and nucleolin C23 (C23) could be related to resistance of leukemia and could provide an important prognostic leukemia indicator [80].

Resistance to chemotherapeutics used in ALL is a major challenge and involves complex cellular processes. Guzmán-Ortiz et al. [81] studied proteome changes in B-lineage pediatric ALL cell line CCRF-SB after adaptation to vincristine, a vinca alkaloid used in ALL therapy [81]. Vincristine, by interaction with tubulin, disrupts the microtubule polymerization, resulting in cell cycle arrest and apoptosis [82]. They found 135 proteins exclusively expressed in the presence of vincristine, indicating that signal transduction and mitochondrial ATP production may serve as potential therapeutic targets. In a previous study, Verrills et al. [83]. reported the proteomic changes of the T-lineage ALL cell line CCRF-CEM after exposition to vincristine. They found that vincristine induced changes in the expression of 39 proteins and that a resistant subline differentially expressed 42 proteins mainly involved in cytoskeleton metabolism regulation of apoptosis, gene, chaperones and ribosomal proteins [83].

Leukemia studies aim to decipher the mechanisms, pathways and the degree to which the proteome impacts leukemia subtypes and to identify whether disease stratification based on proteome features could provide precise targets for therapy. Strategies of phosphoproteomics can be used to profile the activation/deactivation of crucial molecules in signaling pathways which are key to the progression, remission and relapse of leukemia, since leukemogenesis is controlled via the regulation and interaction of signaling cascades [84,85]. A commonly mutated pathway in pediatric cancers is the receptor tyrosine kinase/ras (RTK/RAS) pathway. Mutations in this pathway are identified as possible targets for treatment and are mainly implicated on clonal evolution in high hyperdiploid ALL, a subtype of the most common childhood cancer [86,87]. Mutations of KRAS in signal transduction domains considerably affect the ability of proteins to accomplish their normal cell-signaling functions [87]. In a study by Siekmann et al. patient-derived xenograft ALL (PDX-ALL) models were established with dependencies on fms-like tyrosine kinase 3 (FLT3) and platelet-derived growth factor receptor b (PDGFRB), which were interrogated by phosphoproteomics using iTRAQ mass spectrometry [88]. Phosphoproteomic analyses identified group I PAKs as targets of RTKs in ALL, while PAK inhibition affects in vitro growth and survival of ALL cells [88]. According to the findings of this study, PAKs is identified as a potential downstream target in RTK-dependent childhood ALL, the inhibition of which might assist in preventing the selection or acquisition of resistance mutations toward tyrosine kinase inhibitors [88].

The JAK/STAT pathway have also been implicated in the oncogenesis of many cancers as well as of childhood leukemia [89]. A JAK mutant has been identified in childhood B-cell ALL leading to overactivity in cell proliferation [89]. Somatic mutations in tyrosine-protein phosphatase non-receptor type 11 (PTPN11) lead to hyperactivation of the catalytic activity instead of the normal inhibitory function [90,91]. The Notch signaling pathway is one of the most frequently overactivated signaling pathways in cancer, and mutations in Notch family proteins are detected in a majority of T-cell ALL [92]. Activation of γ-secretase is crucial in the activation of the Notch pathway and inhibitors can be applied to block this activation. These are currently tested in clinical trials [93]. Increased mTOR activity has been implicated in ALL relapses and has been suggested as a therapeutic candidate target [94,95]. The crucial function of proteins on the stimulation of signaling pathways in the course of diagnosis and predicting relapse remains to be elucidated [96]. Knowledge of the proteomic landscape of ALL that emerges from the consequences of genetic and epigenetic events would prove to be valuable in identifying "druggable" target proteins.

High hyperdiploid B-cell ALL and ETV6/RUNX1-positive pediatric ALL are among the most common subtypes of childhood leukemia. In a study by Yang et al. [97]. it has been demonstrated that the characteristic extra chromosomes have an impact on the transcriptome and proteome suggesting that hyperdiploid leukemia cases harbor aberrant chromatin organization that causes genome-wide transcriptional dysregulation [97]. In hyper-diploid cases, 1286 proteins were up-regulated (more important of which were CD44 and FLT3) and 1127 were down-regulated (IGF2BP1 CLiC5 RAG1 RAG2) by proteome HiRIEF LC-Ms/MS analyses. A previous study by Costa et al. [98]. on protein expression in pre-B2 lymphoblastic cells from children with ALL in relation with t(12;21) translocation has identified several proteins of interest, defining a "protein-map" associated to some sub-groups of patients with particular features. The correlation between the proteins' expression and the t(12;21) or its fusion transcript ETV6-RUNX1 still remains to be verified. Nevertheless, this new approach for identification and classification of patient subgroups could lead to interesting therapeutic targets [98].

Children with T-ALL display resistance in glucocorticoid treatment. Serafin et al. identified, by reverse-phase protein arrays, that lymphocyte cell-specific protein-tyrosine kinase (LCK) was aberrantly activated in PPR patients [99]. They also showed that LCK inhibitors, such as dasatinib, bosutinib, nintedanib, and WH-4-023, could induce cell death in GC-resistant T-ALL cells, and remarkably, co-treatment with dexamethasone is capable of reversing GC resistance, even at therapeutic drug concentrations. These results offer a new insight into the biology and treatment of pediatric T-ALL by providing a new targeted therapy option with the use of LCK inhibitors, which could be easily rendered into clinical practice in an attempt to overcome GC resistance and improve the outcome of poor-responder T-ALL pediatric patients [99].

Phosphoproteomics is designed to provide information on pathway activation and signaling networks and offer opportunities for targeted therapy [100]. In a recent MS-based global phosphoproteomic profiling of 11 T-cell ALL cell lines targetable kinases were recognized [101]. Cordo et al. [100]. reported a comprehensive dataset consisting of 21,000 phosphosites on 4896 phosphoproteins, including 217 kinases. Moreover, they identified active Src-family kinases signaling and active cyclin-dependent kinases. They validated putative targets for therapy ex vivo and detected potential combination treatments, such as the inhibition of the INSR/IGF-1R axis to increase the sensitivity to dasatinib treatment. Moreover, since multiple clinical trials are investigating the JAK inhibitor ruxolitinib for the treatment of T-ALL in the presence of JAK mutations, Cordo et al. [100]. showed that ruxolitinib treatment is effective ex vivo in T-ALL cells with elevated JAK kinase activity. Mass spectrometry-based phosphoproteomic studies dedicated to T-ALL may prove to be helpful tools to decipher specific pathological signaling pathways and escape mechanisms. This will ultimately lead to the identification of novel disease-specific or individualized biomarkers [102].

Studies on the comparative analysis between the bone marrow tumor microenvironment and the peripheral blood are very important to decipher the ALL biology. Overarching challenges of the hidden mechanisms behind immature lymphoid cells accumulation in the bone marrow and the mechanisms underlying the chemotherapy effects against B-ALL will shed light on the leukemia biology and the cumulative impact of chemotherapy [103]. A recent study by Brotto et al. [103] highlighted a possible role for transthyretin and IFN-g as mechanisms related to disease remission.

Noteworthy, interesting results were depicted in a recent study by Leo et al. [104]. who performed a comprehensive multi-omic analysis of 49 readily available childhood ALL cell lines, using proteomics, transcriptomics, and pharmacoproteomic characterization. They connected the molecular phenotypes with drug responses to 528 oncology drugs, identifying drug correlations as well as lineage-dependent correlations [104]. Their observations indicate that both conventional lineage and oncogenic traits contribute to proteome-level differences in their cell line panel. Phenotypic profiling supports current clinical practice in leukemia stratification and suggests that MS-based proteomics could be an effective path to discover the drivers contributing to pathogenic phenotypes. They identified the diacylglycerol-analog bryostatin-1 as a therapeutic applicant in the MEF2D-HNRNPUL1 fusion high-risk subtype, for which this drug triggers pro-apoptotic ERK signaling linked to molecular mediators of pre-B cell negative selection [104]. Table 1 summarizes proteomic studies on childhood ALL.

Central nervous system involvement remains one of the major causes of ALL treatment failure [105,106]. Despite the therapeutic advances in ALL, CNS relapse occurs in 3–8% of the children with ALL and is associated with increased morbidity and mortality [107]. In normal physiological conditions, 80% of the protein in the CSF is hematogenic in origin [108]. Thus, protein content changes in CSF provide an attractive approach to study hematological malignancies [109]. Although CSF is obtained by using an invasive method, it is considered as the optimal fluid for diagnosis of CNS infiltration in ALL. Efforts have been made in recent years to detect novel biomarkers of hematologic malignancy in CSF [110]. As demonstrated in a pilot study, gel-free, label-free quantitative proteomics is feasible for profiling of CSF in pediatric leukemia/lymphoma [74,111]. Moreover, in the same study, the expression of antithrombin III and plasminogen decreased over time in one child who developed CNS thrombosis, compared to other subjects [111]. In another prospective pilot study, quantitative proteomics by using LC-MS/MS was used to discover differential expression of CSF protein in newly diagnosed children with leukemia and CNS infiltration versus healthy controls aiming to discover possible prognostic biomarkers [112]. Using LC-MS/MS, 51 proteins were identified to be significantly different between the two groups including 32 proteins that were up-regulated and 19 proteins that were down-regulated. Among them, TIMP1, LGALS3BP, A2M, AHSG, FN1, HRG, and ITIH4 have been associated with cancer, while CF I, C2, and C4A, have been related to complement activity [112]. In another study, Mo et al. implemented label-free LC−MS/MS in order to explore proteomic profiles in patients suffering from ALL with CNS infiltration [113]. Among the 428 unique proteins identified, they quantified 10 altered proteins during treatment [113].

Some of the proteins are likely to play a vital biological role as biomarkers for the development of ALL, with diverse biological functions after induction chemotherapy. It is noteworthy that those altered proteins should be further investigated as predictive markers of ALL with CNS infiltration, some of which may have the prospect of becoming new therapeutic targets in childhood ALL with CNS involvement. Interesting results have been reported from an exploratory study by Yu et al. [71]. who investigated protein dynamics in children with B-cell ALL undergoing chemotherapy by implementing a 4-plex N,N-dimethyl leucine isobaric labeling strategy in a longitudinal study [71]. According to their results, neural cell adhesion molecule (NRCAM), neuronal growth regulator 1, (NEGR1) and secretogranin-3 (SCG3,) were significantly altered at different stages of chemotherapy. All the aforementioned proteins have been related to neurologic disorders and may reflect CNS injury caused by chemotherapy on neuronal membranes and other structures. Thus, they may also be implicated in long-term neurocognitive effects of chemotherapy [71]. Table 2 summarizes the proteomic studies conducted in CSF in relation to ALL.

Table 1. Synopsis of proteomic studies of childhood ALL.

Author/Year/Country	Objective	Sample	Proteomic Approach	Main Results
Jiang N et al. [79] 2011 Singapore	Identify potential prognostic protein biomarkers. Discover promising regulators of PRED-induced apoptosis	Cell Line Bone marrow	2-DE & MALDI-TOF	PCNA was highly predictive of PRED response in patients independent of molecular subtype.
Braoudaki M et al. [77] 2013 Greece	Evaluate differential expression in proteomic profiles of low risk- and high risk-ALL. Characterize candidate biomarkers related to diagnosis, prognosis and patient targeted therapy	Plasma Bone marrow	2-DE & MALDI-TOF	CLUS, CERU, APOE, APOA4, APOA1, GELS, S100A9, AMBP, ACTB, CATA and AFAM proteins play a role in leukemia prognosis Vitronectin and plasminogen: contribute to leukemogenesis. Bicaudal D-related protein 1: biomarker for pediatric ALL therapeutics.
Wang D et al. [74] 2013 China	Compare differential proteins in lymphocytes between children with c-ALL and healthy children. Explore the mechanisms of c-ALL. Find new diagnostic and therapeutic strategies for c-ALL.	Bone marrow	SDS-PAGE MALDI-TOF	15 proteins differentially expressed. 2 high expressions (Glutathione S-transferase P, PHB) 6 low expressions (PRDX4, 60s acidic ribosomal protein P0, Cytoplasmic actin, pyridoxine-5′-phosphate oxidase, Triosephosphate isomerase 1, FLJ26567)
Costa O et al. [98] 2014 France	Compare the lymphoblastes proteome in c-ALL in accordance with the presence of t(12;21).	Bone marrow	2-DE nanoLC Ion trap MS/MS	Over-expression of CNN2, MAT-2β, hnRNPA2, PITPβ, PSMB2, HSPC263 (OTUB1). Under-expression: BUB3, hnRNPE2, PSMB6, CK2a
Cavalcante MS et al. [75] 2016 Brazil	Perform proteomic analysis of serum from pediatric patients with B-ALL Identify candidate biomarker proteins, for use in early diagnosis and evaluation of treatment.	Serum	FPLC nanoUPLC-ESI-MS/MS	Upregulation and candidate biomarkers for early diagnosis: Leucine-rich alpha-2-glycoprotein 1 (LRG1), Clusterin (CLU), thrombin (F2), heparin cofactor II (SERPIND1), alpha-2-macroglobulin (A2M), alpha-2-antiplasmin (SERPINF2), Alpha-1 antitrypsin (SERPINA1), Complement factor B (CFB) and Complement C3 (C3).
Xu G et al. [78] 2017 China	Figure out the critical altered proteins which can indicate the risk rank	Bone marrow	LC-ESI-MS/MS	86 differently expressed proteins in the high-risk B-ALL 35 proteins have directive interactions
Guzmán-Ortiz AL et al. [81] 2017 Mexico	Identify changes in the proteome after adaptation to vincristine.	B-ALL cell line	MS ESI-MS/MS	135 proteins exclusively expressed in the presence of vincristine—represent potential therapeutic targets (Toll receptor signaling pathway, Ras Pathway, B-T cell activation, CCKR signaling map cytokine-mediated signaling pathway, oxidative phosphorylation.)

Table 1. *Cont.*

Author/Year/Country	Objective	Sample	Proteomic Approach	Main Results
Serafin V et al. [99] 2017 Italy	Identification of deregulated signaling pathways to point out new targeted approaches.	Bone marrow Cell lines Primary xenograft (PDX) cells	Reverse-phase protein arrays (RPPA)	Lymphocyte cell-specific protein-tyrosine kinase (LCK) aberrantly activated in PPR patients. Resistance to glucocorticoid treatment in pediatric T-ALL can be reversed by LCK inhibitors in vitro and in vivo. IL-4 overexpression contributes to LCK-induced glucocorticoid resistance.
Siekmann IK et al. [88] 2018 Germany Canada UK	Decipher signaling circuits that link RTK activity with biological output in vivo	Patient-derived xenograft ALL (PDX-ALL) models with dependencies on fms-like tyrosine kinase 3 (FLT3) and platelet-derived growth factor receptor b (PDGFRB)	Phosphoproteomics iTRAQ nano-LC MS/MS	Group I PAKs act as signaling hubs in RTK-dependent pathways in ALL. Inhibition of group I PAKs by FRAX486 augments the antileukemic efficacy of midostaurin in FLT3-driven ALL.
Calderon-Rodríguez SI et al. [73] 2019 Colombia	Study of the plasma proteome of Colombian children diagnosed with B-cell ALL (B-ALL) to determine potential disease markers that reflect processes altered by the presence of the disease or in response to it.	Plasma	Nano-LC-MS/MS	25 proteins were differentially expressed in B-ALL Potential biomarkers that could be used to differentiate unhealthy patients from healthy individuals
Yang M et al. [97] 2019 Sweden Germany UK	Proteogenomic analysis of a series of pediatric BCP-ALL, including high hyperdiploid and diploid/near-diploid ETV6/RUNX1-positive cases, aiming to determine the effects of aneuploidy.	Bone marrow	HiRIEF LC-MS/MS	Proteins differentially expressed between hyperdiploid and ETV6/RUNX1-positive leukemia had higher mRNA-protein correlations. CTCF and cohesin: low expression in hyperdiploid ALL
Broto GE et al. [103] 2020 Brazil	Comparing bone marrow and peripheral blood profiles, before chemotherapy—at diagnosis, and the cumulative effects found after the induction treatment	Bone marrow Peripheral blood B-ALL	Nano-LC-MS/MS	D0, PB characterized as a pro-inflammatory environment, with the involvement of several down-regulated. Coagulation proteins as KNG, plasmin, and plasminogen. D28 characterized by immune response-related processes and the super expression of the transcription factor IRF3 and transthyretin. RUNX1 found in both D0 and D28. IRF3-IFN γ axis induction as a possible mechanism enrolled in disease resolution, transthyretin as an up-regulated protein induced by the induction phase of chemotherapy.

15

Table 1. *Cont.*

Author/Year/Country	Objective	Sample	Proteomic Approach	Main Results
Uzozie A et al. [96] 2021 Canada	Reveal proteome signatures characteristic of leukemic subtypes. Explore how effectively PDX models replicate the primary leukemic proteome.	Cell lines Bone marrow Peripheral blood PDXs	LC-MSMS	Proteome differentiates pediatric B-ALL and T-ALL from non-leukemic cells. The proteome of xenograft ALL closely resemble matched patient proteome. Relapse specific changes in patients are retained in PDXs. Proliferation and immune response processes differ between PDXs and patients. Xenografts recapitulate proteome response to structural genomic changes in patients.
Cordo V et al. [100] 2022 Netherlands	Provide information on pathway activation and signaling networks that offer opportunities for targeted therapy.	T-cell ALL lines PDXs	Reverse phase protein array (RPPA)	21,000 phosphosites on 4896 phosphoproteins, including 217 kinases. Validate putative targets for therapy ex vivo and identify potential combination treatments, such as the inhibition of the INSR/IGF-1R axis to increase the sensitivity to dasatinib treatment.
Yu R et al. [76] 2022 China	Screen serum autoantibodies of pediatric B-ALL, aiming to contribute to the early detection of B-ALL in children.	Pooled B-ALL cell lines (NALM-6, REH and BALL-1 cells)	Serological proteome analysis (SERPA)	α-enolase and VDAC1 were identified as candidate autoantigens in children with B-ALL and potential serological markers.
Leo IR et al. [104] 2022 Sweden	Perform comprehensive multi-omic analyses using proteomics, transcriptomics, and pharmacoproteomic characterization	Childhood ALL cell lines	LC-MS	In-depth proteomic analysis of childhood ALL cell lines covering numerous cytogenetic subtypes quantifying more than 12,000 proteins and 19,000 protein-coding transcripts as well as sensitivity to 528 oncology and investigational drugs. Identify the diacylglycerol-analog bryostatin-1 as a therapeutic candidate in the MEF2D-HNRNPUL1 fusion high-risk subtype ALL

Table 2. Proteomic studies on ALL in CSF.

Author/Year/Country	Proteomic Approach	Main Results
Priola GM et al. [111] 2015 USA	LC-MS/MS	Protein C Inhibitor (SERPINA5) and heparin cofactor II (SERPIND1) changed over the course of therapy. Antithrombin III (ATIII) and plasminogen (PLMN) levels decreased expression over time in one child with CNS thrombosis.
Guo L et al. [112] 2019 China	LC-MS/MS	51 proteins identified, 32 up-regulated and 19 down-regulated including TIMP1, LGALS3BP, A2M, AHSG, FN1, HRG, ITIH4, CF I, C2, C4A.
Mo F et al. [113] 2019 China	LC-MS/MS	428 unique proteins identified, 10 altered proteins during treatment
Yu Q et al. [71] 2020 USA	4-plex N,N dimethyl leucine (DiLeu) isobaric labeling strategy and MS	63 proteins were significantly altered

5. Conclusions

Childhood ALL is a biologically heterogeneous disease characterized by structural alterations, genetic and somatic mutations through a process of complex protein-based signaling network pathway modifications. Changes in protein expression can partially be determined by the analysis of the static genome. Although implementation of next-generation genomic, transcriptomic, and epigenetic sequencing tools unveiled the genetic landscape of childhood ALL, uncovering the underlying dynamic changes at a protein level still remains a challenge.

Proteomics offers complementary information to genomics and transcriptomics by analyzing protein structure, expression, and modification status. Advances in the field of MS enables high-throughput collection of global proteomic profiles representing an opportunity to discover new biological markers and druggable targets. Novel disease-specific biomarkers will provide an additional reference for predicting treatment responses and individual prognosis. Deeper characterization of biomarkers and molecular pathways, especially in patients with relapsed/refractory disease, will ultimately identify precision medicine candidates for application of translational precision therapy.

Funding: This research received no external funding.

Institutional Review Board Statement: Not applicable.

Informed Consent Statement: Not applicable.

Data Availability Statement: Data sharing is not applicable to this article.

Conflicts of Interest: The authors declare no conflict of interest.

References

1. Inaba, H.; Mullighan, C.G. Pediatric Acute Lymphoblastic Leukemia. *Haematologica* **2020**, *105*, 2524–2539. [CrossRef] [PubMed]
2. Iacobucci, I.; Mullighan, C.G. Genetic Basis of Acute Lymphoblastic Leukemia. *J. Clin. Oncol.* **2017**, *35*, 975–983. [CrossRef] [PubMed]
3. Pui, C.-H.; Nichols, K.E.; Yang, J.J. Somatic and germline genomics in paediatric acute lymphoblastic leukaemia. *Nat. Rev. Clin. Oncol.* **2019**, *16*, 227–240. [CrossRef]
4. Jeha, S.; Pei, D.; Choi, J.; Cheng, C.; Sandlund, J.T.; Coustan-Smith, E.; Campana, D.; Inaba, H.; Rubnitz, J.E.; Ribeiro, R.C.; et al. Improved CNS Control of Childhood Acute Lymphoblastic Leukemia without Cranial Irradiation: St Jude Total Therapy Study 16. *J. Clin. Oncol.* **2019**, *37*, 3377–3391. [CrossRef] [PubMed]
5. Borowitz, M.J.; Wood, B.L.; Devidas, M.; Loh, M.L.; Raetz, E.A.; Salzer, W.L.; Nachman, J.B.; Carroll, A.J.; Heerema, N.A.; Gastier-Foster, J.M.; et al. Prognostic significance of minimal residual disease in high risk B-ALL: A report from Children's Oncology Group study AALL0232. *Blood* **2015**, *126*, 964–971. [CrossRef]

6. Wood, B.; Wu, D.; Crossley, B.; Dai, Y.; Williamson, D.; Gawad, C.; Borowitz, M.J.; Devidas, M.; Maloney, K.W.; Larsen, E.; et al. Measurable residual disease detection by high-throughput sequencing improves risk stratification for pediatric B-ALL. *Blood* **2018**, *131*, 1350–1359. [CrossRef]
7. Smith, M.A.; Seibel, N.L.; Altekruse, S.F.; Ries, L.A.; Melbert, D.L.; O'Leary, M.; Smith, F.O.; Reaman, G.H. Outcomes for children and adolescents with cancer: Challenges for the twenty-first century. *J. Clin. Oncol.* **2010**, *28*, 2625–2634. [CrossRef]
8. Kwon, Y.W.; Jo, H.S.; Bae, S.; Seo, Y.; Song, P.; Song, M.; Yoon, J.H. Application of Proteomics in Cancer: Recent Trends and Approaches for Biomarkers Discovery. *Front. Med.* **2021**, *8*, 747333. [CrossRef]
9. Noone, A.M.; Cronin, K.A.; Altekruse, S.F.; Howlader, N.; Lewis, D.R.; Petkov, V.I.; Penberthy, L. Cancer Incidence and Survival Trends by Subtype Using Data from the Surveillance Epidemiology and End Results Program, 1992–2013. *Cancer Epidemiol. Biomark. Prev.* **2017**, *26*, 632–641. [CrossRef]
10. National Cancer Institute. Age-Adjusted and Age-Specific SEER Cancer Incidence Rates, 2014–2018. Available online: https://seer.cancer.gov/csr/1975_2018/results_merged/sect_02_childhood_cancer_iccc.pdf (accessed on 18 April 2021).
11. Lim, J.Y.; Bhatia, S.; Robison, L.L.; Yang, J.J. Genomics of racial and ethnic disparities in childhood acute lymphoblastic leukemia. *Cancer* **2014**, *120*, 955–962. [CrossRef]
12. Wiemels, J. Perspectives on the causes of childhood leukemia. *Chem. Biol. Interact.* **2012**, *196*, 59–67. [CrossRef] [PubMed]
13. Stieglitz, E.; Loh, M.L. Genetic predispositions to childhood leukemia. *Ther. Adv. Hematol.* **2013**, *4*, 270–290. [CrossRef] [PubMed]
14. Buitenkamp, T.D.; Izraeli, S.; Zimmermann, M.; Forestier, E.; Heerema, N.A.; van den Heuvel-Eibrink, M.M.; Pieters, R.; Korbijn, C.M.; Silverman, L.B.; Schmiegelow, K.; et al. Acute lymphoblastic leukemia in children with Down syndrome: A retrospective analysis from the Ponte di Legno study group. *Blood* **2014**, *123*, 70–77. [CrossRef] [PubMed]
15. Mullighan, C.G.; Collins-Underwood, J.R.; Phillips, L.A.; Loudin, M.G.; Liu, W.; Zhang, J.; Ma, J.; Coustan-Smith, E.; Harvey, R.C.; Willman, C.L.; et al. Rearrangement of CRLF2 in B-progenitor- and Down syndrome-associated acute lymphoblastic leukemia. *Nat. Genet.* **2009**, *41*, 1243–1246. [CrossRef]
16. Lilljebjörn, H.; Fioretos, T. New oncogenic subtypes in pediatric B-cell precursor acute lymphoblastic leukemia. *Blood* **2017**, *130*, 1395–1401. [CrossRef]
17. Bastian, L.; Schroeder, M.P.; Eckert, C.; Schlee, C.; Tanchez, J.O.; Kämpf, S.; Wagner, D.L.; Schulze, V.; Isaakidis, K.; Lázaro-Navarro, J.; et al. PAX5 biallelic genomic alterations define a novel subgroup of B-cell precursor acute lymphoblastic leukemia. *Leukemia* **2019**, *33*, 1895–1909. [CrossRef]
18. Gu, Z.; Churchman, M.; Roberts, K.; Li, Y.; Liu, Y.; Harvey, R.C.; McCastlain, K.; Reshmi, S.C.; Payne-Turner, D.; Iacobucci, I.; et al. Genomic analyses identify recurrent MEF2D fusions in acute lymphoblastic leukaemia. *Nat. Commun.* **2016**, *7*, 13331. [CrossRef]
19. Paulsson, K.; Lilljebjörn, H.; Biloglav, A.; Olsson, L.; Rissler, M.; Castor, A.; Barbany, G.; Fogelstrand, L.; Nordgren, A.; Sjögren, H.; et al. The genomic landscape of high hyperdiploid childhood acute lymphoblastic leukemia. *Nat. Genet.* **2015**, *47*, 672–676. [CrossRef]
20. Vora, A.; Goulden, N.; Wade, R.; Mitchell, C.; Hancock, J.; Hough, R.; Rowntree, C.; Richards, S. Treatment reduction for children and young adults with low-risk acute lymphoblastic leukaemia defined by minimal residual disease (UKALL 2003): A randomised controlled trial. *Lancet Oncol.* **2013**, *14*, 199–209. [CrossRef]
21. Hunger, S.P.; Mullighan, C.G. Acute Lymphoblastic Leukemia in Children. *N. Engl. J. Med.* **2015**, *373*, 1541–1552. [CrossRef]
22. Pui, C.H.; Yang, J.J.; Hunger, S.P.; Pieters, R.; Schrappe, M.; Biondi, A.; Vora, A.; Baruchel, A.; Silverman, L.B.; Schmiegelow, K.; et al. Childhood Acute Lymphoblastic Leukemia: Progress Through Collaboration. *J. Clin. Oncol.* **2015**, *3*, 2938–2948. [CrossRef] [PubMed]
23. Holmfeldt, L.; Wei, L.; Diaz-Flores, E.; Walsh, M.; Zhang, J.; Ding, L.; Payne-Turner, D.; Churchman, M.; Andersson, A.; Chen, S.C.; et al. The genomic landscape of hypodiploid acute lymphoblastic leukemia. *Nat. Genet.* **2013**, *45*, 242–252. [CrossRef] [PubMed]
24. Safavi, S.; Olsson, L.; Biloglav, A.; Veerla, S.; Blendberg, M.; Tayebwa, J.; Behrendtz, M.; Castor, A.; Hansson, M.; Johansson, B.; et al. Genetic and epigenetic characterization of hypodiploid acute lymphoblastic leukemia. *Oncotarget* **2015**, *6*, 42793–42802. [CrossRef] [PubMed]
25. Harrison, C.J. Cytogenetics of paediatric and adolescent acute lymphoblastic leukaemia. *Br. J. Haematol.* **2009**, *144*, 147–156. [CrossRef] [PubMed]
26. Greaves, M. Darwin and evolutionary tales in leukemia. The Ham-Wasserman Lecture. *Hematol. Am. Soc. Hematol. Educ. Program.* **2009**, *2009*, 3–12. [CrossRef]
27. Lilljebjörn, H.; Henningsson, R.; Hyrenius-Wittsten, A.; Olsson, L.; Orsmark-Pietras, C.; von Palffy, S.; Askmyr, M.; Rissler, M.; Schrappe, M.; Cario, G.; et al. Identification of ETV6-RUNX1-like and DUX4-rearranged subtypes in paediatric B-cell precursor acute lymphoblastic leukaemia. *Nat. Commun.* **2016**, *7*, 11790. [CrossRef]
28. Felice, M.S.; Gallego, M.S.; Alonso, C.N.; Alfaro, E.M.; Guitter, M.R.; Bernasconi, A.R.; Rubio, P.L.; Zubizarreta, P.A.; Rossi, J.G. Prognostic impact of t(1;19)/TCF3-PBX1 in childhood acute lymphoblastic leukemia in the context of Berlin-Frankfurt-Münster-based protocols. *Leuk. Lymphoma* **2011**, *52*, 1215–1221. [CrossRef]
29. Jeha, S.; Pei, D.; Raimondi, S.C.; Onciu, M.; Campana, D.; Cheng, C.; Sandlund, J.T.; Ribeiro, R.C.; Rubnitz, J.E.; Howard, S.C.; et al. Increased risk for CNS relapse in pre-B cell leukemia with the t(1;19)/TCF3-PBX1. *Leukemia* **2009**, *23*, 1406–1409. [CrossRef]
30. Mullighan, C.G. Molecular genetics of B-precursor acute lymphoblastic leukemia. *J. Clin. Investig.* **2012**, *122*, 3407–3415. [CrossRef]

31. Andersson, A.K.; Ma, J.; Wang, J.; Chen, X.; Gedman, A.L.; Dang, J.; Nakitandwe, J.; Holmfeldt, L.; Parker, M.; Easton, J.; et al. The landscape of somatic mutations in infant MLL-rearranged acute lymphoblastic leukemias. *Nat. Genet.* **2015**, *47*, 330–337. [CrossRef]
32. Brown, P.; Levis, M.; Shurtleff, S.; Campana, D.; Downing, J.; Small, D. FLT3 inhibition selectively kills childhood acute lymphoblastic leukemia cells with high levels of FLT3 expression. *Blood* **2005**, *105*, 812–820. [CrossRef]
33. Brown, P.A.; Kairalla, J.A.; Hilden, J.M.; Dreyer, Z.E.; Carroll, A.J.; Heerema, N.A.; Wang, C.; Devidas, M.; Gore, L.; Salzer, W.L.; et al. FLT3 inhibitor lestaurtinib plus chemotherapy for newly diagnosed KMT2A-rearranged infant acute lymphoblastic leukemia: Children's Oncology Group trial AALL0631. *Leukemia* **2021**, *35*, 1279–1290. [CrossRef] [PubMed]
34. Kang, Z.J.; Liu, Y.F.; Xu, L.Z.; Long, Z.J.; Huang, D.; Yang, Y.; Liu, B.; Feng, J.X.; Pan, Y.J.; Yan, J.S.; et al. The Philadelphia chromosome in leukemogenesis. *Chin. J. Cancer* **2016**, *35*, 48. [CrossRef] [PubMed]
35. Biondi, A.; Gandemer, V.; De Lorenzo, P.; Cario, G.; Campbell, M.; Castor, A.; Pieters, R.; Baruchel, A.; Vora, A.; Leoni, V.; et al. Imatinib treatment of paediatric Philadelphia chromosome-positive acute lymphoblastic leukaemia (EsPhALL2010): A prospective, intergroup, open-label, single-arm clinical trial. *Lancet Haematol.* **2018**, *5*, e641–e652. [CrossRef]
36. Schultz, K.R.; Carroll, A.; Heerema, N.A.; Bowman, W.P.; Aledo, A.; Slayton, W.B.; Sather, H.; Devidas, M.; Zheng, H.W.; Davies, S.M.; et al. Children's Oncology Group. Long-term follow-up of imatinib in pediatric Philadelphia chromosome-positive acute lymphoblastic leukemia: Children's Oncology Group study AALL0031. *Leukemia* **2014**, *28*, 1467–1471. [CrossRef]
37. Roberts, K.G.; Li, Y.; Payne-Turner, D.; Harvey, R.C.; Yang, Y.L.; Pei, D.; McCastlain, K.; Ding, L.; Lu, C.; Song, G.; et al. Targetable kinase-activating lesions in Ph-like acute lymphoblastic leukemia. *N. Engl. J. Med.* **2014**, *371*, 1005–1015. [CrossRef]
38. Ding, Y.Y.; Stern, J.W.; Jubelirer, T.F.; Wertheim, G.B.; Lin, F.; Chang, F.; Gu, Z.; Mulligahn, C.G.; Li, Y.; Harvey, R.C.; et al. Clinical efficacy of ruxolitinib and chemotherapy in a child with Philadelphia chromosome-like acute lymphoblastic leukemia with GOLGA5-JAK2 fusion and induction failure. *Haematologica* **2018**, *103*, e427–e431. [CrossRef]
39. Hu, X.; Li, J.; Fu, M.; Zhao, X.; Wang, W. The JAK/STAT signaling pathway: From bench to clinic. *Sig. Transduct. Target. Ther.* **2021**, *6*, 402. [CrossRef]
40. Dillon, M.; Lopez, A.; Lin, E.; Sales, D.; Perets, R.; Jain, P. Progress on Ras/MAPK Signaling Research and Targeting in Blood and Solid Cancers. *Cancers* **2021**, *13*, 5059. [CrossRef]
41. Stivala, S.; Codilupi, T.; Brkic, S.; Baerenwaldt, A.; Ghosh, N.; Hao-Shen, H.; Dirnhofer, S.; Dettmer, M.S.; Simillion, C.; Kaufmann, B.A.; et al. Targeting compensatory MEK/ERK activation increases JAK inhibitor efficacy in myeloproliferative neoplasms. *J. Clin. Investig.* **2019**, *129*, 1596–1611. [CrossRef]
42. Liu, Y.; Easton, J.; Shao, Y.; Maciaszek, J.; Wang, Z.; Wilkinson, M.R.; McCastlain, K.; Edmonson, M.; Pounds, S.B.; Shi, L.; et al. The genomic landscape of pediatric and young adult T-lineage acute lymphoblastic leukemia. *Nat. Genet.* **2017**, *49*, 1211–1218. [CrossRef] [PubMed]
43. D'Angiò, M.; Valsecchi, M.G.; Testi, A.M.; Conter, V.; Nunes, V.; Parasole, R.; Colombini, A.; Santoro, N.; Varotto, S.; Caniglia, M.; et al. Clinical features and outcome of SIL/TAL1-positive T-cell acute lymphoblastic leukemia in children and adolescents: A 10-year experience of the AIEOP group. *Haematologica* **2015**, *100*, e10–e13. [CrossRef] [PubMed]
44. Girardi, T.; Vicente, C.; Cools, J.; De Keersmaecker, K. The genetics and molecular biology of T-ALL. *Blood* **2017**, *129*, 1113–1123. [CrossRef] [PubMed]
45. Maude, S.L.; Dolai, S.; Delgado-Martin, C.; Vincent, T.; Robbins, A.; Selvanathan, A.; Ryan, T.; Hall, J.; Wood, A.C.; Tasian, S.K.; et al. Efficacy of JAK/STAT pathway inhibition in murine xenograft models of early T-cell precursor (ETP) acute lymphoblastic leukemia. *Blood* **2015**, *125*, 1759–1767. [CrossRef] [PubMed]
46. Kathpalia, M.; Mishra, P.; Bajpai, R.; Bhurani, D.; Agarwal, N. Efficacy and safety of nelarabine in patients with relapsed or refractory T-cell acute lymphoblastic leukemia: A systematic review and meta-analysis. *Ann. Hematol.* **2022**, *101*, 1655–1666. [CrossRef]
47. Teachey, D.T.; Devidas, M.; Wood, B.L.; Chen, Z.; Hayashi, R.J.; Hermiston, M.L.; Annett, R.D.; Archer, J.H.; Asselin, B.L.; August, K.J.; et al. Children's Oncology Group Trial AALL1231: A Phase III Clinical Trial Testing Bortezomib in Newly Diagnosed T-Cell Acute Lymphoblastic Leukemia and Lymphoma. *J. Clin. Oncol.* **2022**, *40*, 2106–2118. [CrossRef]
48. Patrick, K.; Vora, A. Update on biology and treatment of T-cell acute lymphoblastic leukaemia. *Curr. Opin. Pediatr.* **2015**, *27*, 44–49. [CrossRef]
49. Waanders, E.; Gu, Z.; Dobson, S.M.; Antić, Ž.; Crawford, J.C.; Ma, X.; Edmonson, M.N.; Payne-Turner, D.; van de Vorst, M.; Jongmans, M.C.J.; et al. Mutational landscape and patterns of clonal evolution in relapsed pediatric acute lymphoblastic leukemia. *Blood Cancer Discov.* **2020**, *1*, 96–111. [CrossRef]
50. Burke, M.J.; Kostadinov, R.; Sposto, R.; Gore, L.; Kelley, S.M.; Rabik, C.; Trepel, J.B.; Lee, M.J.; Yuno, A.; Lee, S.; et al. Decitabine and Vorinostat with Chemotherapy in Relapsed Pediatric Acute Lymphoblastic Leukemia: A TACL Pilot Study. *Clin. Cancer Res.* **2020**, *26*, 2297–2307. [CrossRef]
51. Place, A.E.; Pikman, Y.; Stevenson, K.E.; Harris, M.H.; Pauly, M.; Sulis, M.L.; Hijiya, N.; Gore, L.; Cooper, T.M.; Loh, M.L.; et al. Phase I trial of the mTOR inhibitor everolimus in combination with multi-agent chemotherapy in relapsed childhood acute lymphoblastic leukemia. *Pediatr. Blood Cancer* **2018**, *65*, e27062. [CrossRef]
52. Hiramatsu, H. Current status of CAR-T cell therapy for pediatric hematologic malignancies. *Int. J. Clin. Oncol.* **2023**, *28*, 729–735. [CrossRef]

53. Rafei, H.; Kantarjian, H.M.; Jabbour, E.J. Targeted therapy paves the way for the cure of acute lymphoblastic leukaemia. *Br. J. Haematol.* **2020**, *188*, 207–223. [CrossRef]
54. Altelaar, A.F.; Munoz, J.; Heck, A.J. Next-generation proteomics: Towards an integrative view of proteome dynamics. *Nat. Rev. Genet.* **2013**, *14*, 35–48. [CrossRef] [PubMed]
55. Macklin, A.; Khan, S.; Kislinger, T. Recent advances in mass spectrometry based clinical proteomics: Applications to cancer research. *Clin. Proteom.* **2020**, *24*, 17. [CrossRef] [PubMed]
56. Liu, Y.; Beyer, A.; Aebersold, R. On the Dependency of Cellular Protein Levels on mRNA Abundance. *Cell* **2016**, *165*, 535–550. [CrossRef] [PubMed]
57. Aebersold, R.; Agar, J.N.; Amster, I.J.; Baker, M.S.; Bertozzi, C.R.; Boja, E.S.; Costello, C.E.; Cravatt, B.F.; Fenselau, C.; Garcia, B.A.; et al. How many human proteoforms are there? *Nat. Chem. Biol.* **2018**, *14*, 206–214. [CrossRef]
58. Melani, R.D.; Gerbasi, V.R.; Anderson, L.C.; Sikora, J.W.; Toby, T.K.; Hutton, J.E.; Butcher, D.S.; Negrão, F.; Seckler, H.S.; Szentić, K.; et al. The Blood Proteoform Atlas: A reference map of proteoforms in human hematopoietic cells. *Science* **2022**, *28*, 411–418. [CrossRef]
59. Ercan, H.; Resch, U.; Hsu, F.; Mitulovic, G.; Bileck, A.; Gerner, C.; Yang, J.-W.; Geiger, M.; Miller, I.; Zellner, M. A Practical and Analytical Comparative Study of Gel-Based Top-Down and Gel-Free Bottom-Up Proteomics Including Unbiased Proteoform Detection. *Cells* **2023**, *12*, 747. [CrossRef]
60. Cunningham, R.; Ma, D.; Li, L. Mass Spectrometry-based Proteomics and Peptidomics for Systems Biology and Biomarker Discovery. *Front. Biol.* **2012**, *1*, 313–335. [CrossRef]
61. Pursiheimo, A.; Vehmas, A.P.; Afzal, S.; Suomi, T.; Chand, T.; Strauss, L.; Poutanen, M.; Rokka, A.; Corthals, G.L.; Elo, L.L. Optimization of Statistical Methods Impact on Quantitative Proteomics Data. *J. Proteome Res.* **2015**, *14*, 4118–4126. [CrossRef]
62. Pietrowska, M.; Wlosowicz, A.; Gawin, M.; Widlak, P. MS-Based Proteomic Analysis of Serum and Plasma: Problem of High Abundant Components and Lights and Shadows of Albumin Removal. *Adv. Exp. Med. Biol.* **2019**, *1073*, 57–76. [PubMed]
63. Dunphy, K.; O'Mahoney, K.; Dowling, P.; O'Gorman, P.; Bazou, D. Clinical Proteomics of Biofluids in Haematological Malignancies. *Int. J. Mol. Sci.* **2021**, *22*, 8021. [CrossRef] [PubMed]
64. Xiao, Z.; Conrads, T.P.; Lucas, D.A.; Janini, G.M.; Schaefer, C.F.; Buetow, K.H.; Issaq, H.J.; Veenstra, T.D. Direct ampholyte-free liquid-phase isoelectric peptide focusing: Application to the human serum proteome. *Electrophoresis* **2004**, *25*, 128–133. [CrossRef] [PubMed]
65. Guo, S.; Jiang, X.; Mao, B.; Li, Q.X. The design, analysis and application of mouse clinical trials in oncology drug development. *BMC Cancer* **2019**, *19*, 718. [CrossRef] [PubMed]
66. Georges, L.M.C.; De Wever, O.; Galván, J.A.; Dawson, H.; Lugli, A.; Demetter, P.; Zlobec, I. Cell Line Derived Xenograft Mouse Models Are a Suitable in vivo Model for Studying Tumor Budding in Colorectal Cancer. *Front. Med.* **2019**, *27*, 139. [CrossRef]
67. Collins, A.T.; Lang, S.H. A systematic review of the validity of patient derived xenograft (PDX) models: The implications for translational research and personalised medicine. *PeerJ* **2018**, *6*, e5981. [CrossRef] [PubMed]
68. Zecha, J.; Gabriel, W.; Spallek, R.; Chang, Y.C.; Mergner, J.; Wilhelm, M.; Bassermann, F.; Kuster, B. Linking post-translational modifications and protein turnover by site-resolved protein turnover profiling. *Nat. Commun.* **2022**, *13*, 165. [CrossRef]
69. Bantscheff, M.; Schirle, M.; Sweetman, G.; Rick, J.; Kuster, B. Quantitative mass spectrometry in proteomics: A critical review. *Anal. Bioanal. Chem.* **2007**, *389*, 1017–1031. [CrossRef]
70. Zhu, W.; Smith, J.W.; Huang, C.M. Mass spectrometry-based label-free quantitative proteomics. *J. Biomed. Biotechnol.* **2010**, *2010*, 840518. [CrossRef]
71. Yu, Q.; Zhong, X.; Chen, B.; Feng, Y.; Ma, M.; Diamond, C.A.; Voeller, J.S.; Kim, M.; DeSantes, K.B.; Capitini, C.M.; et al. Isobaric Labeling Strategy Utilizing 4-Plex N,N-Dimethyl Leucine (DiLeu) Tags Reveals Proteomic Changes Induced by Chemotherapy in Cerebrospinal Fluid of Children with B-Cell Acute Lymphoblastic Leukemia. *J. Proteome Res.* **2020**, *19*, 2606–2616. [CrossRef]
72. Marcus, K.; Lelong, C.; Rabilloud, T. What Room for Two-Dimensional Gel-Based Proteomics in a Shotgun Proteomics World? *Proteomes* **2020**, *8*, 17. [CrossRef] [PubMed]
73. Calderon-Rodríguez, S.I.; Sanabria-Salas, M.C.; Umaña-Perez, A. A comparative proteomic study of plasma in Colombian childhood acute lymphoblastic leukemia. *PLoS ONE* **2019**, *14*, e0221509. [CrossRef] [PubMed]
74. Wang, D.; Lv, Y.Q.; Liu, Y.F.; Du, X.J.; Li, B. Differential protein analysis of lymphocytes between children with acute lymphoblastic leukemia and healthy children. *Leuk. Lymphoma* **2013**, *54*, 381–386. [CrossRef]
75. Cavalcante Mde, S.; Torres-Romero, J.C.; Lobo, M.D.; Moreno, F.B.; Bezerra, L.P.; Lima, D.S.; Matos, J.C.; Moreira Rde, A.; Monteiro-Moreira, A.C. A panel of glycoproteins as candidate biomarkers for early diagnosis and treatment evaluation of B-cell acute lymphoblastic leukemia. *Biomark. Res.* **2016**, *27*, 4. [CrossRef]
76. Yu, R.; Yang, S.; Liu, Y.; Zhu, Z. Identification and validation of serum autoantibodies in children with B-cell acute lymphoblastic leukemia by serological proteome analysis. *Proteome Sci.* **2022**, *20*, 3. [CrossRef] [PubMed]
77. Braoudaki, M.; Lambrou, G.I.; Vougas, K.; Karamolegou, K.; Tsangaris, G.T.; Tzortzatou-Stathopoulou, F. Protein biomarkers distinguish between high- and low-risk pediatric acute lymphoblastic leukemia in a tissue specific manner. *J. Hematol. Oncol.* **2013**, *6*, 52. [CrossRef]
78. Xu, G.; Li, Z.; Wang, L.; Chen, F.; Chi, Z.; Gu, M.; Li, S.; Wu, D.; Miao, J.; Zhang, Y.; et al. Label-free quantitative proteomics reveals differentially expressed proteins in high risk childhood acute lymphoblastic leukemia. *J. Proteom.* **2017**, *150*, 1–8. [CrossRef]

79. Jiang, N.; Kham, S.K.; Koh, G.S.; Suang Lim, J.Y.; Ariffin, H.; Chew, F.T.; Yeoh, A.E. Identification of prognostic protein biomarkers in childhood acute lymphoblastic leukemia (ALL). *J. Proteom.* **2011**, *74*, 843–857. [CrossRef] [PubMed]
80. Hu, J.; Lin, M.; Liu, T.; Li, J.; Chen, B.; Chen, Y. DIGE-based proteomic analysis identifies nucleophosmin/B23 and nucleolin C23 as over-expressed proteins in relapsed/refractory acute leukemia. *Leuk. Res.* **2011**, *35*, 1087–1092. [CrossRef]
81. Guzmán-Ortiz, A.L.; Aparicio-Ozores, G.; Valle-Rios, R.; Medina-Contreras, O.; Patiño-López, G.; Quezada, H. Proteomic changes in a childhood acute lymphoblastic leukemia cell line during the adaptation to vincristine. *Bol. Med. Hosp. Infant. Mex.* **2017**, *74*, 181–192.
82. Risinger, A.L.; Giles, F.J.; Mooberry, S.L. Microtubule dynamics as a target in oncology. *Cancer Treat. Rev.* **2009**, *35*, 255–261. [CrossRef] [PubMed]
83. Verrills, N.M.; Liem, N.L.; Liaw, T.Y.; Hood, B.D.; Lock, R.B.; Kavallaris, M. Proteomic analysis reveals a novel role for the actin cytoskeleton in vincristine resistant childhood leukemia an in vivo study. *Proteomics* **2006**, *6*, 1681–1694. [CrossRef] [PubMed]
84. Kemper, E.K.; Zhang, Y.; Dix, M.M.; Cravatt, B.F. Global profiling of phosphorylation-dependent changes in cysteine reactivity. *Nat. Methods* **2022**, *19*, 341–352. [CrossRef]
85. Floyd, B.M.; Drew, K.; Marcotte, E.M. Systematic Identification of Protein Phosphorylation-Mediated Interactions. *J. Proteome Res.* **2021**, *20*, 1359–1370. [CrossRef] [PubMed]
86. de Smith, A.J.; Ojha, J.; Francis, S.S.; Sanders, E.; Endicott, A.A.; Hansen, H.M.; Smirnov, I.; Termuhlen, A.M.; Walsh, K.M.; Metayer, C.; et al. Clonal and microclonal mutational heterogeneity in high hyperdiploid acute lymphoblastic leukemia. *Oncotarget* **2016**, *7*, 72733–72745. [CrossRef]
87. Malinowska-Ozdowy, K.; Frech, C.; Schönegger, A.; Eckert, C.; Cazzaniga, G.; Stanulla, M.; zur Stadt, U.; Mecklenbräuker, A.; Schuster, M.; Kneidinger, D.; et al. KRAS and CREBBP mutations: A relapse-linked malicious liaison in childhood high hyperdiploid acute lymphoblastic leukemia. *Leukemia* **2015**, *29*, 1656–1667. [CrossRef]
88. Siekmann, I.K.; Dierck, K.; Prall, S.; Klokow, M.; Strauss, J.; Buhs, S.; Wrzeszcz, A.; Bockmayr, M.; Beck, F.; Trochimiuk, M.; et al. Combined inhibition of receptor tyrosine and p21-activated kinases as a therapeutic strategy in childhood ALL. *Blood Adv.* **2018**, *2*, 2554–2567. [CrossRef]
89. Vainchenker, W.; Constantinescu, S.N. JAK/STAT signaling in hematological malignancies. *Oncogene* **2013**, *32*, 2601–2613. [CrossRef]
90. Liu, X.; Qu, C.K. Protein Tyrosine Phosphatase SHP-2 (PTPN11) in Hematopoiesis and Leukemogenesis. *J. Signal Transduct.* **2011**, *2011*, 195239. [CrossRef]
91. Zhou, B.; Lin, W.; Long, Y.; Yang, Y.; Zhang, H.; Wu, K.; Chu, Q. Notch signaling pathway: Architecture, disease, and therapeutics. *Signal Transduct Target Ther.* **2022**, *7*, 95. [CrossRef]
92. Yuan, X.; Wu, H.; Xu, H.; Xiong, H.; Chu, Q.; Yu, S.; Wu, G.S.; Wu, K. Notch signaling: An emerging therapeutic target for cancer treatment. *Cancer Lett.* **2015**, *369*, 20–27. [CrossRef] [PubMed]
93. López-Nieva, P.; González-Sánchez, L.; Cobos-Fernández, M.Á.; Córdoba, R.; Santos, J.; Fernández-Piqueras, J. More Insights on the Use of γ-Secretase Inhibitors in Cancer Treatment. *Oncologist* **2021**, *26*, e298–e305. [CrossRef]
94. Simioni, C.; Martelli, A.M.; Zauli, G.; Melloni, E.; Neri, L.M. Targeting mTOR in Acute Lymphoblastic Leukemia. *Cells* **2019**, *8*, 190. [CrossRef] [PubMed]
95. Pinchinat, A.; Raetz, E. How do mTOR inhibitors fit in the landscape of treatment for relapsed acute lymphoblastic leukemia? *Haematologica* **2022**, *107*, 2292–2294. [CrossRef] [PubMed]
96. Uzozie, A.C.; Ergin, E.K.; Rolf, N.; Tsui, J.; Lorentzian, A.; Weng, S.S.H.; Nierves, L.; Smith, T.G.; Lim, C.J.; Maxwell, C.A.; et al. PDX models reflect the proteome landscape of pediatric acute lymphoblastic leukemia but divert in select pathways. *J. Exp. Clin. Cancer Res.* **2021**, *40*, 96. [CrossRef]
97. Yang, M.; Vesterlund, M.; Siavelis, I.; Moura-Castro, L.H.; Castor, A.; Fioretos, T.; Jafari, R.; Lilljebjörn, H.; Odom, D.T.; Olsson, L.; et al. Proteogenomics and Hi-C reveal transcriptional dysregulation in high hyperdiploid childhood acute lymphoblastic leukemia. *Nat. Commun.* **2019**, *10*, 1519. [CrossRef] [PubMed]
98. Costa, O.; Schneider, P.; Coquet, L.; Chan, P.; Penther, D.; Legrand, E.; Jouenne, T.; Vasse, M.; Vannier, J.P. Proteomic profile of pre-B2 lymphoblasts from children with acute lymphoblastic leukemia (ALL) in relation with the translocation (12; 21). *Clin. Proteom.* **2014**, *11*, 31. [CrossRef]
99. Serafin, V.; Capuzzo, G.; Milani, G.; Minuzzo, S.A.; Pinazza, M.; Bortolozzi, R.; Bresolin, S.; Porcù, E.; Frasson, C.; Indraccolo, S.; et al. Glucocorticoid resistance is reverted by LCK inhibition in pediatric T-cell acute lymphoblastic leukemia. *Blood* **2017**, *130*, 2750–2761. [CrossRef]
100. Cordo', V.; Meijer, M.T.; Hagelaar, R.; de Goeij-de Haas, R.R.; Poort, V.M.; Henneman, A.A.; Piersma, S.R.; Pham, T.V.; Oshima, K.; Ferrando, A.A.; et al. Phosphoproteomic profiling of T cell acute lymphoblastic leukemia reveals targetable kinases and combination treatment strategies. *Nat. Commun.* **2022**, *13*, 1048. [CrossRef]
101. Beekhof, R.; van Alphen, C.; Henneman, A.A.; Knol, J.C.; Pham, T.V.; Rolfs, F.; Labots, M.; Henneberry, E.; Le Large, T.Y.; de Haas, R.R.; et al. INKA, an integrative data analysis pipeline for phosphoproteomic inference of active kinases. *Mol. Syst. Biol.* **2019**, *15*, e8250. [CrossRef]
102. Lawton, M.L.; Emili, A. Mass Spectrometry-Based Phosphoproteomics and Systems Biology: Approaches to Study T Lymphocyte Activation and Exhaustion. *J. Mol. Biol.* **2021**, *433*, 167318. [CrossRef] [PubMed]

103. Broto, G.E.; Corrêa, S.; Trigo, F.C.; Dos Santos, E.C.; Tomiotto-Pelissier, F.; Pavanelli, W.R.; Silveira, G.F.; Abdelhay, E.; Panis, C. Comparative Analysis of Systemic and Tumor Microenvironment Proteomes from Children with B-Cell Acute Lymphocytic Leukemia at Diagnosis and after Induction Treatment. *Front. Oncol.* **2020**, *10*, 550213. [CrossRef] [PubMed]
104. Leo, I.R.; Aswad, L.; Stahl, M.; Kunold, E.; Post, F.; Erkers, T.; Struyf, N.; Mermelekas, G.; Joshi, R.N.; Gracia-Villacampa, E.; et al. Integrative multi-omics and drug response profiling of childhood acute lymphoblastic leukemia cell lines. *Nat. Commun.* **2022**, *13*, 1691. [CrossRef] [PubMed]
105. Baytan, B.; Evim, M.S.; Güler, S.; Güneş, A.M.; Okan, M. Acute Central Nervous System Complications in Pediatric Acute Lymphoblastic Leukemia. *Pediatr. Neurol.* **2015**, *53*, 312–318. [CrossRef]
106. Manley, S.; Keenan, R.; Campbell, H.; Caswell, M.; Pizer, B. No evidence for routine cerebrospinal fluid cytology in detecting asymptomatic central nervous system relapse in children with acute lymphoblastic leukaemia: 20 years' experience of a UK primary treatment centre. *Br. J. Haematol.* **2014**, *164*, 462–464. [CrossRef]
107. Thastrup, M.; Duguid, A.; Mirian, C.; Schmiegelow, K.; Halsey, C. Central nervous system involvement in childhood acute lymphoblastic leukemia: Challenges and solutions. *Leukemia* **2022**, *36*, 2751–2768. [CrossRef]
108. Galicia, N.; Díez, P.; Dégano, R.M.; Guest, P.C.; Ibarrola, N.; Fuentes, M. Proteomic Biomarker Identification in Cerebrospinal Fluid for Leptomeningeal Metastases with Neurological Complications. *Adv. Exp. Med. Biol.* **2017**, *974*, 85–96.
109. Roy, S.; Josephson, S.A.; Fridlyand, J.; Karch, J.; Kadoch, C.; Karrim, J.; Damon, L.; Treseler, P.; Kunwar, S.; Shuman, M.A.; et al. Protein biomarker identification in the CSF of patients with CNS lymphoma. *J. Clin. Oncol.* **2008**, *26*, 96–105. [CrossRef]
110. Carbonara, K.; Andonovski, M.; Coorssen, J.R. Proteomes Are of Proteoforms: Embracing the Complexity. *Proteomes* **2021**, *9*, 38. [CrossRef]
111. Priola, G.M.; Foster, M.W.; Deal, A.M.; Richardson, B.M.; Thompson, J.W.; Blatt, J. Cerebrospinal fluid proteomics in children during induction for acute lymphoblastic leukemia: A pilot study. *Pediatr. Blood Cancer* **2015**, *62*, 1190–1194. [CrossRef]
112. Guo, L.; Ren, H.; Zeng, H.; Gong, Y.; Ma, X. Proteomic analysis of cerebrospinal fluid in pediatric acute lymphoblastic leukemia patients: A pilot study. *OncoTargets Ther.* **2019**, *12*, 3859–3868. [CrossRef] [PubMed]
113. Mo, F.; Ma, X.; Liu, X.; Zhou, R.; Zhao, Y.; Zhou, H. Altered CSF Proteomic Profiling of Paediatric Acute Lymphocytic Leukemia Patients with CNS Infiltration. *J. Oncol.* **2019**, *2019*, 3283629. [CrossRef] [PubMed]

Disclaimer/Publisher's Note: The statements, opinions and data contained in all publications are solely those of the individual author(s) and contributor(s) and not of MDPI and/or the editor(s). MDPI and/or the editor(s) disclaim responsibility for any injury to people or property resulting from any ideas, methods, instructions or products referred to in the content.

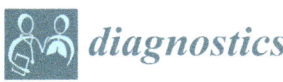

Systematic Review

The Prognostic Significance of BRAF Gene Analysis in Children and Adolescents with Papillary Thyroid Carcinoma: A Systematic Review and Meta-Analysis

Eleni P Kotanidou [1], Styliani Giza [1], Vasiliki Rengina Tsinopoulou [1], Kosmas Margaritis [1], Anastasia Papadopoulou [1], Eleni Sakellari [1], Savvas Kolanis [1], Eleni Litou [1], Anastasios Serbis [2] and Assimina Galli-Tsinopoulou [1,*]

[1] Unit of Pediatric Endocrinology and Metabolism, 2nd Department of Pediatrics, School of Medicine, Faculty of Health Sciences, Aristotle University of Thessaloniki, AHEPA University Hospital, Stilponos Kyriakidi 1, 54636 Thessaloniki, Greece
[2] Department of Pediatrics, School of Medicine, Faculty of Health Sciences, University of Ioannina, 45500 Ioannina, Greece
* Correspondence: agalli@auth.gr; Tel.: +30-2310-994801

Abstract: Thyroid cancer represents the prominent endocrine cancer in children. Papillary thyroid cancer (PTC) constitutes its most frequent (>90%) pediatric histological type. Mutations energizing the mitogen-activated-protein kinase (MAPK) pathway are definitely related to PTC. Its most common genetic alteration is in proto-oncogene B-Raf (BRAF). Mutated BRAF is proposed as a prognostic tool in adult PTC. We conducted a systematic review and meta-analysis evaluating the association of mutated BRAF gene and prognostic clinicopathological characteristics of PTC in children/adolescents. Systematic search for relevant studies included PubMed, MEDLINE, Scopus, clinicaltrials.gov and Cochrane Library. Pooled estimates of odds ratios for categorical data and mean difference for continuous outcomes were calculated using random/fixed-effect meta-analytic models. BRAFV600E mutation presents a pooled pediatric/adolescent prevalence of 33.12%. Distant metastasis is significantly associated with mutated BRAF gene (OR = 0.32, 95% CI = 0.16–0.61, p = 0.001). Tumor size (MD = −0.24, 95% CI = −0.62–0.135, p = 0.21), multifocality (OR = 1.13, 95% CI = 0.65–2.34, p = 0.74), vascular invasion (OR = 1.17, 95% CI = 0.67–2.05, p = 0.57), lymph node metastasis (OR = 0.92, 95% CI = 0.63–1.33, p = 0.66), extra-thyroid extension (OR = 0.78, 95% CI = 0.53–1.13, p = 0.19) and tumor recurrence (OR = 1.66, 95% CI = 0.68–4.21, p = 0.376) presented no association or risk with BRAF mutation among pediatric/adolescent PTC. Mutated BRAF gene in children and adolescents is less common than in adults. Mutation in BRAF relates significantly to distant metastasis among children/adolescents with PTC.

Keywords: children; adolescents; papillary thyroid cancer; proto-oncogene B-raf gene (BRAF); prognosis

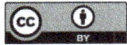

1. Introduction

Thyroid cancer represents the principal endocrine cancer in pediatric and adolescent population, with a female predominance of 4:1 [1]. Although rare, accounting for about 4% of pediatric malignancies, a rapid increase in incidence has been documented, almost globally [2]. The most common histological type recognized in >90% of cases is papillary thyroid cancer (PTC) [3].

It has long been supported that pediatric and adult patients with thyroid cancer have distinct characteristics in terms of initial presentation, clinical course, and mortality. Children and adolescents are often diagnosed with more advanced disease, exhibiting an increased rate of lymph node and distant metastases and often have persistent or recurrent disease [4]. Paradoxically, the prognosis is more favorable in children than in adults, as evidenced by the high overall survival rate of 97.70% from 1975 to 2005, which has been further advanced to 99.27% from 2006 to 2016, according to the Surveillance, Epidemiology and End Results (SEER) database [5].

This phenomenon may be explained on a molecular basis, as the two populations also have different genetic features. Point mutations activating the mitogen-activated protein kinase (MAPK) pathway play an important role. Among them, the most common genetic alteration of PTC in adults is located in the proto-oncogene B-Raf (BRAF) gene and consists of a T to A transversion (T1799A), resulting in a valine to glutamate substitution at residue 600 (V600E) of the BRAF protein. However, recorded mutation prevalence rates range from 27% to 83% among different populations [4]. Since there is a lack of definitive evidence on the clinicopathological significance of BRAF V600E in adult PTC, several meta-analyses have been conducted to elucidate its role in the diagnosis, management and prognosis of aggressive PTC cases. Various associations have been reported between the presence of BRAF V600E mutation and demographic data or risk factors, such as tumor size, multifocality, lymph node metastasis, vascular invasion, extra-thyroid extension, and advanced stage of tumor node metastasis [6–10].

In the pediatric population, BRAF V600E, although prevalent, is recognized at a lower rate compared to adults. In sporadic pediatric PTC, the BRAF V600E mutation ranged between 0 and 63% in different studies [11–19]. Furthermore, the BRAF V600E mutation is not clearly associated with distinct negative clinicopathological features and does not predict an unfavourable course, in contrast to adult PTC [12,13,18,20]. In the recently published European Thyroid Association Guidelines for the management of pediatric thyroid nodules and differentiated thyroid cancer (DTC), the authors recommend that the molecular gene analysis for the presence of BRAF V600E mutation in a fine-needle aspiration (FNA) specimen may be useful for diagnosis of PTC and therefore may be incorporated into the diagnostic work-up [21]. However, the use of BRAFV600E as a molecular marker in pediatric and adolescent PTC remains controversial.

Mutant BRAF is proposed to serve as a diagnostic and prognostic tool and may be a promising target for molecular therapy [22]. The real incidence and evidence of the actual effect of BRAF mutation in pediatric PTCs remains controversial in different studies. In this context, we conducted a systematic review of available evidence and a meta-analysis of data published over the past two decades to evaluate the association of BRAF gene mutations and PTC in children and adolescents, their prognostic role in terms of clinicopathological characteristics, and relationship with survival outcome.

2. Materials and Methods

The current systematic review and meta-analysis was designed following a predefined protocol, according to the Preferred Reporting Items for Systematic Reviews and Meta-Analysis (PRISMA) guidelines, which is registered in the PROSPERO database under the identification number: PROSPERO 2022 CRD42022358663.

2.1. Eligibility Criteria

The present systematic review included all original studies that reported a molecular study of proto-oncogene BRAF gene, in children and adolescents, aged up to 21 years, with a histopathological diagnosis of PTC. Studies were included only if they reported clinical or laboratory characteristics of PTC and/or assessed the overall survival of their participants. According to our predefined eligibility criteria, the diagnosis of PTC needed to be confirmed in all included individuals by either tumor biopsy or FNA biopsy, while BRAF genetic analysis could be reported by any available molecular method, such as Sanger analysis or direct sequencing. Relevant studies published in the last 20 years were identified. Language was restricted to English. No limitation of publication status was implied.

Exclusion criteria, in order to minimize potential publication bias and duplication of results, referred to studies including patients older than 21 years of age, data from univariate analyses if the HR was the primary outcome, studies involving other than PTC carcinomas, review articles, case reports, presentations, conference proceedings, editorials, expert opinions, research using big data (e.g., using SEER study data) and in vitro studies.

2.2. Study Outcomes

The main outcome of the present study was to investigate the difference in the prevalence of known prognostic factors between children and adolescents with PTC and a mutated BRAF gene compared to PTC patients without BRAF gene alterations. More specifically, the primary outcomes combined differences in the prevalence of the following tumor variables: multifocality, vascular invasion, extra-thyroid extension (ETE), presence of lymph node metastasis (LNM), distant metastases, and tumor recurrence. Data on differences in diametric tumor size and data regarding gender (male/female) distribution were also compared between BRAF positive and negative patients. The secondary outcome was the absolute overall survival difference of PTC patients with BRAF gene mutations compared to PTC patients without BRAF gene mutations.

2.3. Information Sources

Relevant studies over the past 20 years, evaluating the association of BRAF mutations with prognostic factors for PTC in children and adolescents, were identified by searching the following databases: PubMed, Ovid Medical Literature Analysis and Retrieval System Online (MEDLINE), SCOPUS, the US registry of clinical trials [www.clinicaltrials.com (accessed on 30 September 2022)] Cochrane Central Register of Controlled Trials and Cochrane reviews. Search was performed on September 2022, using a combination of relevant terms in the English language, such as "BRAF gene", "B-raf gene", "proto-oncogene B-raf gene", "papillary thyroid cancer", "children", "adolescents", "young adults". Two reviewers independently selected studies according to the inclusion criteria, while a third independent reviewer was available to address any discrepancies. Bibliographies from review articles were thoroughly examined to identify relevant studies, ensuring that papers and articles not selected in the initial search were also included.

2.4. Screening, Data Collection and Analysis

Conducted with a pilot-tested form by two reviewers and verified by a third using a predefined datasheet, data collection was performed. Two authors, E.P.K. and S.G., with expertise in systematic review, screened all titles and abstracts for eligibility, in a completely independent manner. Full texts were reviewed by the two reviewers and discrepancies were resolved with the involvement of a third reviewer, A.G.T. Reasons for exclusion were recorded for all studies excluded in the title, abstract or full text level of the review process. Data were extracted from full texts of the studies on a predefined worksheet. Two authors (A.P. and E.L.) extracted the following from the included articles: first author, country, publication years, study type, recruitment period, sample size, sample origin, method of BRAF analysis, BRAF V600E mutations, PTC-related risk factors. Age, gender, tumor size, vascular invasion, LNM, ETE, lymph node metastasis and distant metastasis were concluded as the predefined risk factors for PTC patients. The survival rate after any timepoint in retrospective, or in the present in prospective, studies was also recorded. Finally, funding sources and authors' conflict of interest were recorded and included. Any disagreements were resolved by a third investigator (E.P.K.).

2.5. Quality Assessment of Included Studies

Quality assessment of the included studies was conducted by two reviewers (E. S. and V.R.T.) using the Critical Appraisal Checklist JBI Tool for Analytical Cross-Sectional Studies, developed by the JBI, Faculty of Health and Medical Sciences at the University of Adelaide [23]. The tool consists of eight different questions that assess the methodological quality of each study, determining the extent to which the possibility of bias has been addressed in its design, conduction and analysis. Each question was rated by the two reviewers as green for "Yes", red for "No", or yellow for "Unclear". Discrepancies were resolved by discussion.

2.6. Measures of Effect

Effect measures used in the synthesis and presentation of results were set as follows: continuous outcomes as mean difference and 95% CI; dichotomous outcomes as odds ratio and 95% CI.

2.7. Data Synthesis

Data synthesis was performed with random-effects model, and two-tailed statistical significance was defined as a *p*-value < 0.05. For statistical analysis, the Comprehensive Meta-Analysis, v3.0 software (Biostat, Englewood, NJ, USA), was employed. The magnitude of the effect of each study was calculated by the OR, or briefly by the weighted mean difference (WMD) of the 95% CI briefly. In addition, heterogeneity was quantified using the I^2 statistic. When $I^2 < 50\%$, a fixed-effects model was applied; otherwise, a random-effects model was used. The Begg funnel plot was used to control for potential publication bias.

3. Results

3.1. Study Selection and Characteristics

The initial systematic screening of the available evidence resulted in a total of 817 studies. Among them, 267 records were excluded as duplicates; 12 records were excluded due to language other than English; 22 records were excluded as reviews and editorials; 22 records were excluded as case reports; 149 records were excluded as they concerned adult populations; 245 records were excluded since they reported mixed adult and child/adolescent population data, without subgroup analyses; six records were excluded since they did not mention the exact age of the population; 35 records were excluded as they did not report any of the outcomes of the present review; nine records were excluded due to populations with cancer type other than PTC; 13 records were excluded as basic science studies. Finally, a total of 37 studies that met our selection criteria were included in our meta-analysis. The selection flowchart of the research is presented in Figure 1.

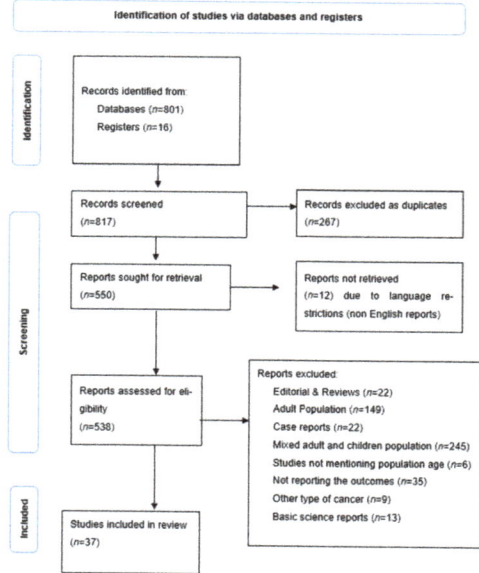

Figure 1. Systematic review flow chart of records identification and study screening.

Basic characteristics of the included studies and the associated factors examined are included in Table 1. Data regarding the methodology applied in the molecular analysis of the BRAF gene in included studies are presented in Supplementary Table S1, in combination with details regarding funding of the studies.

Table 1. Included studies' characteristics.

No	Authors, Year	Study Type	Recruitment (Country, Time)	Sample Size (n)	Sample Origin	Age (Years)	Gender (Boys/Girls)	BRAF Mutations Prevalence (%)	
								BRAF V600E	Other
1	Alzahrani [17], 2017	RC	Middle East, 1998–2015	79	registry	8–18	11/68	24	
2	Ballester [24], 2016	RCrS	USA, 2009–2014	25	clinical	10–19	6/19	40	
3	Buryk [25], 2013	RCaS	USA, 2009–2012	5	clinical	12–15	1/4	40	
4	Cordioli [16], 2017	RC	Brazil, NR	35	clinical	4–18	9/26	8.6	
5	Espadinha [26], 2009	C	Portugal, 2000–2007	15	clinical	5–21	4/11	7	
6	Franko [27], 2022	RC	USA, 1989–2019	122	clinical	<18	NR	21.3	0.75 (T599del)
7	Geng [18], 2017	RC	China, 1994–2014	48	clinical	3–14	19/29	35.4	
8	Gertz [15], 2016	RCrS	USA, 2008–2012	14	registry	8–18	5/9	31	7 (c.1799_1801 delTGA)
9	Givens [13], 2014	RCrS	USA, 1999–2012	19	registry	3–18	NR	36.8	
10	Hardee [20], 2017	RCrS	USA, 2003–2015	50	registry	<21	15/35	48	
11	Henke [12], 2014	RCrs	USA, 1973–2005	27	registry	6–21	6/21	63	
12	Hess [28], 2022	RCrS	USA, 2010–2019	27	clinical	9.1–18.7	4/23	33.3	
13	Kumagai [11], 2004	C	Japan/Ukraine, 1962–1995	44	registry	<17	NR		6.81 (T1796A)
14	Kure [29], 2019	RC	Japan, 2009–2017	14	registry	13–21	0/14	14.3	
15	Kurt [30], 2012	C	Turkey, 1995–2010	2	registry	14–20	1/1	50	
16	Lee [31], 2021	RCrS	Korea, 1983–2020	106	clinical/registry	4.3–19.8	22/84	38.7	
17	Li [7], 2022	RC	China, 2018–2021	169	clinical	6–18	40/129	57.4	
18	Macerola [32], 2021	RC	Italy, 2014–2020	163	registry	8–18	47/116	36.2	0.6 (K599I)
19	Mitsutake [33], 2015	RC	Japan, 2013–2014	67	clinical	9–22	NR	64.2	
20	Mollen [34], 2022	RCrS	USA, 2001–2017	62	clinical	4.2–18.9	47/15	30.6	
21	Mostufi-Moab [19], 2018	RCrS	USA, 1989–2012	62	registry	2–18	NR	19.4	
22	Newfield [35], 2022	RC	USA, 2001–2015	39	registry	<18	NR	28.2	2.6 (K601E)
23	Nies [36], 2021	RC	USA, 1946–2019	94	registry	10–16	NR	8.5	
24	Oishi [37], 2017	CC	Japan, 1991–2013	81	registry	6–20	7/74	54	
25	Onder [38], 2016	RC	Turkey, 1995–2015	50	registry	6–18	9/41	30	
26	Passon [39], 2015	RC	Italy, NR	2	clinical	17–19	0/2	0	
27	Pekova [40], 2019	RC	Czech Rep, 2003–2017	83	clinical	14.2 ± 3.4	24/59	18.1	
28	Pessôa-Pereira [41], 2019	RC	Brazil, 2006–2012	5	registry	12–20	0/5	20	
29	Poyrazoglu [42], 2017	RC	Turkey, 1983–2015	75	clinical	1.3–17.8	24/51	25	
30	Prasad ML [14], 2016	RCrS	USA, 2009–2015	28	clinical	6–18	8/20	48	
31	Rogounovitch [43], 2021	RC	Belarus, 2001–2007	34	registry	4–14	12/22	14.7	0 (K601E)
32	Romittii [44], 2012	RCrS	Brazil, NR	3	registry	10–18	0/3	0	
33	Şenyürek [45], 2022	RC	Turkey, 1995–2020	55	registry	5–18	15/55	33	
34	Sisdeli L [46], 2019	RC	Brazil, 1993–2017	80	registry	<18	NR	15	
35	Stenman [47], 2021	RC	Sweden, 1992–2021	5	registry	9–15	2/3	20	
36	Vasko V [48], 2005	RCrS	Ukraine, 1999–2004	4	clinical	14–20	2/2	25	
37	Zou M [49], 2014	RC	Saudi Arabia, 1987–2006	6	clinical	12–21	1/5	16.7	

NR: not reported, RC: retrospective cohort, C: cohort, RCaS: retrospective case series, RCrS: retrospective cross sectional, CC: case control. Age in presented as min-max or mean ± standard deviation.

3.2. Prevalence of BRAF Mutation

The most prevalent mutation of BRAF gene molecular analyses across all studies was BRAF V600E mutation, with reported prevalence rates ranging from 0% to 64.2% among pediatric and adolescent populations. Other reported genetic alterations of BRAF gene were BRAF c.1799_1801delTGA, BRAF T1796A, BRAF T599del, BRAF K599I, and BRAF K601E, with extreme modest frequency rates compared to V600E (Table 1).

Overall, BRAFV600E mutation was confirmed among a group of 596 individuals from a totality of 1799 children and adolescents with PTC in this systematic review and meta-analysis, resulting in a pooled BRAFV600E prevalence of 33.12% (Tables 1 and 2).

Table 2. Tumor Characteristics among PTC patients according to BRAF analysis.

No	Author, Year	Total Study Sample (n)	BRAF Mutation Status (+/−)	Sample per BRAF Group (n)	Tumor Size (cm) or (f*)	Multifocality (%)	Vascular Invasion (%)	LNM (%)	ETE (%)	DM (%)	Tumor Recurrence (%)
1	Alzahrani [17], 2017	79	+	19	2.8 ± 1.4	50	40	86.7	35.7	0	52.6
			−	60	3.3 ± 1.6	53.8	51.4	82.8	46.2	15	33.9
2	Ballester [24], 2016	25	+	10	NR	NR	NR	50	NR	NR	NR
			−	15	NR	NR	NR	46.7	NR	NR	NR
3	Buryk [25], 2013	5	+	2	2.7 ± 0.56	NR	NR	100	NR	NR	NR
			−	3	1.7 ± 0.17	NR	NR	33.3	NR	NR	NR
4	Cordioli [16], 2017	35	+	3	4.6 ± 1.25	NR	NR	100	0	0	NR
			−	16	2.9 ± 1.48	NR	NR	88.2	64.7	35.2	NR
5	Espadinha [26], 2009	15	+	1	NR	NR	NR	0	NR	NR	NR
			−	14	NR	NR	NR	NR	NR	NR	NR
6	Franko [27], 2022	122	+	26	* <2 cm = 11, 2–4 cm = 5, >4 cm = 10	NR	30.7	72	46.1	0	NR
			−	96	NR	NR	NR	NR	NR	NR	NR
7	Geng [18], 2017	48	+	17	* <2 cm = 2, 2–4 cm = 11, >4 cm = 4	20	NR	64.7	16.0	36.6	20
			−	31	* 2–4 cm = 17, >4 cm = 14	80	NR	80.6	84.0	63.4	80
8	Gertz [15], 2016	14	+	4	1.7 ± 1.2	NR	33.3	NR	25	0	NR
			−	9	2.7 ± 2.4	NR	33.3	NR	22.2	0	NR
9	Givens [13], 2014	19	+	7	2.08 ± 1.21	NR	NR	NR	60	0	16.7
			−	12	2.22 ± 1.78	NR	NR	NR	62.5	41.7	12.5
10	Hardee [20], 2017	50	+	24	* <2cm = 18, 2–4 cm = 2, >4 cm = 4	NR	NR	58	0	NR	21
			−	26	* <2cm = 13, 2–4 cm = 5, >4 cm = 7	NR	NR	69%	4	NR	8
11	Henke [12], 2014	27	+	17	NR	NR	NR	64.7	70.6	5.9	NR
			−	10	NR	NR	NR	60	50	0	NR
12	Hess [28], 2022	27	+	9	1.37 ± 1.09	NR	NR	42.8	NR	NR	NR
			−	18	3.22 ± 2.04	NR	NR	68.75	NR	NR	NR
13	Kumagai [11], 2004	44	+	3	1.56 ± 0.87	NR	NR	33.3	NR	0	NR
			−	NR	NR	NR	NR	NR	NR	NR	NR
14	Kure [29], 2019	14	+	2	1.25 ± 0.77	NR	50	33.3	0	0	NR
			−	12	2.34 ± 1.79	NR	50	66.6	8.3	8.33	NR
15	Kurt [30], 2012	2	+	1	NR	NR	NR	100	100	0	NR
			−	1	NR	32.5	NR	0	0	0	NR
16	Lee [31], 2021	106	+	41	1.40 ± 1.00	41.5	NR	68.4	60.5	2.5	16.2
			−	65	2.10 ± 1.30	23.7	NR	76.2	75.8	43.18	46.6
17	Li [7], 2022	169	+	97	1.55 ± 1.03	50	NR	14.4	24.7	2.1	2
			−	72	2.49 ± 1.18	NR	NR	8.3	36.1	4.1	8.3
18	Macerola [32], 2021	163	+	59	NR	NR	NR	NR	NR	NR	NR
			−	104	NR	NR	NR	NR	NR	NR	NR
19	Mitsutake [33], 2015	67	+	43	1.22 ± 0.68	NR	NR	14.2	58.1	0	NR
			−	20	1.83 ± 0.95	NR	NR	20	35	10.5	NR
20	Mollen [34], 2022	62	+	19	NR	NR	NR	NR	NR	NR	NR
			−	43	NR	NR	NR	NR	NR	NR	NR

Table 2. Cont.

No	Author, Year	Total Study Sample (n)	BRAF Mutation Status (+/−)	Sample per BRAF Group (n)	Tumor Size (cm) or (f*)	Multifocality (%)	Vascular Invasion (%)	LNM (%)	ETE (%)	DM (%)	Tumor Recurrence (%)
21	Mostufi-Moab [19], 2018	62	+	12	1.10–4.00	NR	NR	63.6	NR	0	NR
			−	50	NR	NR	NR	NR	NR	NR	NR
22	Newfield [35], 2022	39	+	11	2.67 ± 1.98	NR	54.5	81.8	NR	0	NR
			−	18	2.70 ± 1.44	NR	50	50	NR	7.14	NR
23	Nies [36], 2021	94	+	8	2.90 (2.3–3.2)	NR	NR	100	NR	100	NR
			−	86	3.50 (2.3–5.5)	NR	NR	NR	NR	100	NR
24	Oishi [37], 2017	81	+	44	3.20 ± 1.8	NR	NR	98	36	0	NR
			−	37	2.80 ± 1.3	NR	NR	81	44	8	NR
25	Onder [38], 2016	50	+	15	2.12 ± NR	93.3	NR	60	13.3	0	33.3
			−	35	2.26 ± NR	57.14	NR	61.5	8.57	14.2	5.7
26	Passon [39], 2015	2	+	0	NR	NR	NR	0	NR	0	NR
			−	2	NR	NR	NR	0	NR	0	NR
27	Pekova [40], 2019	83	+	15	2.00 ± 1.06	53.3	20	46.6	40	0	20
			−	68	2.22 ± 1.36	55.8	24.3	76.47	54.4	14.7	8.8
28	Pessôa-Pereira [41], 2019	5	+	1	1 ± 0	0	0	0	0	0	NR
			−	4	2.32 ± 1.39	75	25	50	0	0	NR
29	Poyrazoglu [42], 2017	75	+	14	* ≤1 cm = 3 >1 cm = 11	85.7	50	57.1	42.8	7.1	NR
			−	42	* ≤1 cm = 16 >1 cm = 26	42.8	40.5	38	28.6	9.5	NR
30	Prasad ML [14], 2016	28	+	13	1.44 ± 1.04	23.1	23.1	38.4	7.7	0	NR
			−	14	2.21 ± 1.13	50	NR	71.4	NR	14.3%	NR
31	Rogounovitch [43], 2021	34	+	5	1.44 ± 0.34	0	100	100	0	0	NR
			−	29	1.6 ± 0.9	NR	NR	NR	NR	NR	NR
32	Romittii [44], 2012	3	+	-	-	-	-	-	-	-	-
			−	1	10.5 ± 0	NR	NR	NR	NR	0	NR
33	Şenyürek [45], 2022	55	+	18	1.50 (0.6–5)	83.3	55.5	33.3	25	0	33.3
			−	37	1.40 (0.4–5)	56.7	32.4	35.1	21.6	8.1	2.7
34	Sisdeli L [46], 2019	80	+	12	3.35 ± 1.38	NR	NR	75	NR	25	NR
			−	68	2.64 ± 1.58	NR	NR	NR	NR	NR	NR
35	Stenman [47], 2021	5	+	1	4.20 ± 0	0	NR	100	100	NR	100
			−	4	4.57 ± 2.12	50	NR	100	75	25	50
36	Vasko V [48], 2005	4	+	3	2.36 ± 0.55	0	NR	NR	NR	NR	NR
			−	1	1.50 ± 0	0	NR	NR	NR	NR	NR
37	Zou M [49], 2014	6	+	1	NR	NR	NR	0	NR	0	NR
			−	3	NR	NR	NR	44.4	NR	0	NR

NR: not reported, LNM lymph node metastasis, ETE extra-thyroid extension, DM distant metastasis. Tumor size data are presented as mean ± standard deviation or median (min–max) in most included studies. * Tumor size data presented as categorical variable (f = number of participants per tumor size group).

3.3. BRAF Mutation and Gender

A random-effects model was applied to analyze the data of relevance among mutated BRAF and gender ($p = 0.65$, $I^2 = 11.6\%$). Prevalence of BRAFV600E mutation in female PTC patients was relatively higher than that in male PTC patients, without reaching significance (OR = 0.91, 95% CI = 0.62–1.33) (Figure 2).

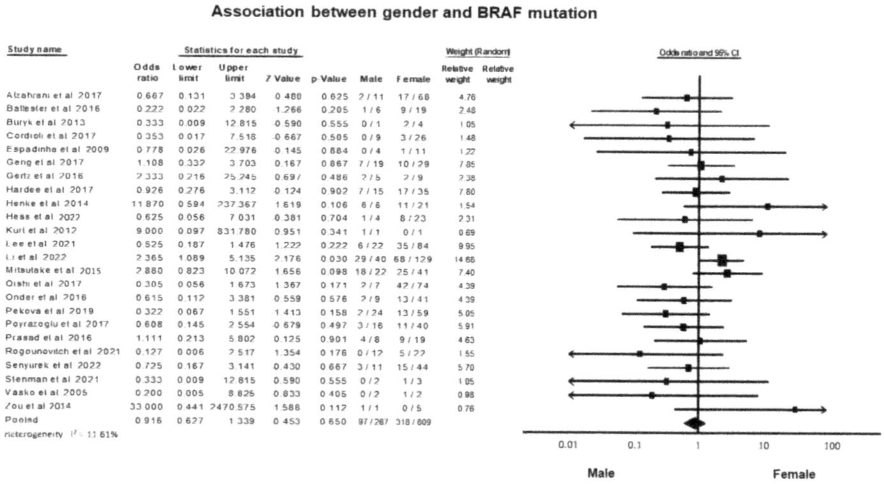

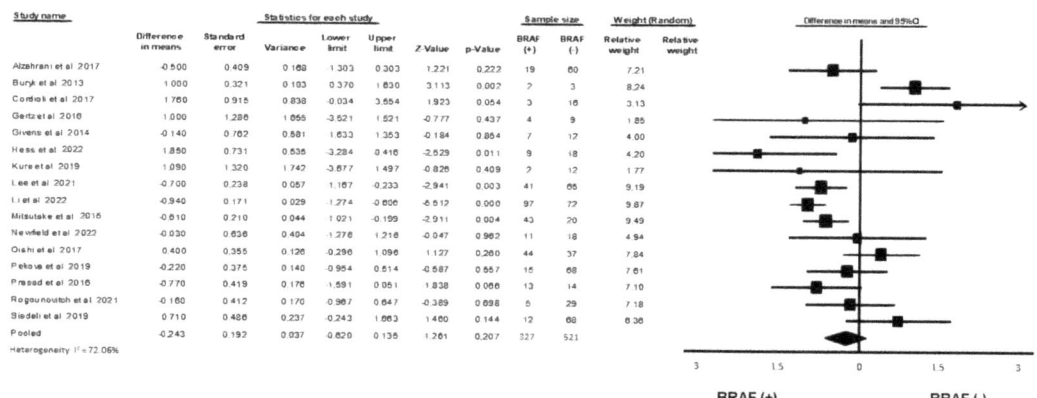

Figure 2. BRAF mutation and Gender correlation forest plot [7,12,14–18,20,24–26,28,30,31,33,37,38, 40,42,43,45,47–49].

3.4. BRAF Mutation and Tumor Size

A random-effects model on continuous data was applied to explore the effect of the presence of BRAF mutation to the size of PTC as expressed by the actual tumor diameter ($p = 0.21$, $I^2 = 72.06\%$). Meta-analysis revealed that tumor size was not significantly associated with BRAF mutation in children and adolescent patients with PTC (Mean Difference = -0.24, 95% CI = -0.62–0.135, St. error = 0.192) (Figure 3).

Figure 3. BRAF mutation and tumor size forest plot [7,13–17,25,28,29,31,33,35,37,40,43,46].

3.5. BRAF Mutation and Multifocality

A random-effects model was applied to analyze dichotomous data on the presence of multifocality in PTC ($p = 0.74$, $I^2 = 68.19\%$). According to our findings, tumor multifocality was not associated with BRAF gene mutation in pediatric and adolescent PTC (Table 2, OR = 1.13, 95% CI = 0.65–2.34) (Figure 4).

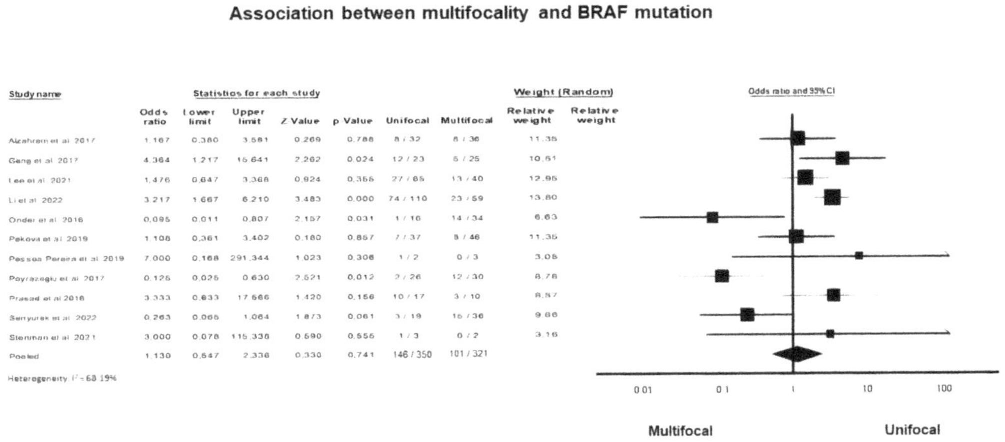

Association between multifocality and BRAF mutation

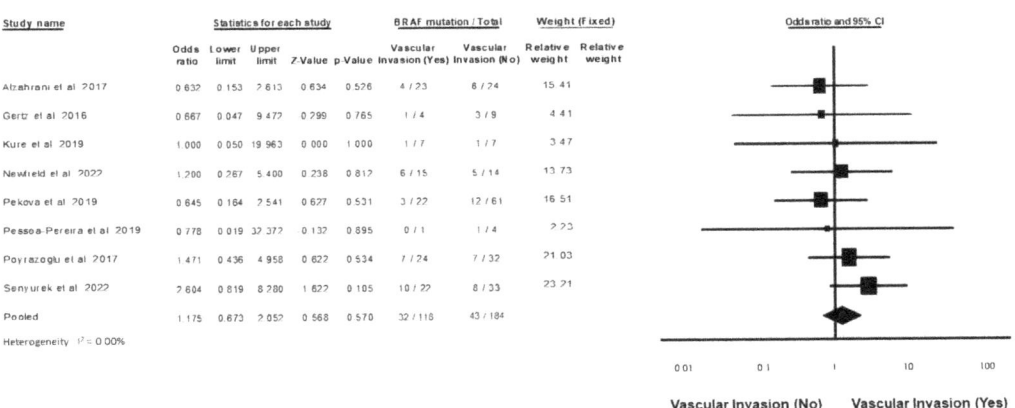

Figure 4. BRAF mutation and Multifocality forest plot [7,14,17,18,31,38,40–42,45,47].

3.6. BRAF Mutation and Vascular Invasion

A fixed-effects model was applied to analyze the presence of vascular invasion in PTC ($p = 0.57$, $I^2 = 0\%$). Pooled data of the present meta-analysis prove that the presence of vascular invasion in children and adolescents with PTC, does not exert a significantly higher risk for BRAF mutation (OR = 1.17, 95% CI = 0.67–2.05) (Figure 5).

Figure 5. BRAF mutation and Vascular invasion forest plot [15,17,29,35,40–42,45].

3.7. BRAF Mutation and Lymph Node Metastasis (LNM)

Data on the presence or not of Lymph Node Metastasis (LNM) upon diagnosis of PTC in children and adolescents was analyzed after the application of a random-effects model ($p = 0.66$, $I^2 = 20.83\%$). LNM is not associated with mutated or absence of BRAF in PTC children and adolescents (OR = 0.92, 95% CI = 0.63–1.33) (Figure 6).

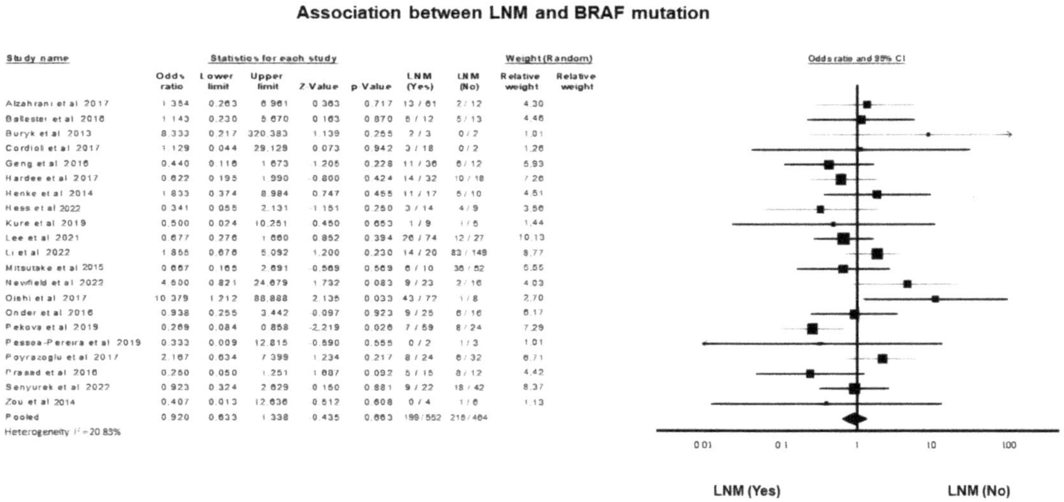

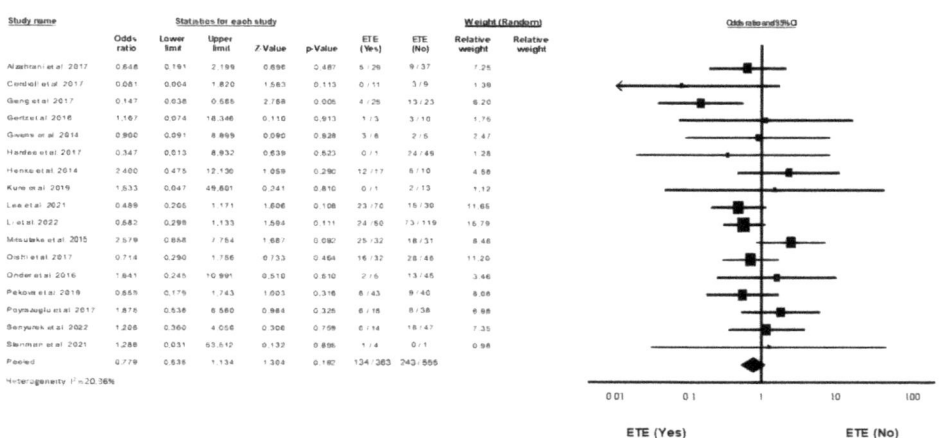

Figure 6. BRAF mutation and LNM forest plot [7,12,14,16–18,20,24,25,28,29,31,33,35,37,38,40–42,45,49].

3.8. BRAF Mutation and Extrathyroidal Extension (ETE)

A random-effects model was applied in order to meta-analyze categorical data on the presence or not of extrathyroidal extension of the PTC tumor in our study pooled population ($p = 0.19$, $I^2 = 20.36\%$). ETE is not significantly related to a higher rate of carrying a mutated BRAF gene among pediatric and adolescent patients with PTC (OR = 0.78, 95% CI = 0.53–1.13) (Figure 7).

Figure 7. BRAF mutation and ETE forest plot [7,12,13,15–18,20,29,31,33,37,38,40,42,45,47].

3.9. Distant Metastasis in BRAF Mutation

A fixed-effects model was selected to analyze the correlation between the presence of BRAF mutation and the emerge of distant metastasis after PTC ($p = 0.001$, $I^2 = 0\%$). It was found that distant metastasis is significantly associated with the presence of a mutated BRAF gene in children and adolescents with PTC (OR = 0.32, 95% CI = 0.16–0.61) (Figure 8).

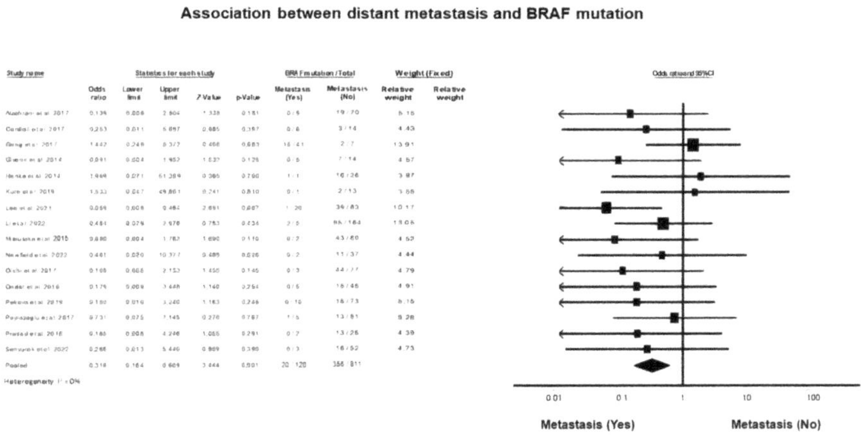

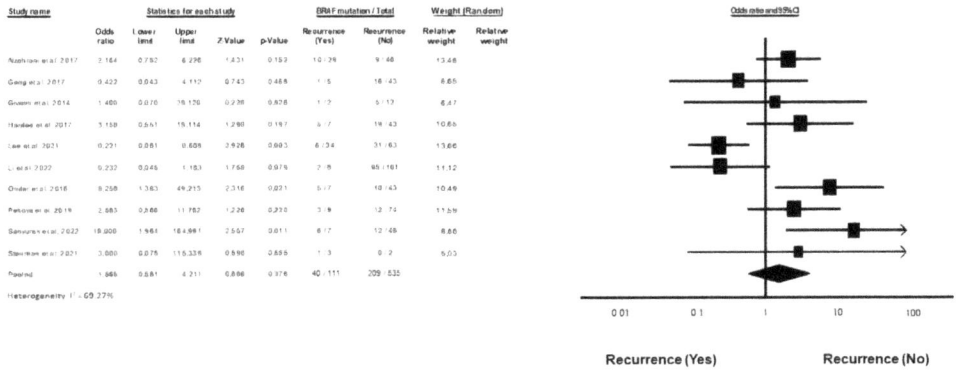

Figure 8. BRAF mutation and Distant Metastasis Forest plot [7,12–14,16–18,29,31,33,35,37,38,40,42,45].

3.10. Tumor Recurrence and BRAF Mutation

A random-effects model was utilized to analyze data regarding tumor recurrence rates and the presence of a mutated BRAF gene in children and adolescents with PTC ($p = 0.376$, $I^2 = 69.27\%$). It was found that BRAF mutation is not associated with tumor recurrence in the studied population (OR = 1.66, 95% CI = 0.68–4.21) (Figure 9).

Figure 9. BRAF mutation and Tumor Recurrence Forest plot [7,13,17,18,20,31,38,40,45,47].

3.11. BRAF Mutation and Survival Rate

Survival rate appeared as a variable reported in very few pediatric and adolescent studies. According to the present analyses, only a few records were identified as measuring survival at different time-points. Nies et al. report an overall 5-year survival rate of 98.5% in their small BRAF mutated cohort group [36]. In the same study, follow-up time ranged from 0.8–65 years, and thus authors report a 20-, 25-, and 30-year overall survival rate at 93.5%, 90.6%, and 86.8%, respectively [36]. Hardee et al. report a 100% survival rate in their cohort, with a follow- up time frame ranging from 10 to 42 years, as they recorded survival in year 2015 [20]. Mollen et al. reported a 100% survival rate in a median follow-up time of 6-years [34]. Finally, Henke et al. also report 100% overall survival during a 13.4 year study period [12]. It is obvious that, in pediatric protocols, recording survival is of poor scientific interest and is largely expected to reach the maximum (100%). The ten-year survival rate, usually reported in adult oncology, constitutes an outcome that was fairly reported in the childhood or adolescent cohorts, reflecting its difficulty in interpretation.

3.12. Assessment of Quality and Biases of the Included Studies

Quality assessment of included studies was performed using the JBI tool, consisting of eight different items, each of which scored 1 if the statement was 'Yes' (green sign) and 0 if the statement was 'No' (red sign), or 'Unclear' or 'Not applicable' (yellow sign) (Figure 10). The vast majority of studies assessed were considered as high quality (54.5%). More precisely, 35.13% scored seven out of eight points and 18.91% were graded with eight out of eight points, based upon the JBI quality assessment tool. Fifteen studies out of thirty-seven were at moderate risk related to quality assessment (40.53%), scoring five out of eight points (21.62%) and six out of eight (18.91%). Only a small percentage of studies (5.4%) recorded as low quality [13,24], since they confronted issues with domains regarding the criteria used for measurement of condition, identification of confounding factors and strategies to deal with them.

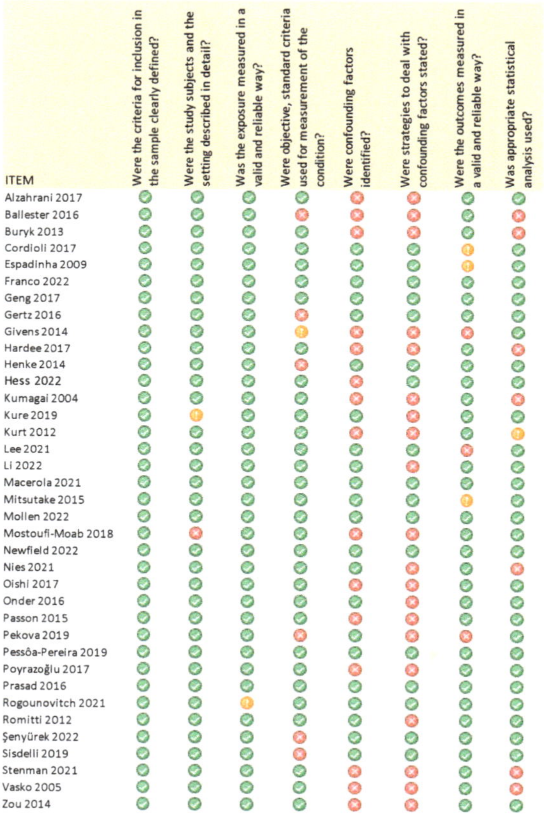

Figure 10. Risk of bias summary; authors' judgements on each risk of bias item for each included study [7,11–20,24–49].

The domain "inclusion criteria definition" was the only item of the JBI tool which all studies succeeded in scoring. Most of the studies met difficulties in scoring the items "identification of confounding factors" and "strategies statement to deal with cofounding factors". Accordingly, the least scored domain was "strategies to deal with confounding factors", in which 20 out of 37 studies scored zero (54%).

4. Discussion

The discrete clinical behaviour of pediatric and adult PTC seems also to derive from distinct differences at the molecular level. An essential factor promoting the factor of tumorigenesis is the activation of the MAPK pathway through genetic alterations of its components. Among them, BRAF gene holds a key role, almost exclusively through the V600E mutation, which is recognized as the most frequent oncogenic variant in adult PTC. Due to its high prevalence, BRAF V600E has gained special research interest as to whether it could serve to identify patients with a potential for an aggressive clinical course. This research query has been extensively explored by meta-analyses of studies concerning adult PTC cases [6–10]. The present study consists of the first coordinated attempt to systematically review and meta-analyse all available evidence on pediatric and/or adolescent PTC, in order to elucidate any association of BRAF gene mutations with the clinicopathological features and the long-term outcome in the age of interest (<21 years). Except for the profoundly lower frequency of BRAF V600E in children and adolescents with PTC compared to adults, only distant metastasis upon diagnosis was as unfavourable prognostic factors that was associated with the BRAF V600E mutation. Furthermore, the excellent prognosis can only be hypothesized, due to the scarce data on survival rate, not allowing further analysis.

The mutation of great interest in the literature was BRAF V600E, which has consistently emerged as the most prevalent alteration of the BRAF gene. The predominance of V600E mutation in the longitudinal analyses of BRAF is recorded both during the first years of the specific loci study, two decades ago, through classical molecular techniques [11], and recently through advanced techniques such as high-resolution melt analysis [32] and next generation sequencing [27,35]. The widely varying prevalence from 0% [39] to 64.2% [33] in different protocols, resulted in a pooled prevalence of 33.12% among individuals < 21 years of age. Thus, it is shown that pediatric cohorts exhibit a lower frequency of BRAF V600E mutation frequency than adult series, where the overall estimated prevalence was 74.63% [10], almost 2-fold more, ranging between 25.4–89% [50,51]. The great difference in mutation rates among studies may be attributed to the variable heterogenous proportion of children and adolescents included. Two studies found that patients with BRAFV600E mutation positive tumors were significantly older than the BRAF V600E negative patients [20,46]. In contrast, Geng et al. [18] reported that the presence of BRAFV600E mutation was associated with age at diagnosis of less than ten years. However, most studies failed to support any association between age and BRAFV600E [12,13,38]. It seems reasonable to hypothesize that, in studies including more adolescents than children, the prevalence increases, to "catch up" with that series of adult patients only. It is questionable whether this significantly different frequency of BRAF V600E between pediatric and adult populations may be implicated in their distinct clinicopathological characteristics and prognosis.

The gender distribution among PTC patients presents a well-known dimorphism, both in adults and in children or adolescents. Girls are more frequently diagnosed with PTC than boys by a ratio of 4:1. On the other hand, the BRAF V600E mutation is found more prevalent in male PTC patients. However, the relationship between BRAF V600E mutation and gender did not reach the level of statistical significance in this pooled data ($p = 0.06$). This finding is in accordance with the results of several other protocols [17,18,20,37,38,42,45,52]. Only two studies describe an association of the BRAF V600E mutation with the male gender [7,12]. It seems clear that the great female predominance among PTC patients in all age groups, opposed to the association of the BRAF V600E mutation with male gender in some studies, cannot be attributed to this genetic alteration according to the currently available data.

Regarding the intrinsic morphological features of a tumor, the diametrical tumor size, expressed in metric data, was not found to be significantly associated with a mutated BRAF variant. Our finding is in accordance with the vast majority of studies investigating the relationship between the presence of BRAFV600E mutation presence and tumor size [12,13,17,18,20,37,42,45]. Sisdelli et al. [46] supported an association of BRAF V600E mutation with larger tumor diameter, while Li et al. found the BRAFV600E mutation more frequent in patients with smaller tumor size [7]. Tumor size is the first element that guides the management algorithm of a thyroid nodule management and, thus, appears as an important variable in the risk stratification of a PTC by TNM grading. Diameters larger than 1 cm are defined as the precursor for a more aggressive oncogenic behaviour [1,21], independently of the BRAF V600E mutation. It is obvious that differences in the reporting of tumor size over time are significantly correlated with the improvement of ultrasound diagnostic ability, combined with higher qualifications and awareness among health professionals.

Multifocality, as another aggressive locoregional prognostic factor, was not found to be associated with BRAF gene mutation. Eleven studies were included in the meta-analysis and the data are not only scarce but also divergent. Our results are in agreement with those of three studies [17,45], while two other studies found a negative correlation with BRAFV600E mutations identified more frequently in patients lacking multifocal tumor [7,18]. Only in the study by Onder et al. was BRAFV600E mutation more frequently present in cases with multifocal tumors [38], while Şenyürek et al. [45] reached a borderline positive association ($p = 0.052$).

Turning to parameters indicative of extra-thyroid disease, we did not demonstrate any association of BRAF gene mutation with vascular invasion, as did other researchers [12,13,17,42]. High quality data on the effect of BRAF gene mutation on vascular invasion is lacking in the literature, perhaps due to the limited recording of vascular invasion as an independent prognostic parameter by investigators. ETE did not exhibit any difference in rate based on the presence or absence of the BRAF mutation. Similarly, previous studies reported no effect of BRAF V600E alteration on ETE [13,17,37,38,42]. Paradoxically, Geng et al. reported a negative correlation of BRAF V600E variant with ETE [18]. Furthermore, BRAF V600E mutation status was not associated with LNM. According to our results, most studies failed to support any association [13,17,18,20,38,42]. BRAF V600E was significantly more frequent in the BRAF V600E positive PCT patients, studied only by Li et al. and Oishi et al. [7,37].

Finally, in addition to the extent of the disease at diagnosis, another important parameter that determines long-term outcome is tumor recurrence. However, only one study described a positive association between BRAF mutation status and risk for recurrence [38]. The absence of an association between tumor recurrence and mutated BRAF is also only supported by scarce data [17,18]. Pooling of the available evidence in this study did not confirm any relevance between recurrence and BRAF mutations, due to very few and heterogenous data.

In the present meta-analysis, mutated BRAF was significantly associated with the presence of distant metastasis at diagnosis. Distant metastasis at diagnosis is usually considered an indicator of rapid growth of the primary tumor and a consistent reflection of poor disease prognosis. Data regarding the relation between BRAF mutation and the presence of distant metastasis are reported to be largely contradictory in the literature for both children and adults. In the majority of the cohorts investigated in the present meta-analysis, the prevalence of distant metastasis at diagnosis was low, as the total metastatic PCT events at diagnosis were pooled at the raw number of only 120 individuals.

According to our finding, the probability of detecting a mutated BRAF allele at diagnosis was significantly lower (OR:0.316) among patients with distant metastasis compared with those without metastatic disease. In adult PCT, it has been demonstrated by meta-analyses that BRAF mutation is also emerging as negatively associated with the presence of metastasis, but without reaching significance [10]. The validity of our finding is further firmly supported by the fact that heterogeneity was not evident in the pool of the available pediatric data (0%). It is highly significant that an emerging value for the molecular status BRAF is apparent, in terms of predicting the clinical course of PCT in children and adolescents.

An end point in the management of patients with PCT is the assessment of long-term survival, even in the pediatric population. The positive or negative effect of a prognostic factor ideally reflects the survival rate. The analysis of survival rates as a mathematic outcome is characterized by a specific burden, in order to obtain a reliable to estimate when based on retrospective data. The population subject to "loss of follow-up" during transition to adult health care professionals also complicates the derived survival outcomes, as systematic, long-term follow-up of pediatric patients with PTC is prone to missing data, especially when research in conducted out of a registry. In the available literature, the overall survival rate is estimated ≥98.5% and reached 100% in the four studies that conducted follow-up for 5.8–19.5 (4.5–52.8), 5.5–38.8, 10–42 and 6 years, respectively [12,20,34,36]. Interestingly, Hanke et al. did not find any difference in progression-free survival (PFS) at 10 years based on BRAF V600E mutational status [12].

Furthermore, Nies et al. observed that extrapulmonary metastatic disease was recorded in all cases that died, hypothesizing that BRAF V600E positive patients had smaller tumor sizes and a delayed diagnosis of metastasis due to the poor sensitivity of radioactive iodine (RAI) scans [36]. However, it is noteworthy that, even in the presence of metastatic disease, in a large series of 1433 pediatric patients with PTC, long-term follow-up has shown 5-, 15-, and 30-yr survival rates of 98%, 97%, and 91%, respectively [53]. It is obvious that future high quality cohort data, through registry implementation, could longitudinally address the question of the association between BRAF status and distinct survival rates among pediatric PTC survivors.

The meta-analytic approach to adult PTC data [6–10] has reached conclusions which are not parallel to the findings of the present study and, thus, may seem unexpected. It is noteworthy that, in the present analysis, BRAF mutation was not associated with potential aggressive prognostic factors or the overall survival rate of pediatric PTC patients, except for the presence of distant metastasis. In contrast to our findings, adult data suggest that the presence of BRAF V600E is significantly associated with a cluster of tumor prognostic factors (tumor diameter, lymph node metastasis, multifocality, vascular invasion and extrathyroid extension) [10]. Applying the rationale that children "are not just small adults", this study provides evidence that BRAF gene analysis could also be applied during childhood PCT, as a marker for the prognosis of distant metastatic disease.

Thus, this meta-analysis could support the hypothesis that BRAF mutation status may provide part of the explanation for the different biomolecular behaviour of PTC in adult and pediatric populations. Moreover, it also justifies the increased interest in the study of fusions that are found to be more prevalent and associated with aggressive potential and unfavorable events. Franco et al. found that patients with RET/NTRK fusions had exhibited worse outcomes than those with BRAF-mutant disease [27]. Even BRAF fusions, reported in 2.7% of PTC pediatric cases [4], were associated with younger age [46] and aggressive disease, as implied by more frequent ETE, LNM and DM, as well as with requirement for higher RAI treatment doses [40].

Although this meta-analysis included 37 studies, and a total of 1799 PTC pediatric patients with PTC, to investigate all PTC prognostic factors in relation to BRAF mutational status on risk stratification of pediatric patients, there were some limitations that should be acknowledged. The studies included populations of different demographic and racial characteristics, affected by a wide spectrum of environmental factors, and who received a variety of methods of diagnosis and molecular analysis. All these parameters increased the heterogeneity of the sample and reflected the burden of drawing firm conclusions in mathematical random effects models. In addition, several studies were performed in a small number of patients, analysing only some of the outcomes reviewed here. Furthermore, the present study did not analyze different therapeutic strategies in PTC and the evaluation of different treatment approaches in pediatric and adolescent PTC was out of the scope of the present protocol. Finally, most of the data meta-analyzed in the present study originated from cross-sectional and retrospective previous studies, thus complicating the ability to demonstrate causality.

5. Conclusions

In conclusion, BRAF V600E mutation is less common in children and adolescents than in adults. Its prognostic potential lies in its significant negative relationship with the presence of distant metastasis. No significant correlation between BRAF mutational status and gender, tumor size, multifocality, lymph node metastasis, extrathyroidal extension, vascular invasion, tumor recurrence or survival rate is evident among children and adolescents with PTC. Further research is needed in order to describe in more detail its role in the risk stratification and management of pediatric and adolescent patients with PTC, and to establish guidelines. However, it remains a target for molecular therapy and immunomodulation with BRAF inhibitors.

Supplementary Materials: The following supporting information can be downloaded at: https://www.mdpi.com/article/10.3390/diagnostics13061187/s1, Table S1: Included studies characteristics regarding methods of molecular analysis and funding sources/competing interest.

Author Contributions: Conceptualization, A.G.-T.; methodology, A.G.-T., E.P.K. and S.G.; protocol, S.K., E.P.K., S.G. and A.G.-T.; validation E.P.K., S.G., A.P. and E.L.; resources, E.P.K. and S.G.; data acquisition, A.P. and E.L.; software, K.M.; data analysis, E.P.K., S.G. and K.M.; investigation, E.P.K. and S.G.; quality assessment, V.R.T. and E.S., writing—original draft preparation, E.P.K., S.G., V.R.T., A.P., E.L., E.S., K.M., S.K., A.S. and A.G.-T.; writing—review and editing, A.G.-T., A.S., E.P.K. and S.G.; visualization, K.M.; supervision, A.G.-T.; funding acquisition, A.G.-T. All authors have read and agreed to the published version of the manuscript.

Funding: This research received no external funding.

Institutional Review Board Statement: Not applicable.

Informed Consent Statement: Not applicable.

Data Availability Statement: The data used to support the findings of this study are publicly available and listed in the supplementary material of this article.

Conflicts of Interest: The authors declare no conflict of interest.

References

1. Francis, G.L.; Waguespack, S.G.; Bauer, A.J.; Angelos, P.; Benvenga, S.; Cerutti, J.M.; Dinauer, C.A.; Hamilton, J.; Hay, I.D.; Luster, M.; et al. Management Guidelines for Children with Thyroid Nodules and Differentiated Thyroid Cancer. *Thyroid* **2015**, *25*, 716–759. [CrossRef] [PubMed]
2. Vaccarella, S.; Lortet-Tieulent, J.; Colombet, M.; Davies, L.; Stiller, C.A.; Schüz, J.; Togawa, K.; Bray, F.; Franceschi, S.; Dal Maso, L.; et al. Global Patterns and Trends in Incidence and Mortality of Thyroid Cancer in Children and Adolescents: A Population-Based Study. *Lancet Diabetes Endocrinol.* **2021**, *9*, 144–152. [CrossRef]
3. Bernier, M.O.; Withrow, D.R.; Berrington de Gonzalez, A.; Lam, C.J.K.; Linet, M.S.; Kitahara, C.M.; Shiels, M.S. Trends in Pediatric Thyroid Cancer Incidence in the United States, 1998–2013. *Cancer* **2019**, *125*, 2497–2505. [CrossRef] [PubMed]
4. Rangel-Pozzo, A.; Sisdelli, L.; Cordioli, M.I.V.; Vaisman, F.; Caria, P.; Mai, S.; Cerutti, J.M. Genetic Landscape of Papillary Thyroid Carcinoma and Nuclear Architecture: An Overview Comparing Pediatric and Adult Populations. *Cancers* **2020**, *12*, 3146. [CrossRef]
5. Zhang, B.; Wu, W.; Shang, X.; Huang, D.; Liu, M.; Zong, L. Incidence and Prognosis of Thyroid Cancer in Children: Based on the SEER Database. *Pediatr. Surg. Int.* **2022**, *38*, 445–456. [CrossRef] [PubMed]
6. Tufano, R.P.; Teixeira, G.V.; Bishop, J.; Carson, K.A.; Xing, M. BRAF Mutation in Papillary Thyroid Cancer and Its Value in Tailoring Initial Treatment: A Systematic Review and Meta-Analysis. *Medicine* **2012**, *91*, 274–286. [CrossRef]
7. Li, C.; Lee, K.C.; Schneider, E.B.; Zeiger, M.A. BRAF V600E Mutation and Its Association with Clinicopathological Features of Papillary Thyroid Cancer: A Meta-Analysis. *J. Clin. Endocrinol. Metab.* **2012**, *97*, 4559–4570. [CrossRef]
8. Wang, Z.; Chen, J.Q.; Liu, J.L.; Qin, X.G. Clinical Impact of BRAF Mutation on the Diagnosis and Prognosis of Papillary Thyroid Carcinoma: A Systematic Review and Meta-Analysis. *Eur. J. Clin. Investig.* **2016**, *46*, 146–157. [CrossRef]
9. Song, J.Y.; Sun, S.R.; Dong, F.; Huang, T.; Wu, B.; Zhou, J. Predictive Value of BRAFV600E Mutation for Lymph Node Metastasis in Papillary Thyroid Cancer: A Meta-Analysis. *Curr. Med. Sci.* **2018**, *38*, 785–797. [CrossRef]
10. Wei, X.; Wang, X.; Xiong, J.; Li, C.; Liao, Y.; Zhu, Y.; Mao, J. Risk and Prognostic Factors for BRAFV600E Mutations in Papillary Thyroid Carcinoma. *Biomed. Res. Int.* **2022**, *2022*, 9959645. [CrossRef]

11. Kumagai, A.; Namba, H.; Saenko, V.A.; Ashizawa, K.; Ohtsuru, A.; Ito, M.; Ishikawa, N.; Sugino, K.; Ito, K.; Jeremiah, S.; et al. Low Frequency of BRAFT1796A Mutations in Childhood Thyroid Carcinomas. *J. Clin. Endocrinol. Metab.* **2004**, *89*, 4280–4284. [CrossRef] [PubMed]
12. Henke, L.E.; Perkins, S.M.; Pfeifer, J.D.; Ma, C.; Chen, Y.; Dewees, T.; Grigsby, P.W. BRAF V600E Mutational Status in Pediatric Thyroid Cancer. *Pediatr. Blood Cancer* **2014**, *61*, 1168–1172. [CrossRef] [PubMed]
13. Givens, D.J.; Buchmann, L.O.; Agarwal, A.M.; Grimmer, J.F.; Hunt, J.P. BRAF V600E Does Not Predict Aggressive Features of Pediatric Papillary Thyroid Carcinoma. *Laryngoscope* **2014**, *124*, E389–E393. [CrossRef] [PubMed]
14. Prasad, M.L.; Vyas, M.; Horne, M.J.; Virk, R.K.; Morotti, R.; Liu, Z.; Tallini, G.; Nikiforova, M.N.; Christison-Lagay, E.R.; Udelsman, R.; et al. NTRK Fusion Oncogenes in Pediatric Papillary Thyroid Carcinoma in Northeast United States. *Cancer* **2016**, *122*, 1097–1107. [CrossRef] [PubMed]
15. Gertz, R.J.; Nikiforov, Y.; Rehrauer, W.; McDaniel, L.; Lloyd, R.V. Mutation in BRAF and Other Members of the MAPK Pathway in Papillary Thyroid Carcinoma in the Pediatric Population. *Arch. Pathol. Lab Med.* **2016**, *140*, 134–139. [CrossRef] [PubMed]
16. Cordioli, M.I.C.V.; Moraes, L.; Bastos, A.U.; Besson, P.; de Alves, M.T.S.; Delcelo, R.; Monte, O.; Longui, C.; Cury, A.N.; Cerutti, J.M. Fusion Oncogenes Are the Main Genetic Events Found in Sporadic Papillary Thyroid Carcinomas from Children. *Thyroid* **2017**, *27*, 182–188. [CrossRef]
17. Alzahrani, A.S.; Murugan, A.K.; Qasem, E.; Alswailem, M.; Al-Hindi, H.; Shi, Y. Single Point Mutations in Pediatric Differentiated Thyroid Cancer. *Thyroid* **2017**, *27*, 189–196. [CrossRef]
18. Geng, J.; Wang, H.; Liu, Y.; Tai, J.; Jin, Y.; Zhang, J.; He, L.; Fu, L.; Qin, H.; Song, Y.; et al. Correlation between BRAF V600E Mutation and Clinicopathological Features in Pediatric Papillary Thyroid Carcinoma. *Sci. China Life Sci.* **2017**, *60*, 729–738. [CrossRef]
19. Mostoufi-Moab, S.; Labourier, E.; Sullivan, L.; Livolsi, V.; Li, Y.; Xiao, R.; Beaudenon-Huibregtse, S.; Kazahaya, K.; Scott Adzick, N.; Baloch, Z.; et al. Molecular Testing for Oncogenic Gene Alterations in Pediatric Thyroid Lesions. *Thyroid* **2018**, *28*, 60–67. [CrossRef]
20. Hardee, S.; Prasad, M.L.; Hui, P.; Dinauer, C.A.; Morotti, R.A. Pathologic Characteristics, Natural History, and Prognostic Implications of BRAFV600E Mutation in Pediatric Papillary Thyroid Carcinoma. *Pediatr. Dev. Pathol.* **2017**, *20*, 206–212. [CrossRef]
21. Lebbink, C.A.; Links, T.P.; Czarniecka, A.; Dias, R.P.; Elisei, R.; Izatt, L.; Krude, H.; Lorenz, K.; Luster, M.; Newbold, K.; et al. 2022 European Thyroid Association Guidelines for the Management of Pediatric Thyroid Nodules and Differentiated Thyroid Carcinoma. *Eur. Thyroid J.* **2022**, *11*, e220146. [CrossRef] [PubMed]
22. Poulikakos, P.I.; Sullivan, R.J.; Yaeger, R. Molecular Pathways and Mechanisms of BRAF in Cancer Therapy. *Clin. Cancer Res.* **2022**, *28*, 4618–4628. [CrossRef]
23. Moola, S.; Munn, Z.; Tufanaru, C.; Aromataris, E.; Sears, K.; Sfetcu, R.; Currie, M.; Lisy, K.; Qureshi, R.; Mattis, P.; et al. Chapter 7: Systematic Reviews of Etiology and Risk. In *JBI Manual for Evidence Synthesis*; JBI: North Adelaide, SA, Australia, 2020. [CrossRef]
24. Ballester, L.Y.; Sarabia, S.F.; Sayeed, H.; Patel, N.; Baalwa, J.; Athanassaki, I.; Hernandez, J.A.; Fang, E.; Quintanilla, N.M.; Roy, A.; et al. Integrating Molecular Testing in the Diagnosis and Management of Children with Thyroid Lesions. *Pediatr. Dev. Pathol.* **2016**, *19*, 94–100. [CrossRef]
25. Buryk, M.A.; Monaco, S.E.; Witchel, S.F.; Mehta, D.K.; Gurtunca, N.; Nikiforov, Y.E.; Simons, J.P. Preoperative Cytology with Molecular Analysis to Help Guide Surgery for Pediatric Thyroid Nodules. *Int. J. Pediatr. Otorhinolaryngol.* **2013**, *77*, 1697–1700. [CrossRef] [PubMed]
26. Espadinha, C.; Santos, J.R.; Sobrinho, L.G.; Bugalho, M.J. Expression of Iodine Metabolism Genes in Human Thyroid Tissues: Evidence for Age and BRAFV600E Mutation Dependency. *Clin. Endocrinol.* **2009**, *70*, 629–635. [CrossRef]
27. Franco, A.T.; Ricarte-Filho, J.C.; Isaza, A.; Jones, Z.; Jain, N.; Mostoufi-Moab, S.; Surrey, L.; Laetsch, T.W.; Li, M.M.; DeHart, J.C.; et al. Fusion Oncogenes Are Associated With Increased Metastatic Capacity and Persistent Disease in Pediatric Thyroid Cancers. *J. Clin. Oncol.* **2022**, *40*, 1081–1090. [CrossRef] [PubMed]
28. Hess, J.R.; Newbern, D.K.; Beebe, K.L.; Walsh, A.M.; Schafernak, K.T. High Prevalence of Gene Fusions and Copy Number Alterations in Pediatric Radiation Therapy-Induced Papillary and Follicular Thyroid Carcinomas. *Thyroid* **2022**, *32*, 411–420. [CrossRef]
29. Kure, S.; Ishino, K.; Kudo, M.; Wada, R.; Saito, M.; Nagaoka, R.; Sugitani, I.; Naito, Z. Incidence of BRAF V600E Mutation in Patients with Papillary Thyroid Carcinoma: A Single-Institution Experience. *J. Int. Med. Res.* **2019**, *47*, 5560–5572. [CrossRef]
30. Kurt, B.; Yalçln, S.; Alagöz, E.; Karsllıoğlu, Y.; Yigit, N.; Günal, A.; Deveci, M.S. The Relationship of the BRAF(V600E) Mutation and the Established Prognostic Factors in Papillary Thyroid Carcinomas. *Endocr. Pathol.* **2012**, *23*, 135–140. [CrossRef]
31. Lee, Y.A.; Lee, H.; Im, S.W.; Song, Y.S.; Oh, D.Y.; Kang, H.J.; Won, J.K.; Jung, K.C.; Kwon, D.; Chung, E.J.; et al. NTRK and RET Fusion-Directed Therapy in Pediatric Thyroid Cancer Yields a Tumor Response and Radioiodine Uptake. *J. Clin. Investig.* **2021**, *131*, e144847. [CrossRef]
32. Macerola, E.; Proietti, A.; Poma, A.M.; Ugolini, C.; Torregrossa, L.; Vignali, P.; Basolo, A.; Materazzi, G.; Elisei, R.; Santini, F.; et al. Molecular Alterations in Relation to Histopathological Characteristics in a Large Series of Pediatric Papillary Thyroid Carcinoma from a Single Institution. *Cancers* **2021**, *13*, 3123. [CrossRef] [PubMed]
33. Mitsutake, N.; Fukushima, T.; Matsuse, M.; Rogounovitch, T.; Saenko, V.; Uchino, S.; Ito, M.; Suzuki, K.; Suzuki, S.; Yamashita, S. BRAFV600E Mutation Is Highly Prevalent in Thyroid Carcinomas in the Young Population in Fukushima: A Different Oncogenic Profile from Chernobyl. *Sci. Rep.* **2015**, *5*, 16976. [CrossRef] [PubMed]

34. Mollen, K.P.; Shaffer, A.D.; Yip, L.; Monaco, S.E.; Huyett, P.; Viswanathan, P.; Witchel, S.F.; Duvvuri, U.; Simons, J.P. Unique Molecular Signatures Are Associated with Aggressive Histology in Pediatric Differentiated Thyroid Cancer. *Thyroid* 2022, *32*, 236–244. [CrossRef]
35. Newfield, R.S.; Jiang, W.; Sugganth, D.X.; Hantash, F.M.; Lee, E.; Newbury, R.O. Mutational Analysis Using next Generation Sequencing in Pediatric Thyroid Cancer Reveals BRAF and Fusion Oncogenes Are Common. *Int. J. Pediatr. Otorhinolaryngol.* 2022, *157*, 111121. [CrossRef] [PubMed]
36. Nies, M.; Vassilopoulou-Sellin, R.; Bassett, R.L.; Yedururi, S.; Zafereo, M.E.; Cabanillas, M.E.; Sherman, S.I.; Links, T.P.; Waguespack, S.G. Distant Metastases From Childhood Differentiated Thyroid Carcinoma: Clinical Course and Mutational Landscape. *J. Clin. Endocrinol. Metab.* 2021, *106*, E1683–E1697. [CrossRef]
37. Oishi, N.; Kondo, T.; Nakazawa, T.; Mochizuki, K.; Inoue, T.; Kasai, K.; Tahara, I.; Yabuta, T.; Hirokawa, M.; Miyauchi, A.; et al. Frequent BRAF V600E and Absence of TERT Promoter Mutations Characterize Sporadic Pediatric Papillary Thyroid Carcinomas in Japan. *Endocr. Pathol.* 2017, *28*, 103–111. [CrossRef]
38. Onder, S.; Ozturk Sari, S.; Yegen, G.; Sormaz, I.C.; Yılmaz, I.; Poyrazoglu, S.; Sanlı, Y.; Giles Senyurek, Y.; Kapran, Y.; Mete, O. Classic Architecture with Multicentricity and Local Recurrence, and Absence of TERT Promoter Mutations Are Correlates of BRAF (V600E) Harboring Pediatric Papillary Thyroid Carcinomas. *Endocr. Pathol.* 2016, *27*, 153–161. [CrossRef]
39. Passon, N.; Bregant, E.; Sponziello, M.; Dima, M.; Rosignolo, F.; Durante, C.; Celano, M.; Russo, D.; Filetti, S.; Damante, G. Somatic Amplifications and Deletions in Genome of Papillary Thyroid Carcinomas. *Endocrine* 2015, *50*, 453–464. [CrossRef]
40. Pekova, B.; Dvorakova, S.; Sykorova, V.; Vacinova, G.; Vaclavikova, E.; Moravcova, J.; Katra, R.; Vlcek, P.; Sykorova, P.; Kodetova, D.; et al. Somatic Genetic Alterations in a Large Cohort of Pediatric Thyroid Nodules. *Endocr. Connect* 2019, *8*, 796. [CrossRef]
41. Pessôa-Pereira, D.; da Medeiros, M.F.S.; Lima, V.M.S.; da Silva, J.C.; de Cerqueira, T.L.O.; da Silva, I.C.; Fonseca, L.E.; Sampaio, L.J.L.; de Lima, C.R.A.; Ramos, H.E. Association between BRAF (V600E) Mutation and Clinicopathological Features of Papillary Thyroid Carcinoma: A Brazilian Single-Centre Case Series. *Arch. Endocrinol. Metab.* 2019, *63*, 97–106. [CrossRef]
42. Poyrazoğlu, Ş.; Bundak, R.; Baş, F.; Yeğen, G.; Şanlı, Y.; Darendeliler, F. Clinicopathological Characteristics of Papillary Thyroid Cancer in Children with Emphasis on Pubertal Status and Association with BRAFV600E Mutation. *J. Clin. Res. Pediatr. Endocrinol.* 2017, *9*, 185–193. [CrossRef]
43. Rogounovitch, T.I.; Mankovskaya, S.V.; Fridman, M.V.; Leonova, T.A.; Kondratovitch, V.A.; Konoplya, N.E.; Yamashita, S.; Mitsutake, N.; Saenko, V.A. Major Oncogenic Drivers and Their Clinicopathological Correlations in Sporadic Childhood Papillary Thyroid Carcinoma in Belarus. *Cancers* 2021, *13*, 3374. [CrossRef]
44. Romitti, M.; Wajner, S.M.; Zennig, N.; Goemann, I.M.; Bueno, A.L.; Meyer, E.L.S.; Maia, A.L. Increased Type 3 Deiodinase Expression in Papillary Thyroid Carcinoma. *Thyroid* 2012, *22*, 897–904. [CrossRef] [PubMed]
45. Şenyürek, Y.G.; İşcan, Y.; Sormaz, İ.C.; Poyrazoğlu, Ş.; Tunca, F. The Role of American Thyroid Association Pediatric Thyroid Cancer Risk Stratification and BRAFV600E Mutation in Predicting the Response to Treatment in Papillary Thyroid Cancer Patients ≤18 Years Old. *J. Clin. Res. Pediatr. Endocrinol.* 2022, *14*, 196. [CrossRef] [PubMed]
46. Sisdelli, L.; Cordioli, M.I.C.V.; Vaisman, F.; Moraes, L.; Colozza-Gama, G.A.; Alves, P.A.G.; Araújo, M.L.; Alves, M.T.S.; Monte, O.; Longui, C.A.; et al. AGK-BRAF Is Associated with Distant Metastasis and Younger Age in Pediatric Papillary Thyroid Carcinoma. *Pediatr. Blood Cancer* 2019, *66*, e27707. [CrossRef]
47. Stenman, A.; Backman, S.; Johansson, K.; Paulsson, J.O.; Stålberg, P.; Zedenius, J.; Christofer Juhlin, C. Pan-Genomic Characterization of High-Risk Pediatric Papillary Thyroid Carcinoma. *Endocr. Relat. Cancer* 2021, *28*, 337. [CrossRef] [PubMed]
48. Vasko, V.; Hu, S.; Wu, G.; Xing, J.C.; Larin, A.; Savchenko, V.; Trink, B.; Xing, M. High Prevalence and Possible de Novo Formation of BRAF Mutation in Metastasized Papillary Thyroid Cancer in Lymph Nodes. *J. Clin. Endocrinol. Metab.* 2005, *90*, 5265–5269. [CrossRef]
49. Zou, M.; Baitei, E.Y.; Alzahrani, A.S.; Binhumaid, F.S.; Alkhafaji, D.; Al-Rijjal, R.A.; Meyer, B.F.; Shi, Y. Concomitant RAS, RET/PTC, or BRAF Mutations in Advanced Stage of Papillary Thyroid Carcinoma. *Thyroid* 2014, *24*, 1256–1266. [CrossRef]
50. Celik, M.; Bulbul, B.Y.; Ayturk, S.; Durmus, Y.; Gurkan, H.; Can, N.; Tastekin, E.; Ustun, F.; Sezer, A.; Guldiken, S. The Relation between BRAFV600E Mutation and Clinicopathological Characteristics of Papillary Thyroid Cancer. *Med. Glas (Zenica)* 2020, *17*, 30–34. [CrossRef]
51. Jung, Y.Y.; Yoo, J.H.; Park, E.S.; Kim, M.K.; Lee, T.J.; Cho, B.Y.; Chung, Y.J.; Kang, K.H.; Ahn, H.Y.; Kim, H.S. Clinicopathologic Correlations of the BRAFV600E Mutation, BRAF V600E Immunohistochemistry, and BRAF RNA in Situ Hybridization in Papillary Thyroid Carcinoma. *Pathol. Res. Pract.* 2015, *211*, 162–170. [CrossRef]
52. Iwadate, M.; Mitsutake, N.; Matsuse, M.; Fukushima, T.; Suzuki, S.; Matsumoto, Y.; Ookouchi, C.; Mizunuma, H.; Nakamura, I.; Nakano, K.; et al. The Clinicopathological Results of Thyroid Cancer With BRAFV600E Mutation in the Young Population of Fukushima. *J. Clin. Endocrinol. Metab.* 2020, *105*, dgaa573. [CrossRef] [PubMed]
53. Hogan, A.R.; Zhuge, Y.; Perez, E.A.; Koniaris, L.G.; Lew, J.I.; Sola, J.E. Pediatric Thyroid Carcinoma: Incidence and Outcomes in 1753 Patients. *J. Surg. Res.* 2009, *156*, 167–172. [CrossRef] [PubMed]

Disclaimer/Publisher's Note: The statements, opinions and data contained in all publications are solely those of the individual author(s) and contributor(s) and not of MDPI and/or the editor(s). MDPI and/or the editor(s) disclaim responsibility for any injury to people or property resulting from any ideas, methods, instructions or products referred to in the content.

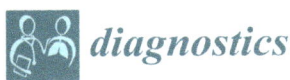

Review

Sarcoma Botryoides: Optimal Therapeutic Management and Prognosis of an Unfavorable Malignant Neoplasm of Female Children

Chrysoula Margioula-Siarkou [1], Stamatios Petousis [1,*], Aristarchos Almperis [1], Georgia Margioula-Siarkou [1], Antonio Simone Laganà [2], Maria Kourti [3], Alexios Papanikolaou [1] and Konstantinos Dinas [1]

1. Gynaecologic Oncology Unit, 2nd Department of Obstetrics and Gynaecology, Aristotle University of Thessaloniki, Hippokration General Hospital, 54642 Thessaloniki, Greece
2. Unit of Gynecologic Oncology, ARNAS "Civico–Di Cristina–Benfratelli", Department of Health Promotion, Mother and Child Care, Internal Medicine and Medical Specialties (PROMISE), University of Palermo, 90127 Palermo, Italy
3. 3rd Department of Pediatrics, Aristotle University of Thessaloniki, Hippokration General Hospital, 54642 Thessaloniki, Greece
* Correspondence: petousisstamatios@gmail.com

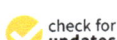

Citation: Margioula-Siarkou, C.; Petousis, S.; Almperis, A.; Margioula-Siarkou, G.; Laganà, A.S.; Kourti, M.; Papanikolaou, A.; Dinas, K. Sarcoma Botryoides: Optimal Therapeutic Management and Prognosis of an Unfavorable Malignant Neoplasm of Female Children. *Diagnostics* **2023**, *13*, 924. https://doi.org/10.3390/diagnostics13050924

Academic Editor: Edward J. Pavlik

Received: 22 December 2022
Revised: 5 February 2023
Accepted: 14 February 2023
Published: 1 March 2023

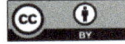

Copyright: © 2023 by the authors. Licensee MDPI, Basel, Switzerland. This article is an open access article distributed under the terms and conditions of the Creative Commons Attribution (CC BY) license (https://creativecommons.org/licenses/by/4.0/).

Abstract: Embryonal rhabdomyosarcoma (ERMS) is a rare malignancy and occurs primarily in the first two decades of life. Botryoid rhabdomyosarcoma is an aggressive subtype of ERMS that often manifests in the genital tract of female infants and children. Due to its rarity, the optimal treatment approach has been a matter of debate. We conducted a search in the PubMed database and supplemented it with a manual search to retrieve additional papers eligible for inclusion. We retrieved 13 case reports and case series, from which we summarized that the current trend is to approach each patient with a personalized treatment plan. This consists of a combination of local debulking surgery and adjuvant or neoadjuvant chemotherapy (NACT). Effort is made in every approach to avoid radiation for the sake of preserving fertility. Radical surgeries and radiation still have a role to play in extensive disease and in cases of relapse. Despite the rarity and aggressiveness of this tumor, disease-free survival and overall prognosis is excellent, especially when it is diagnosed early, compared with other subtypes of rhabdomyosarcoma (RMS). We conclude that the practice of a multidisciplinary approach is appropriate, with favorable outcomes; however, larger-scale studies need to be organized to have a definite consensus on optimal management.

Keywords: sarcoma botryoides; fertility-sparing surgery; embryonal rhabdomyosarcoma; genital tract; prognosis; treatment; local debulking; neoadjuvant chemotherapy; radiation

1. Introduction

Rhabdomyosarcoma (RMS) is the most common soft tissue tumor of early childhood and young adulthood, accounting for 4 to 6% of all malignancies in this age group, with boys being affected 1.5 times more frequently than girls. The primary sites of origin are in the region of the head and neck (35–40%), followed by the genitourinary tract (25%) [1–6]. There are three major histologic subtypes of RMS described in the literature: embryonal, alveolar, and pleomorphic/undifferentiated, with embryonal rhabdomyosarcoma (ERMS) being the most common subtype (2/3 of genitourinary cases) [7]. This last one can be further classified into the classic subtype, the spindle cell subtype, and the botryoid subtype [8]. The botryoid subtype of ERMS is suggested to be the most common according to the literature. This specific rare type of tumor has an embryologic origin in the skeletal muscle cells and arises from the mucosal surfaces on the walls of hollow organs, such as the vagina, bladder, biliary tract, and nasopharynx of infants, or, more rarely, the uterine cervix [3]. Sarcoma botryoides most usually affects young people; however, it can also present in some rare cases in the elderly. It also seems that botryoid sarcoma arising from the vagina tends to develop in very young girls during infancy and early childhood [9,10]. Cervical and uterine tumors, on the other hand, primarily develop in older females with a peak incidence in the second decade [11]. The name botryoides originates from the ancient Greek root bórty(s), which indicates the appearance of "a bunch of grapes". The typical presentation of the tumor is a nodular, grape-like mass protruding from the vagina, which should alarm every doctor since an early diagnosis is paramount to preventing death and preserving fertility in this delicate age. In the last decades, there has been a paradigm shift in the treatment of patients, including a multidisciplinary approach consisting of a variety of surgical procedures, radiation therapy, and systemic chemotherapy [1,12].

The main purpose of the present manuscript is to provide a comprehensive narrative review of the literature and summarize the main outcomes regarding the optimal therapeutic management and prognosis of this rare neoplasm of female childhood.

2. Methods

A literature search was performed in September 2022 through the PubMed, Scopus, and Web of Science databases. The main objective of the present study was to identify any type of research article reporting outcomes about therapeutic management and/or prognosis of cases diagnosed with botryoid sarcoma. The literature search was focused on the period 1990–2022. An electronic search was conducted by using the terms "botryoid sarcoma" [tiab] or botryoid rhabdomyosarcoma [tiab].

Observational cohort studies, both prospective and retrospective; case series; case reports; and narrative and systematic reviews that reported on the management and the prognosis of botryoid sarcoma were included in the present review. Studies were included irrespective of stage of disease at initial diagnosis and use of adjuvant therapy. The exclusion criteria concerned studies with incomplete data that did not permit definitive conclusions, non-English studies, and published abstracts without available full text.

The main outcomes of interest to identify in the included studies were age at diagnosis, primary location of the tumor, main symptom, size, stage, presence of metastases, treatment, status after treatment, diagnosis of relapse, treatment of relapse, follow up in months, and outcome as well as the main immunohistochemistry biomarkers used for final diagnosis.

Systematic search initially identified 221 papers potentially eligible for inclusion in the present analysis. After adjusting for inclusion and exclusion criteria, there were finally 13 case series or case reports included in the present review.

3. Results

3.1. Management

According to the literature search, female patients with a diagnosis of botryoides sarcoma are most commonly admitted to the hospital due to abnormal vaginal bleeding or a "grape-like" polypoid or prolapsing mass protruding from the vaginal introitus. In some cases, additional symptoms have also been described such as leukorrhea and malodorous discharge [13]. In addition, clinicians must be aware of characteristics of this unusual disease, especially the common sites of origin (vagina, bladder, etc.), the aggressiveness of the tumor, and the clinical manifestations, to avoid misdiagnosis and mismanagement, since benign polyps in the vagina or cervix are relatively uncommon in children. Furthermore, some authors also suggest that any polypoidal mass spotted in a child should be considered as botryoid RMS unless proven otherwise, given the fact that this kind of tumor can rightly be suspected in the majority of cases, and, thus, contributing to a more favorable management of the patient [14]. The initial workup usually includes imaging procedures, with first being ultrasound, followed by MRI of the primary site and regional lymph nodes, which is the best imaging method for RMS, given its superior ability to depict soft tissue changes. A computerized tomography (CT) scan and bone marrow biopsy can also provide assistance in assessing any metastatic manifestation from RMS [15], since the primary sites of metastasis in genitourinary RMSs are the lungs and the bone marrow [2,15]. According to the literature, a risk-specific approach to staging is recommended, based on the Intergroup

Rhabdomyosarcoma Study Group (IRSG) clinical categorization method [16] and the TNM staging approach for rhabdomyosarcoma [8] in order to determine the patient's clinical risk group; this will consequently stratify the treatment. Additionally, Borinstein et al. [17], in a recently published consensus article, included the tumor's PAX/FOXO1 fusion status (positive/negative) in the risk stratification of patients, since the expression of this fusion gene is associated with dismal outcomes. Molecular testing (e.g., FISH, reverse transcription PCR, or next-generation sequencing) can readily identify PAX/FOXO1 fusions, and because results may impact treatment decisions, it was recommended by these sarcoma experts to test for FOXO1 fusions on all patients with alveolar or embryonal histology. For the diagnosis of botryoid-variant RMS, three crucial criteria have been proposed that must be fulfilled: a polypoid appearance of the lesion, an origin below a mucous membrane-covered surface, and the presence of a cambium layer [18]. However, the gold standard for the diagnosis is histopathology and post-surgery immunohistochemistry, although, in some cases, the diagnosis is achieved by preoperative histopathology or intraoperative frozen section [19]. The optimal management of botryoid RMS is a debatable matter for gynecologists. Until the 1970s, radical surgery with pelvic exenteration was regarded as the treatment of choice. Over the years, the Intergroup Rhabdomyosarcoma Study Group (IRSG) had an important impact on changing that practice, so that the frequency of radical surgery was progressively reduced from 100% in the first IRSG study to 13% in the fourth IRSG study [20–22]. Surgical treatment has evolved from radical exenterations to local surgical resection in appropriate candidates along with other treatment modalities that are offered such as multi-agent adjuvant or neoadjuvant chemotherapy with or without radiotherapy. Exenterative surgery still plays a role in treating persistent or recurrent tumors [1,23]. In recent years, the effective treatment for sarcoma botryoides has been considered local control of vaginal and cervical tumor with fertility-sparing methods such as polypectomy, conization, local excisions, and robot-assisted radical trachelectomy [24]. Cases were found in the literature in which vaginectomy and buccal mucosa vaginoplasty was implemented as local therapy for pediatric vaginal rhabdomyosarcoma in the spirit of local control for genitourinary RMS with the purpose of avoiding radiation. Due to the fact that about half of the cases of botryoid sarcoma affect the vagina, adequate local control is paramount in the treatment of these patients, as suggested by the high recurrence rates observed in these patients when treated with chemotherapy alone [25]. Given the high incidence of micrometastatic disease that leads to relapse in patients treated only with local therapy, all RMS patients (where possible) were treated with adjuvant chemotherapy. The current trend, as seen in the majority of cases presented in Table 1, is to begin with multi-agent NACT as the first step to downstage the tumor and then proceed with excision with a safe margin of 1 cm to 2 cm, followed by 6–12 cycles of adjuvant chemotherapy to limit the chance of recurrence. Standardized schemes of chemotherapy are based on protocols created by the IRSG. The most widely used regimen of chemotherapy for children and young adults is the combination of vincristine, actinomycin D, and cyclophosphamide (VAC), usually given in 6 to 12 cycles [26]. The recommendations of Borinstein et al. [11], who proposed a treatment algorithm based on the risk group and the gene fusion status of the patient with RMS, are consistent with this practice. The management of this tumor poses a great challenge since it mostly occurs at a young age, when the preservation of hormonal, sexual, and reproductive function is fundamental. This makes fertility-sparing procedures more enticing while radiation and radical excision are not routinely preferred. Nevertheless, they still play an important role and should be reserved for cases of relapse and for the treatment of gross residual disease following surgery or chemotherapy. This approach is further encouraged by the results of the studies performed by the IRSG, which stated that the 5-year survival among patients with nonmetastatic disease was not statistically different among those who underwent versus among those who did not undergo postoperative radiation therapy. These conclusions omitted the irrefutably negative effects of radiation on maintaining the fertility of the young [8]. While surgery can be considered for lesions that can be resected with minimal morbidity, radiotherapy is often used to treat the primary tumor site, if not initially treated, and to treat metastatic sites when such therapy is feasible. Furthermore, it can be observed that there are patients who complete therapy for RMS and frequently are not able to achieve complete radiographic response by cross-sectional imaging, although their PET scans are often normal. This finding is likely due to tumor scarring or differentiation. At this point, it is suggested that resection or biopsy of a residual tumor is not recommended except for the cases in which they are enlarging or causing pain, because the extent of the tumor response does not predict survival. These cases that remain PET avid are challenging to manage, and the decision whether to biopsy or resect a residual PET-avid tumor must be made on a case-by-case basis, weighing the risks of morbidity versus the benefit.

Table 1. Characteristics and treatment of female patients with botryoid sarcoma [18,25,27–36].

Paper	Age (Months/Years)	Entry Year	Site	Symptom	Size	Stage CG/TNM	Metastases	Treatment	STATUS after Treatment	Relapse	Treatment of Relapse	Follow Up	Immunohistochemistry
Pańczak K et al., 2017 [27]	4 months	2017	Vagina	Vaginal bleeding and a mass protruding from the vagina, clitoromegaly	2.5 cm × 2.3 cm × 4.3 cm			Chemotherapy (VAI x7) + vaginoscopic resection R0 + VAI x2 + (adriamycin, cyclophosphamide, carboplatin, topotecan, trofosfamide, idarubicin, vincristine, and etoposide) × 3	Recurrence of vaginal RMS, qualified for radical surgery (vaginal resection)	Yes, after 14 months	Radical surgery (vaginal resection)		Desmin, myogenin (myogenic factor 4), myogenic differentiation 1, Wilms' tumor gene expression, and Ki-67 protein in about 90% of cells
van Sambeeck SJ et al., 2014 [28]	17 months	2014	Vagina	Abnormal vaginal bleeding and vaginal tissue loss with a "grape bunch" appearance	6.9 × 3.7 × 4.1 cm		No distant metastases	Chemotherapy VAI x9, radical surgery or radiotherapy was omitted		Yes, 6 months	Chemotherapy and brachytherapy	Complete remission for almost 1 year	Focal positivity for desmin and myogenin
Rodrigo L. P. Romao et al., 2017 [29]	30 months	2017	Vagina			Stage I/group III		VAC + subtotal vaginectomy (24 weeks) with vaginal reconstruction with buccal mucosa grafts				34 months	Fusion negative
ALSaleh N et al., 2017 [30]	18 months	2017	Uterus, cervix, and vagina	Vaginal bleeding (8 mo) and a mass protruding through the introitus (12 mo) + difficult micturition	10 × 6 cm		Without abdominal or pelvic lymphadenopathy	Chemo VAC x10; after remission: total abdominal hysterectomy, bilateral salpingectomy with upper vaginectomy, ureterolysis, and bilateral ovarian transposition (oopexy) + VAC x5		No		12 months disease free on remission with no complaints	

Table 1. *Cont.*

Paper	Age (Months/Years)	Entry Year	Site	Symptom	Size	Stage CG/TNM	Metastases	Treatment	STATUS after Treatment	Relapse	Treatment of Relapse	Follow Up	Immunohistochemistry
Imawan D K Et al., 2019 [31]	36 months	2019	Cervix	Protruding mass in vagina, with a tendency to bleed	10 cm × 10 cm			Tumor excision		Yes, after 3 months	Wide excision with a 2 cm margin of healthy tissue without intra-operative biopsy + VAC x6	18 months post chemother-apy → still in remission, alive and well 44 months after	(+) Anti-desmin and anti-myogenin antibody
May T et al., 2018 [32]	24 months	2018	Cervix	Mass protruding through the vaginal introitus	10 × 4.0 × 4.5 cm	Stage I, group III rhab-domyosar-coma		Vaginal portion of the mass was resected + chemo (alternating vincristine, dactinomycin, and cyclophos-phamide/vincristine and irinotecan) × 2 + radical trachelectomy + chemo × 12		No		12 months disease free on remission with no complaints	
Neha B et al., 2015 [18]	14 years old	2007	Cervix	Mass protruding from the introitus and white discharge that was occasionally blood-stained				Radical hysterectomy + VAC x6				8 months after surgery, acquired a varicella zoster virus, died due to septic shock and multiple organ failure	
Yasmin F et al., 2015 [33]	7 months	2015	Cervix	Protruding mass in the vaginal area for 7 days	9.5 × 7.4 × 10 cm³			Surgery (subtotal hysterectomy) and chemotherapy (5 cycles, no explanation about the regimen)		Yes (2 months after chemother-apy)	Total hysterectomy and chemother-apy × 5 (no further explanation, advised for × 14)		

Table 1. Cont.

Paper	Age (Months/Years)	Entry Year	Site	Symptom	Size	Stage CG/TNM	Metastases	Treatment	STATUS after Treatment	Relapse	Treatment of Relapse	Follow Up	Immunohistochemistry
Bouchard-Fortier G et al., 2016 [34]	14 years old	2016	Cervix	Mass protruding through the vagina accompanied by uterine bleeding	5.3 × 2.9 × 6.7 cm			Robotic-assisted radical trachelectomy + 35 of 43 weeks of VAC alternating with vincristine and irinotecan				No evidence of disease 10 months following diagnosis	ERMS with diffuse anaplastic features and heterologous (cartilage) differentiation
Bouchard-Fortier G et al., 2016 [34]	20 years old	2016	Cervix	Heavy vaginal bleeding and a mass protruding through the vaginal introitus	5.9 × 3.9 × 2.9 cm			Hysteroscopy + cervical conization (after the mass had detached) + 4 cycles of VAC followed by 4 cycles of VA				No evidence of disease 25 months from diagnosis	
Bouchard-Fortier G et al., 2016 [34]	21 years old	2016	Cervix	One-year history of abnormal uterine bleeding	3.3 × 1.7 × 2.8 cm			6 cycles of VAC + LEEP + robotic-assisted radical trachelectomy and placement of an abdominal cerclage				No evidence of disease 21 months after diagnosis	
Bell S G et al., 2021 [35]	17 years old	2021	Cervix	One-year history of an enlarging mass protruding from the introitus associated with vaginal bleeding				Underwent polypectomy of the mass using electrocautery, and suture margins were negative. + 6× cycles of vincristine, actinomycin-D, and cyclophosphamide					

Table 1. Cont.

Paper	Age (Months/Years)	Entry Year	Site	Symptom	Size	Stage CG/TNM	Metastases	Treatment	STATUS after Treatment	Relapse	Treatment of Relapse	Follow Up	Immunohistochemistry
Melo A et al., 2012 [36]	20 years old	2012	Cervix	Postcoital vaginal bleeding over 1 year			No distant metastases	radical surgery, excision of the upper third of the vagina + adjuvant chemotherapy, consisting of 4 cycles of IVA pattern+ Mesna and further 5 cycles of vincristine and actinomycin.		No		At 3 years after diagnosis, patient remains in complete remission and without clinical signs of ovarian failure	Cell positiveness for actin, vimentin, Myo D1 and desmin
Michlitsch J G et al., 2017 [25]	11 months	2017	Vagina	Tumor fragments were passed per vagina		Stage 1, group IIa	No distant metastases	Partial vaginectomy, converted to a total vaginectomy + VAC therapy				38 months of follow up, patient remains disease free with no evidence of local or distant recurrence	
Michlitsch J G et al., 2017 [25]	30 months	2017	Vagina	Exophytic vaginal mass		Stage 2, group III tumor	No distant metastases	VAC therapy + surgical resection and reconstruction (at 24 weeks)				Disease-free at 41 months following diagnosis, with no evidence of recurrence	
Michlitsch J G et al., 2017 [25]	24 months	2017	Vagina	Vaginal bleeding			No distant metastases	VAC therapy + total vaginectomy with reconstruction (at week 20)				Disease-free at 43 months with no evidence of recurrence	
Michlitsch J G et al., 2017 [25]	25 months	2017	Vagina	Protruding vaginal mass			No distant metastases	VAC therapy + anterior vaginal resection of roughly 180-degree circumference and vaginal reconstruction				Disease-free at 16 months with no evidence of recurrence	

VAC—vincristine, actinomycin D, cyclophosphamide; VAI—vincristine, actinomycin D, ifosfamide; LEEP—loop electrosurgical excision procedure.

3.2. Prognosis

As with most malignancies, the key prognostic factor for the prognosis of botryoid RMS is the extent of disease and early disease stage at diagnosis. Overall, soft tissue sarcomas tend to have a dismal prognosis with a high recurrence risk for all stages, ranging from 45 to 73% (40% recurrence in the lung, 13% in the pelvic area). Furthermore, a great number of patients present with recurrence within the first 2 years after primary therapy [37,38]. However, despite its malignancy and rarity, botryoid sarcoma is associated with a very favorable prognosis (95% survival at 5 years), which has seen a dramatic improvement in recent years through the utilization of multidisciplinary treatment [12]. As indicated by the included studies, the majority of cases do not present distal metastases, which also attributes to the favorable outcomes. Several studies over the years indicated the dramatically improved prognosis, with Raney RB Jr et al. [39] highlighting the 5-year overall survival rates of 87% in patients with early-stage disease and Raney RB et al. [40] reporting overall survival rates up to 97%. Hawkins DS et al. [41] demonstrated that lesions arising from the cervix, which are more common among children than among adult patients, appear to have a better prognosis than the ones arising from other parts of the female genital tract. Nonetheless, although patients with recurrent RMS tend to have poor long-term prognosis, the 5-year survival rate after recurrence for botryoid ERMS versus other embryonal tumors is more favorable, reaching 64% vs. 26%, respectively [42]. It is obvious that long-term follow up is necessary to guarantee adequate oncological and functional results.

4. Discussion

RMS is a rare tumor in childhood and adolescence, accounting for 4–6% of pediatric cancers. The female genital tract is considered the prognostically favorable site, given the improved outcomes during the last several decades. Botryoid sarcoma accounts for the majority of cases of the most common RMS histologic subtype: embryonal RMS. It is found under the mucosal surface of body orifices such as the vagina, bladder, and cervix and accounts for around 10% of all RMS cases. Until today, no clear risk factor for botryoid sarcoma could be identified with certainty due to the low number of published cases. The vast majority of cases occur sporadically. Data from a number of literature reports mention the following risk factors: aging, a certain race (African-American women have double the incidence of White Americans), 5 or more years of tamoxifen prescription, and history of radiation exposure. However, the parity, age of menarche, and menopause were not identified to affect the occurrence of RMS [43]. Chemical exposure, maternal age greater than 30 years, low socioeconomic position, and environmental factors all led to the development of RMS, according to one study [44].

4.1. Molecular Pathways Involved in Botryoid Sarcoma

The pathophysiology behind the formation of sarcoma botryoides remains unknown until today. The greater percentage of children who present with this malignancy have no antecedent risk factors. However, it is more likely to develop in individuals with familial diseases that induce mutations in genes responsible for cell proliferation and death (such as Li–Fraumeni syndrome). Despite the mainly sporadic character of the malignancy, a small portion of cases have been associated with genetic diseases such Li–Fraumeni cancer susceptibility syndrome, familial pleuropulmonary tumor, neurofibromatosis Type I, and Beckwith–Wiedemann syndrome. However, the incidence may be higher in patients diagnosed with RMS before the age of 3 [3,45]. Specific gene alterations such as KRAS activation and p53 inactivation have been linked to the presentation of RMS. Most embryonal rhabdomyosarcomas, in particular, have a point mutation in exon 6 of the p53 gene on chromosome 17. In a family, the heterozygous p53 germline mutation was reported as the source of the Li–Fraumeni cancer susceptibility syndrome, which presents as a cluster of soft tissue cancers (including sarcomas). Dehner et al. [46] also reported a connection between the blastoma family and pleuropulmonary tumors, as well as confirming

DICER1 autosuggest, implying that RMS in children must be treated in a broader context to account for the possibility of pleuropulmonary blastoma familial tumor predisposition syndrome [47–49]. The identification of DICER1 mutation is notable since it is found in 60% of Sertoli–Leydig cancers, and germline mutations found in Dicer1 increase the possibility of developing rare cancers. Mousavi and Akhavan [14] revealed the occurrence of cervical sarcoma botryoides in two sisters, suggesting that hereditary factors may play a role in the development of sarcoma botryoides [50–52]. Malignant mixed Mullerian tumor, widely known as carcinosarcoma, can develop exophytically from the uterine wall or cervix and have a sarcomatous gross and microscopic appearance. Nevertheless, malignant mixed Mullerian tumors usually tend to affect older people, in contrast with ERMS [53]. For the time being, it seems reasonable at a minimum to strongly consider referral to genetic counseling for patients who are younger at diagnosis, whose tumors have anaplastic features, or who have a significant family history of malignancy.

4.2. Diagnostic Approach

According to the literature, the diagnosis of this tumor is difficult to make, but as far as the management of this tumor is concerned, there are a variety of approaches in the treatment armamentarium, ranging from extreme, radical procedures to more conservative ones. Nuclear MRI is the gold standard for determining where the tumor originates from (whether it is in the endometrium, myometrium, or cervix) as well as the spread and involvement of neighboring structures. Because of its rarity and high-risk, malignant nature originating in the embryonic mesenchyme, botryoid sarcoma should be suspected in young-age females with vaginal bleeding or a prolapsed mass, since typically the tumor develops behind the mucosal membrane of the organs, forcing the growth to take on a characteristic grape-like form. The importance of histology in RMS prognosis cannot be overstated. Although there are three types of RMS (embryonal, alveolar, and undifferentiated), the embryonal type is the more prevalent and has a better prognosis than the alveolar type, which is rare and has a worse prognosis [18]. The Intergroup Rhabdomyosarcoma Studies (IRS) classifies RMS based on (i) the main site, (ii) tumor size, (iii) lymph node involvement, (iv) surrounding tissue infiltration, and (v) the occurrence of metastases [54]. The stage is established using two systems: the Intergroup Rhabdomyosarcoma Study Group clinical categorization method (Table 2) [16] and the TNM staging approach for rhabdomyosarcoma (Table 3) [8]. Table 2 reports the Intergroup Rhabdomyosarcoma Study Group clinical classification system for rhabdomyosarcoma. It is actually a classification of rhabdomyosarcoma cases into four clinical groups, based on the extent of disease, resectability, and margin status.

Table 2. Intergroup Rhabdomyosarcoma Study Group Clinical Classification System for Rhabdomyosarcoma.

Clinical Group	Extent of Disease, Resectability, and Margin Status
I	A: localized tumor, confined to site of origin, completely resected.
I	B: localized tumor, infiltrating beyond site of origin, completely resected.
II	A: localized tumor, gross total resection, but with microscopic residual disease.
II	B: locally extensive tumor (spread to regional lymph nodes), completely resected.
III	A: localized or locally extensive tumor, gross residual disease after biopsy only.
III	B: localized or locally extensive tumor, gross residual disease after major resection ($\geq$50% debulking).
IV	Any size primary tumor, with or without regional lymph node involvement, with distant metastases, irrespective of surgical approach to primary tumor.

Table 3. TNM Staging System for Rhabdomyosarcoma.

Stage	Sites	T	Tumor Size Designation	N	M
I	Orbit Head and neck * Genitourinary † Biliary tract	T1 or T2	a or b	Any N	M0
II	Bladder or prostate Extremity Cranial parameningeal Other ‡	T1 or T2	a	N0 or Nx	M0
III	Bladder or prostate Extremity Cranial parameningeal Other ‡	T1 or T2	a	N1	M0
IV	All	T1 or T2	a or b	N0 or N1	M1

T1, tumor confined to the anatomic site; T2, tumor extension; a, ≤5 cm in diameter; b, >5 cm in diameter; N0, nodes not clinically involved; N1, nodes clinically involved; Nx, clinical status of nodes unknown; M0, no distant metastases; M1, distant metastases present. * Excluding parameningeal sites. † Nonbladder and nonprostate. ‡ Includes trunk, retroperitoneum, etc., excluding biliary tract.

4.3. Therapeutic Modalities

It is of paramount importance to organize a personalized treatment plan, considering the extent of the disease and the fertility preservation. The management of botryoid rhabdomyosarcoma poses a great challenge for gynecologists. In the past, the traditional treatment for these types of tumors involved exenterative procedures, but today, modalities such as fertility-sparing methods, e.g., polypectomy, conization, local excisions, and robot-assisted radical trachelectomy, are offered and are the ones mostly implemented for the preservation of the reproductive ability. In the last decades, a variety of procedures have been added to the options of pediatric genitourinary and anorectal reconstruction. Buccal mucosa grafts are now widely employed in both adult and pediatric urology for urethral reconstruction with acceptable results. Recent reports have established that buccal mucosa vaginoplasty leads to good outcomes in patients with Mayer–Rokitansky–Kuster–Hauser syndrome (MRKH—agenesis of the Mullerian structures and vagina), complete androgen insensitivity syndrome, and repair of urogenital sinus, as far as cosmetic and functionality results are concerned. Evidence suggests that the grafts retain favorable characteristics over time and adapt well to rapid growth demands such as those imposed by puberty. Harvesting the graft is straightforward and associated with minimal morbidity. In addition, buccal grafts greatly resemble the vaginal tissue that they are to replace. Nevertheless, as with every newly introduced procedure, long-term follow up is necessary to assess the oncological outcomes since it does not represent a standard of care but rather an intervention that holds promise as a viable option with minimal esthetic impact.

It was the first IRGS trial (1972 and 1978) that recommended systematic chemotherapy following extensive surgery such as radical hysterectomy or pelvic exenteration for ERMS of the genital tract [54]. The second IRGS trial (1978–1984) suggested NACT for the first time to minimize the extent of the tumor, allowing for a less radical surgery [39]. Multi-agent adjuvant chemotherapy with or without the addition of radiotherapy plays a substantial role in the effective management of sarcoma botryoides, apart from the surgical resection of the tumor. In clinical practice, there are standardized schemes of chemotherapy that can be used preoperatively to minimize the volume of the tumor or after surgical resection to limit the chances of recurrence. The most frequently used regimen of chemotherapy for children and young adults with nonmetastatic disease is the triplet of vincristine, actinomycin D, and cyclophosphamide (VAC), and it is based on the protocols of IRSG [26]. Unfortunately, there are several toxic effects that are associated with chemotherapy, and sometimes it is not well tolerated by the patients who undergo it. The most usual side effects of cyclophosphamide that are well documented are bone marrow suppression and subsequently susceptibility to infections, hemorrhage cystitis, cardiotoxicity, and gastrointestinal disturbances. Vincristine on the other hand promotes the production of severe neurotoxicity in patients and less commonly myelosuppression, alopecia, and SIADH.

Other regimens consist of VAC plus VAI (vincristine, actinomycin D, and ifosfamide or VIE (vincristine, ifosfamide, and etoposide) plus VAC for 12 months. A randomized controlled trial by Amdt et al. compared the VAC regimen and the combination of vincristine, topotecan, and cyclophosphamide for the treatment of moderated-risk rhabdomyosarcoma. The results suggest that topotecan was not indicated to be more efficient than actinomycin D, with 68% and 73% 4-year survival rates, respectively. Irinotecan is another drug that is currently under examination for its efficacy in the treatment of pediatric rhabdomyosarcoma when combined with the VAC regimen [55].

Surgery and/or radiation still play an important role in the management of high-risk RMS with oligometastatic disease to minimize treatment failures. Aggressive surgical local control most of the time offers the advantage of sparing these young patients radiation-associated complications. However, it should be kept in mind that surgical resection is not without its own possible complications, including wound infections, fistulas, and stenosis [56]. In case of widespread metastases at presentation, local control is often postponed until later in treatment and may be customized to focus on the most symptomatic or critical sites. In almost all of these advanced cases, palliative treatment remains the only option. Although the outcome is not always favorable for the patients, the prognosis of botryoid sarcomas has dramatically improved in recent years through the combination of chemotherapy, radiotherapy, and/or surgery. Similar to the case for most other cancers, the prognosis depends on the tumor size, the histological variant, and the depth to which the disease has spread to adjacent structures at the time of diagnosis. It appears that there is a more favorable prognosis for tumors arising from the cervix compared with the ones arising from other parts of the female genital tract. Generally, the 5-year survival rate for sarcoma botryoides is 83%, 70%, 52%, and 25% for clinical stages I–IV, respectively. Unfortunately, despite the advances in therapeutic modalities, there are several reports of tumor recurrences, with the pelvis being the most common region for primary recurrence. Surprisingly, the 5-year overall survival was equally excellent, reaching 87% in nonmetastatic tumors [57]. Consistent with these results was the publication of Brand et al. [58], in which the patients' survival rate was 80% at 68 months with the use of multimodality therapy (conservative surgery combined with chemotherapy). The identification of nodal metastases through imaging is critically important in the treatment of RMS, and tissue sampling must be performed for all patients with clinically or radiographically suspicious lymphadenopathy. In conclusion, we believe that a combination of debulking surgery, chemotherapy, and in cases of treatment-resistant tumor or remaining disease, radiation therapy demonstrates an appropriate approach in well-selected patients with botryoid sarcoma. This approach provides excellent oncologic outcomes and a low complication rate, taking into account the tumor's location, stage, and the patient's overall characteristics. Nevertheless, since most of the data come from case reports, larger studies with longer follow-up must be conducted in order to determine the most effective treatment guidelines.

4.4. Limitations and Advantages

The present summative review is, to the best of our knowledge, the first one trying to summarize the main literature outcomes about therapeutic management and prognosis. The main limitation of the present manuscript is the fact that it is a narrative review only summarizing results of relatively low-level evidence, such as retrospective series and case reports, as no prospective RCTs or large prospective cohorts were identified through the literature search. However, despite the fact that the level of evidence is low, this is relatively reasonable because the rarity of the disease poses reasonable difficulties in the conduct of level-I evidence studies. Furthermore, as our review finally summarized the main conclusions about the therapeutic modalities and prognostic outcomes, this might be the initial step to organize prospective observational cohorts, rather than multicenter ones, in an attempt to globalize the standards of practice and, thereafter, improve the outcomes of such a demanding clinical entity.

Author Contributions: C.M.-S. was a major contributor in writing the manuscript. C.M.-S., S.P., A.A. and G.M.-S. were responsible for the collection of the relevant literature. A.S.L., M.K., A.P. and K.D. revised the manuscript critically for important intellectual content. All authors have read and agreed to the published version of the manuscript.

Funding: This research received no external funding.

Institutional Review Board Statement: Not applicable.

Informed Consent Statement: Not applicable.

Data Availability Statement: No new data were created or analyzed in this study. Data sharing is not applicable to this article.

Conflicts of Interest: The authors declare no conflict of interest.

References

1. Harel, M.; Ferrer, F.A.; Shapiro, L.H.; Makari, J.H. Future Directions in Risk Stratification and Therapy for Advanced Pediatric Genitourinary Rhabdomyosarcoma. *Urol Oncol.* **2016**, *34*, 103–115. [CrossRef] [PubMed]
2. Ghaemmaghami, F.; Karimi Zarchi, M.; Ghasemi, M. Lower Genital Tract Rhabdomyosarcoma: Case Series and Literature Review. *Arch. Gynecol. Obs.* **2008**, *278*, 65–69. [CrossRef] [PubMed]
3. Villella, J.A.; Bogner, P.N.; Jani-Sait, S.N.; Block, A.M.W.; Lele, S. Rhabdomyosarcoma of the Cervix in Sisters with Review of the Literature. *Gynecol. Oncol.* **2005**, *99*, 742–748. [CrossRef] [PubMed]
4. Ibrahim, U.; Saqib, A.; Mohammad, F.; Ding, J.; Salman, B.; Collado, F.K.; Dhar, M. Embryonal Rhabdomyosarcoma of the Cervix: A Rare Disease at an Uncommon Age. *Cureus* **2017**, *9*, e1864. [CrossRef]
5. Minard-Colin, V.; Walterhouse, D.; Bisogno, G.; Martelli, H.; Anderson, J.; Rodeberg, D.A.; Ferrari, A.; Jenney, M.; Wolden, S.; De Salvo, G.; et al. Localized Vaginal/Uterine Rhabdomyosarcoma-Results of a Pooled Analysis from Four International Cooperative Groups. *Pediatr. Blood Cancer* **2018**, *65*, e27096. [CrossRef] [PubMed]
6. Jayi, S.; Bouguern, H.; Fdili, F.Z.; Chaara, H.; Chbani, L.; Hafidi, I.; Kamaoui, I.; Arifi, S.; Mellas, N.; Bouhafa, T.; et al. Embryonal Rhabdomyosarcoma of the Cervix Presenting as a Cervical Polyp in a 16-Year-Old Adolescent: A Case Report. *J. Med. Case Rep.* **2014**, *8*, 241. [CrossRef]
7. Parham, D.M.; Barr, F.G. Classification of Rhabdomyosarcoma and Its Molecular Basis. *Adv. Anat. Pathol.* **2013**, *20*, 387–397. [CrossRef]
8. Kriseman, M.L.; Wang, W.-L.; Sullinger, J.; Schmeler, K.M.; Ramirez, P.T.; Herzog, C.E.; Frumovitz, M. Rhabdomyosarcoma of the Cervix in Adult Women and Younger Patients. *Gynecol. Oncol.* **2012**, *126*, 351–356. [CrossRef]
9. Hettmer, S.; Wagers, A.J. Muscling in: Uncovering the Origins of Rhabdomyosarcoma. *Nat. Med.* **2010**, *16*, 171–173. [CrossRef]
10. Li, R.F.; Gupta, M.; McCluggage, W.G.; Ronnett, B.M. Embryonal Rhabdomyosarcoma (Botryoid Type) of the Uterine Corpus and Cervix in Adult Women: Report of a Case Series and Review of the Literature. *Am. J. Surg. Pathol.* **2013**, *37*, 344–355. [CrossRef]
11. Behtash, N.; Mousavi, A.; Tehranian, A.; Khanafshar, N.; Hanjani, P. Embryonal Rhabdomyosarcoma of the Uterine Cervix: Case Report and Review of the Literature. *Gynecol. Oncol.* **2003**, *91*, 452–455. [CrossRef] [PubMed]
12. Newton, W.A.; Gehan, E.A.; Webber, B.L.; Marsden, H.B.; van Unnik, A.J.; Hamoudi, A.B.; Tsokos, M.G.; Shimada, H.; Harms, D.; Schmidt, D. Classification of Rhabdomyosarcomas and Related Sarcomas. Pathologic Aspects and Proposal for a New Classification–an Intergroup Rhabdomyosarcoma Study. *Cancer* **1995**, *76*, 1073–1085. [CrossRef] [PubMed]
13. Gödtel, R.; Schäfer, A. [Sarcoma botryoides of the cervix uteri as cause for haemorrhages in childbed (author's transl)]. *Geburtshilfe Frauenheilkd* **1978**, *38*, 485–487. [PubMed]
14. Mousavi, A.; Akhavan, S. Sarcoma Botryoides (Embryonal Rhabdomyosarcoma) of the Uterine Cervix in Sisters. *J. Gynecol. Oncol.* **2010**, *21*, 273–275. [CrossRef] [PubMed]
15. Kim, E.E.; Valenzuela, R.F.; Kumar, A.J.; Raney, R.B.; Eftekari, F. Imaging and Clinical Spectrum of Rhabdomyosarcoma in Children. *Clin. Imaging* **2000**, *24*, 257–262. [CrossRef]
16. Fletcher, C.D.M.; Bridge, J.A.; Hogendoorn, P.C.W.; Mertens, F. *WHO Classification of Tumours of Soft Tissue and Bone*; IARC: Lyon, France, 2013.
17. Borinstein, S.C.; Steppan, D.; Hayashi, M.; Loeb, D.M.; Isakoff, M.S.; Binitie, O.; Brohl, A.S.; Bridge, J.A.; Stavas, M.; Shinohara, E.T.; et al. Consensus and Controversies Regarding the Treatment of Rhabdomyosarcoma. *Pediatr. Blood Cancer* **2018**, *65*, e26809. [CrossRef]
18. Neha, B.; Manjunath, A.P.; Girija, S.; Pratap, K. Botryoid Rhabdomyosarcoma of the Cervix: Case Report with Review of the Literature. *Sultan Qaboos Univ. Med. J.* **2015**, *15*, e433–e437. [CrossRef]

19. Giuntoli, R.L.; Metzinger, D.S.; DiMarco, C.S.; Cha, S.S.; Sloan, J.A.; Keeney, G.L.; Gostout, B.S. Retrospective Review of 208 Patients with Leiomyosarcoma of the Uterus: Prognostic Indicators, Surgical Management, and Adjuvant Therapy. *Gynecol. Oncol.* **2003**, *89*, 460–469. [CrossRef]
20. Maurer, H.M.; Beltangady, M.; Gehan, E.A.; Crist, W.; Hammond, D.; Hays, D.M.; Heyn, R.; Lawrence, W.; Newton, W.; Ortega, J. The Intergroup Rhabdomyosarcoma Study-I. A Final Report. *Cancer* **1988**, *61*, 209–220. [CrossRef]
21. Crist, W.M.; Anderson, J.R.; Meza, J.L.; Fryer, C.; Raney, R.B.; Ruymann, F.B.; Breneman, J.; Qualman, S.J.; Wiener, E.; Wharam, M.; et al. Intergroup Rhabdomyosarcoma Study-IV: Results for Patients with Nonmetastatic Disease. *J. Clin. Oncol.* **2001**, *19*, 3091–3102. [CrossRef]
22. Andrassy, R.J.; Wiener, E.S.; Raney, R.B.; Hays, D.M.; Arndt, C.A.; Lobe, T.E.; Lawrence, W.; Anderson, J.R.; Qualman, S.J.; Crist, W.M. Progress in the Surgical Management of Vaginal Rhabdomyosarcoma: A 25-Year Review from the Intergroup Rhabdomyosarcoma Study Group. *J. Pediatr. Surg.* **1999**, *34*, 731–734; discussion 734–735. [CrossRef] [PubMed]
23. Balat, O.; Balat, A.; Verschraegen, C.; Tornos, C.; Edwards, C.L. Sarcoma Botryoides of the Uterine Endocervix: Long-Term Results of Conservative Surgery. *Eur. J. Gynaecol. Oncol.* **1996**, *17*, 335–337. [PubMed]
24. Yang, J.; Yang, J.; Yu, M.; Yuan, Z.; Cao, D.; Keng, S. Clinical Study on Female Genital Tract Rhabdomyosarcoma in Childhood: Changes During 20 Years in One Center. *Int. J. Gynecol. Cancer* **2017**, *27*, 311–314. [CrossRef] [PubMed]
25. Jennifer, G.M.; Rodrigo, L.P.; Romao Joseph, M.; Gleason Luis, H.; Braga, L.A.; Abha, G.; Armando, J.L. Local control for vaginal botryoid rhabdomyosarcoma with pre-rectal transperineal surgical resection and autologous buccal graft vaginal replacement: A novel, minimally invasive, radiation-sparing approach. *J. Pediatr. Surg.* **2018**, *53*, 1374–1380. [CrossRef]
26. Raney, R.B.; Maurer, H.M.; Anderson, J.R.; Andrassy, R.J.; Donaldson, S.S.; Qualman, S.J.; Wharam, M.D.; Wiener, E.S.; Crist, W.M. The Intergroup Rhabdomyosarcoma Study Group (IRSG): Major Lessons From the IRS-I Through IRS-IV Studies as Background for the Current IRS-V Treatment Protocols. *Sarcoma* **2001**, *5*, 9–15. [CrossRef]
27. Pańczak, K.; Gawron, D.; Sosnowska, P.; Kapczuk, K.; Mańkowski, P. Vaginoscopic Resection for Vaginal Rhabdomyosarcoma during Early Infancy: A Case Report. *J. Minim. Invasive Gynecol.* **2018**, *25*, 533–536. [CrossRef]
28. van Sambeeck, S.J.; Mavinkurve-Groothuis, A.; Flucke, U.; Dors, N. Sarcoma Botryoides in an Infant. *Case Rep.* **2014**, *2014*, bcr2013202080. [CrossRef]
29. Romao, R.L.P.; Lorenzo, A.J. Vaginectomy and Buccal Mucosa Vaginoplasty as Local Therapy for Pediatric Vaginal Rhabdomyosarcoma. *Urology* **2017**, *102*, 222–224. [CrossRef]
30. ALSaleh, N.; ALwadie, H.; Gari, A. Rhabdomyosarcoma of the Genital Tract in an 18-Month-Old Girl. *J. Surg. Case Rep.* **2017**, *2017*. [CrossRef]
31. Imawan, D.K.; Oesman, W.S.; Yuseran, H.; Mustokoweni, S.; Kania, N.; Harsono, A.A.H.; Alkaff, F.F. Recurrent Cervical Sarcoma Botryoides in a 3-Year-Old Female: Approach in a Limited Resource Setting. *Am. J. Case Rep.* **2019**, *20*, 838–843. [CrossRef]
32. May, T.; Allen, L.; Hogen, L.; King, C.; Lorenzo, A.J.; Browne-Farmer, C.; Gupta, A.; Shaikh, F. Laparoscopic Radical Trachelectomy for Embryonal Rhabdomyosarcoma of the Cervix in a 2-Year-Old Girl. *Obstet. Gynecol.* **2018**, *132*, 1486–1490. [CrossRef] [PubMed]
33. Yasmin, F.; Ahmed, M.A.U.; Begum, T.; Ahmed, T.; Baki, M.A. A Case Report of Rhabdomyosarcoma of Uterine Cervix in a 7-Month-Old Child. *Birdem Med. J.* **2017**, *7*, 242–244. [CrossRef]
34. Bouchard-Fortier, G.; Kim, R.H.; Allen, L.; Gupta, A.; May, T. Fertility-Sparing Surgery for the Management of Young Women with Embryonal Rhabdomyosarcoma of the Cervix: A Case Series. *Gynecol. Oncol. Rep.* **2016**, *18*, 4–7. [CrossRef] [PubMed]
35. Bell, S.G.; Konney, T.O.; Appiah-Kubi, A.; Tawiah, A.; Amo-Antwi, K.; Annan, J.J.K.; Lawrence, E.R.; Lieberman, R.; Johnston, C. Two Rare Presentations of Embryonal Rhabdomyosarcoma of the Cervix in Teenagers at a Low-Resource Teaching Hospital in Ghana: A Case Series. *Gynecol. Oncol. Rep.* **2021**, *36*, 100750. [CrossRef] [PubMed]
36. Melo, A.; Amorim-Costa, C.; Pires, M.C.; Fernandes, D.; Soares, M.; CambÃo, M.; Petiz, A. Botryoid Rhabdomyosarcoma of the Uterine Cervix. *J. Obstet. Gynaecol.* **2012**, *32*, 709–711. [CrossRef]
37. Walterhouse, D.; Watson, A. Optimal Management Strategies for Rhabdomyosarcoma in Children. *Paediatr. Drugs* **2007**, *9*, 391–400. [CrossRef] [PubMed]
38. Herzog, C.E. Overview of Sarcomas in the Adolescent and Young Adult Population. *J. Pediatr. Hematol. Oncol.* **2005**, *27*, 215–218. [CrossRef]
39. Raney, R.B.; Gehan, E.A.; Hays, D.M.; Tefft, M.; Newton, W.A.; Haeberlen, V.; Maurer, H.M. Primary Chemotherapy with or without Radiation Therapy and/or Surgery for Children with Localized Sarcoma of the Bladder, Prostate, Vagina, Uterus, and Cervix. A Comparison of the Results in Intergroup Rhabdomyosarcoma Studies I and II. *Cancer* **1990**, *66*, 2072–2081. [CrossRef]
40. Raney, R.B.; Walterhouse, D.O.; Meza, J.L.; Andrassy, R.J.; Breneman, J.C.; Crist, W.M.; Maurer, H.M.; Meyer, W.H.; Parham, D.M.; Anderson, J.R. Results of the Intergroup Rhabdomyosarcoma Study Group D9602 Protocol, Using Vincristine and Dactinomycin with or without Cyclophosphamide and Radiation Therapy, for Newly Diagnosed Patients with Low-Risk Embryonal Rhabdomyosarcoma: A Report from the Soft Tissue Sarcoma Committee of the Children's Oncology Group. *J. Clin. Oncol.* **2011**, *29*, 1312–1318. [CrossRef]
41. Hawkins, D.S.; Chi, Y.-Y.; Anderson, J.R.; Tian, J.; Arndt, C.A.S.; Bomgaars, L.; Donaldson, S.S.; Hayes-Jordan, A.; Mascarenhas, L.; McCarville, M.B.; et al. Addition of Vincristine and Irinotecan to Vincristine, Dactinomycin, and Cyclophosphamide Does Not Improve Outcome for Intermediate-Risk Rhabdomyosarcoma: A Report From the Children's Oncology Group. *J. Clin. Oncol.* **2018**, *36*, 2770–2777. [CrossRef]

42. Pappo, A.S.; Anderson, J.R.; Crist, W.M.; Wharam, M.D.; Breitfeld, P.P.; Hawkins, D.; Raney, R.B.; Womer, R.B.; Parham, D.M.; Qualman, S.J.; et al. Survival after Relapse in Children and Adolescents with Rhabdomyosarcoma: A Report from the Intergroup Rhabdomyosarcoma Study Group. *J. Clin. Oncol.* **1999**, *17*, 3487–3493. [CrossRef] [PubMed]
43. Koivisto-Korander, R.; Butzow, R.; Koivisto, A.-M.; Leminen, A. Clinical Outcome and Prognostic Factors in 100 Cases of Uterine Sarcoma: Experience in Helsinki University Central Hospital 1990-2001. *Gynecol. Oncol.* **2008**, *111*, 74–81. [CrossRef]
44. Grufferman, S.; Wang, H.H.; DeLong, E.R.; Kimm, S.Y.; Delzell, E.S.; Falletta, J.M. Environmental factors in the etiology of rhabdomyosarcoma in childhood. *J. Natl. Cancer Inst.* **1982**, *68*, 107–113.
45. Sardinha, M.G.P.; Ramajo, F.M.; Ponce, C.C.; Marques, C.F.; Bittencourt, C.M.F.; Caldano, F.G.; Moço, J.M.F.L.; de Lacquila Yano, O.; Reis, P.M.d.R.; Malaguti, V.S.; et al. Uterine Cavity Embryonal Rhabdomyosarcoma. *Autops. Case Rep.* **2019**, *9*, e2019104. [CrossRef]
46. Dehner, L.P.; Jarzembowski, J.A.; Hill, D.A. Embryonal rhabdomyosarcoma of the uterine cervix: A report of 14 cases and a discussion of its unusual clinicopathological associations. *Mod. Pathol.* **2012**, *25*, 602–614. [CrossRef]
47. Schultz, K.A.P.; Nelson, A.; Harris, A.K.; Finch, M.; Field, A.; Jarzembowski, J.A.; Wilhelm, M.; Mize, W.; Kreiger, P.; Conard, K.; et al. Pleuropulmonary Blastoma-like Peritoneal Sarcoma: A Newly Described Malignancy Associated with Biallelic DICER1 Pathogenic Variation. *Mod. Pathol.* **2020**, *33*, 1922–1929. [CrossRef]
48. Palazzo, J.P.; Gibas, Z.; Dunton, C.J.; Talerman, A. Cytogenetic Study of Botryoid Rhabdomyosarcoma of the Uterine Cervix. *Virchows Arch A Pathol. Anat. Histopathol.* **1993**, *422*, 87–91. [CrossRef]
49. Pötzsch, C.; Voigtländer, T.; Lübbert, M. P53 Germline Mutation in a Patient with Li-Fraumeni Syndrome and Three Metachronous Malignancies. *J. Cancer Res. Clin. Oncol.* **2002**, *128*, 456–460. [CrossRef]
50. Robertson, J.C.; Jorcyk, C.L.; Oxford, J.T. DICER1 Syndrome: DICER1 Mutations in Rare Cancers. *Cancers* **2018**, *10*, 143. [CrossRef] [PubMed]
51. Ramaswamy, R.; Ali, E.; Ghalib, S.S.; Mukattash, G. Hemoperitoneum Due to Ruptured Botryoid Sarcoma of the Uterus in Young Girl. *J. Indian Assoc. Pediatr. Surg.* **2021**, *26*, 262–264. [CrossRef] [PubMed]
52. Dural, O.; Kebudi, R.; Yavuz, E.; Yilmaz, I.; Buyukkapu Bay, S.; Schultz, K.A.P.; Hill, D.A. DICER1-Related Embryonal Rhabdomyosarcoma of the Uterine Corpus in a Prepubertal Girl. *J. Pediatr. Adolesc. Gynecol.* **2020**, *33*, 173–176. [CrossRef]
53. McCluggage, W.G. Mullerian adenosarcoma of the female genital tract. *Adv. Anat. Pathol.* **2010**, *17*, 122–129. [CrossRef] [PubMed]
54. Hays, D.M.; Shimada, H.; Raney, R.B.; Tefft, M.; Newton, W.; Crist, W.M.; Lawrence, W.; Ragab, A.; Maurer, H.M. Sarcomas of the Vagina and Uterus: The Intergroup Rhabdomyosarcoma Study. *J. Pediatr. Surg.* **1985**, *20*, 718–724. [CrossRef] [PubMed]
55. Ning, Z.; Liu, X.; Qin, G.; Wei, L.; Li, X.; Shen, J. Evaluation of clinical efficacy of Chemotherapy for Rhabdomyosarcoma in children. *Pak. J. Med. Sci.* **2020**, *36*, 1069–1074. [CrossRef] [PubMed]
56. Michalkiewicz, E.L.; Rao, B.N.; Gross, E.; Luo, X.; Bowman, L.C.; Pappo, A.S.; Kaste, S.C.; Hudson, M.M.; Greenwald, C.A.; Jenkins, J.J.; et al. Complications of Pelvic Exenteration in Children Who Have Genitourinary Rhabdomyosarcoma. *J. Pediatr. Surg.* **1997**, *32*, 1277–1282. [CrossRef] [PubMed]
57. Arndt, C.A.; Donaldson, S.S.; Anderson, J.R.; Andrassy, R.J.; Laurie, F.; Link, M.P.; Raney, R.B.; Maurer, H.M.; Crist, W.M. What Constitutes Optimal Therapy for Patients with Rhabdomyosarcoma of the Female Genital Tract? *Cancer* **2001**, *91*, 2454–2468. [CrossRef] [PubMed]
58. Brand, E.; Berek, J.S.; Nieberg, R.K.; Hacker, N.F. Rhabdomyosarcoma of the Uterine Cervix. Sarcoma Botryoides. *Cancer* **1987**, *60*, 1552–1560. [CrossRef]

Disclaimer/Publisher's Note: The statements, opinions and data contained in all publications are solely those of the individual author(s) and contributor(s) and not of MDPI and/or the editor(s). MDPI and/or the editor(s) disclaim responsibility for any injury to people or property resulting from any ideas, methods, instructions or products referred to in the content.

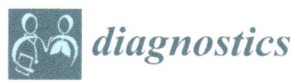

Review

Predictive Factors for Pediatric Craniopharyngioma Recurrence: An Extensive Narrative Review

Anastasios Serbis [1,2], Vasiliki Rengina Tsinopoulou [2], Anastasia Papadopoulou [2], Savvas Kolanis [2], Eleni I. Sakellari [2], Kosmas Margaritis [2], Eleni Litou [2], Stergianna Ntouma [2], Styliani Giza [2], Eleni P. Kotanidou [2] and Assimina Galli-Tsinopoulou [2,*]

[1] Department of Pediatrics, School of Medicine, University of Ioannina, St. Niarhcos Avenue, 45500 Ioannina, Greece
[2] Unit of Pediatric Endocrinology and Metabolism, 2nd Department of Pediatrics, School of Medicine, Faculty of Health Sciences, Aristotle University of Thessaloniki, AHEPA University Hospital, Stilponos Kyriakidi 1, 54636 Thessaloniki, Greece
* Correspondence: agalli@auth.gr; Tel.: +30-2310-994801

Abstract: Despite being classified as benign tumors, craniopharyngiomas (CPs) are associated with significant morbidity and mortality due to their location, growth pattern, and tendency to recur. Two types can be identified depending on age distribution, morphology, and growth pattern, adamantinomatous and papillary. The adamantinomatous CP is one of the most frequently encountered central nervous system tumors in childhood. Our aim was to review the relevant literature to identify clinical, morphological, and immunohistochemical prognostic factors that have been implicated in childhood-onset CP recurrence. Lack of radical surgical removal of the primary tumor by an experienced neurosurgical team and radiotherapy after a subtotal excision has been proven to significantly increase the recurrence rate of CP. Other risk factors that have been consistently recognized in the literature include younger age at diagnosis (especially <5 years), larger tumor size at presentation, cystic appearance, difficult tumor location, and tight adherence to surrounding structures, as well as the histological presence of whorl-like arrays. In addition, several other risk factors have been studied, albeit with conflicting results, especially in the pediatric population. Identifying risk factors for CP recurrence is of utmost importance for the successful management of these patients in order to ultimately ensure the best prognosis.

Keywords: craniopharyngioma; recurrence; risk factors; children; adolescents; youth

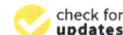

Citation: Serbis, A.; Tsinopoulou, V.R.; Papadopoulou, A.; Kolanis, S.; Sakellari, E.I.; Margaritis, K.; Litou, E.; Ntouma, S.; Giza, S.; Kotanidou, E.P.; et al. Predictive Factors for Pediatric Craniopharyngioma Recurrence: An Extensive Narrative Review. *Diagnostics* 2023, 13, 1588. https://doi.org/10.3390/diagnostics13091588

Academic Editor: Sang Kun Lee

Received: 14 March 2023
Revised: 20 April 2023
Accepted: 27 April 2023
Published: 28 April 2023

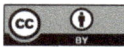

Copyright: © 2023 by the authors. Licensee MDPI, Basel, Switzerland. This article is an open access article distributed under the terms and conditions of the Creative Commons Attribution (CC BY) license (https://creativecommons.org/licenses/by/4.0/).

1. Introduction

Craniopharyngiomas (CPs) are rare epithelial tumors that arise along the path of the craniopharyngeal duct [1,2]. The World Health Organization (WHO) classifies them as grade I tumors due to their lack of histological signs of malignancy [3], although malignant transformation has been reported in rare cases [4]. Histologically, there are two main CP subtypes, namely, adamantinomatous and papillary, which differ in age distribution, frequency, biology, and clinical outcome [2,5–7]. Adamantinomatous CP predominantly affects subjects younger than 14 years of age and is, therefore, considered the "pediatric" type, accounting for 5–10% of central nervous system (CNS) tumors in this age group [5,7].

Despite recent advances in its diagnostic and therapeutic approach, CP is still a tumor that is difficult to treat, with significant neurological, endocrinological, and visual complications [8], which can lead to poor quality of life for patients and their families [9], and with an excess mortality rate compared to the general population [10,11]. Both morbidity and mortality of CPs are related not only to the primary tumor itself but also to its tendency to recur, even after radical surgical excision [12], with an average time of 3 years from treatment to recurrence [13–15].

The quest for reliable markers that could identify those CP patients at increased recurrence risk has been extensive over the past 40 years [16,17]. For example, it is well established that the radical surgical removal of the primary tumor by an experienced neurosurgical team and the use of radiotherapy (RT) significantly reduce the recurrence rate of CP [1,13,18–22]. Other risk factors that have been consistently recognized in the literature include younger age [23–25], larger tumor size, difficult location, and tight adherence to surrounding structures [26–28,28,29], as well as the histological presence of whorl-like arrays [30,31]. In addition, clinical risk factors, albeit with conflicting results, include the presence of hydrocephalus or other signs of increased intracranial pressure (ICP) [1,16,32], visual disturbances [30,32], and hypothalamic [24,33] involvement. Similarly, several studies of CP molecular features had conflicting results, such as Ki-67, p53 gene, vascular endothelial growth factor [VEGF], and cathepsins [34,35,35–39]. Finally, the presence of calcifications in the primary tumor has been linked with an increased recurrence rate [40–42], while the treatment of the patient with recombinant human growth hormone [GH] shows little or no risk [43–45].

We aimed to perform a narrative review of the literature focusing on risk factors that increase the likelihood of recurrence of childhood CP published since the early 1980s. Only two relevant systematic reviews have been conducted in adults, which concluded that there is a need for further studies on CP recurrence markers [16,17].

2. Materials and Methods

In the present study, conducting a narrative review was chosen on the grounds that, even if a systematic review is of paramount importance in gathering and critically synthesizing all relevant literature on a given topic, narrative reviews are complementary to the research process since they constitute a comprehensive and objective analysis of the current knowledge on a topic, such as CP recurrence.

The literature search on PubMed/Medline database was conducted referring to manuscripts/studies published between 1 January 1980, and 31 January 2023, to identify relevant papers using the following keywords: "craniopharyngioma", "risk factors", "regrowth", "recurrence", "pediatric", "child", "adolescent". Exclusion criteria were the following: non-English papers; studies comprised exclusively adult study populations or studies in which the age of participants was not clearly defined; editorials and letters to the editor; studies that examined risk factors for other CNS cancer types, and studies of poor quality, e.g., with inappropriate statistical methods, or inadequate patient or treatment data description and follow-up. Clinical case reports, clinical case series, observational studies, and systematic reviews were all included in the initial evaluation. Duplicates and relevance were initially evaluated based on the title and abstract screening. Full-text articles from all relevant studies were retrieved and reviewed. Additional relevant papers that were identified through a manual search of the references from the retrieved articles were also included.

3. Results

The initial literature search identified 608 records, of which 212 were excluded as duplicates. In addition, 47 reports were not available in the English language and were equally excluded. After the manual check of the reference list of the retrieved reports, 73 additional records were deemed relevant (Figure 1). Among the 422 reports that were retrieved and reviewed in total, 307 were excluded for reasons presented in detail in the screening flowchart (Figure 1). In the end, 115 articles were considered pertinent and were included in the current review.

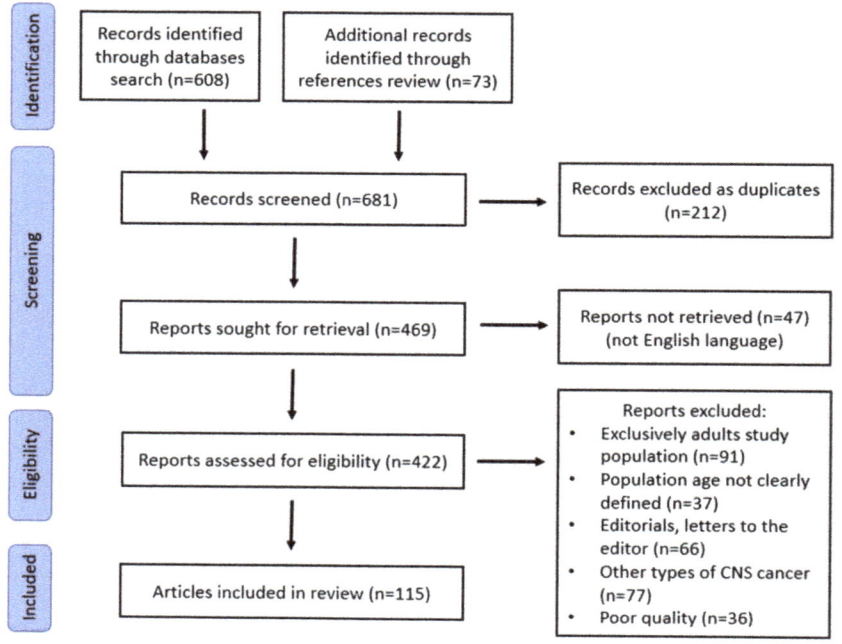

Figure 1. Flowchart of narrative review of the literature (record identification, eligibility, and final inclusion).

4. Discussion

4.1. Epidemiological Characteristics and Recurrence

Regarding the patient's personal history and morphological features of the disease, younger age has been linked in several studies with a higher rate of CP recurrence. For example, in an early large study that included 173 patients (45% children aged <16 years) with CP treated with external RT either alone or following surgery, adjusted for other risk factors for death, and after 12 years of median follow-up, the CP recurrence risk increased in parallel to age of presentation. More specifically, the relative risk was 1.0 for the age group < 16 years, 0.58 for the age group of 16–39, and 0.40 for patients 40 years and older [25]. In a more recent study from France with 171 patients (65 with childhood-onset and 106 adult-onset CP), diagnosis before the age of 10 years was an independent risk factor for recurrence [24]. In addition, it was associated with a higher incidence of obesity, blindness, and panhypopituitarism, and with developmental complications, since among the early onset group, only 40.7% of patients had adequate school performance or professional life compared to 72.4% of patients with later onset of the disease [24].

Similar were the results of a smaller, more recent study by Šteňo et al. [46], which included 38 children and 63 adults with CP treated with RT and/or surgery and were followed for a mean of >10 years. This study showed that the recurrence rate was higher in children compared to adults (39.5% vs. 22.2%, respectively), and this difference persisted even for patients with radical tumor excision (36.7% vs. 14%, respectively). Some studies have identified an even younger age (<5 years) to be an independent risk factor for CP recurrence [23,40,47]. The larger tumor size at presentation and its adhesion to the surrounding structures, as well as a more aggressive behavior of CP in younger patients, could explain the higher rate of CP recurrence in childhood-onset CP. In addition, delayed or nonuse of RT, especially in earlier studies, has been implicated in higher CP recurrence rates in children [16,23,24]. Nevertheless, a few studies have not found an association between CP recurrence risk and younger age [32,48,49].

Male sex has been associated in some studies with an increased risk of CP recurrence. For example, in their large retrospective study, Gautier et al. [24] found that CP recurrence was more common in male subjects. Similarly, Mortini et al. found that the male sex was an independent risk factor for recurrence in a group of adult and pediatric patients [22]. On the contrary, several authors have found no correlation between the male sex and the risk of CP recurrence either in adults or in children [14,29,30,48,49]. Since no plausible pathomechanism has been suggested to explain this male–female difference in recurrence rate and relevant data are inconsistent and scarce, especially in the pediatric population, a strong association between the male sex and increased recurrence risk cannot be established [16].

4.2. Morphological Features of the Tumor and Recurrence Rate

Several morphological features of CP, such as size, location, adherence to surrounding tissues, as well as its consistency, have been studied in relation to its recurrence risk (Table 1). Firstly, large tumor size at presentation (>3–5 cm) has been identified as an independent risk factor. As an example, in an early study with 61 children (median age 7.5 years) treated for CP in Boston between 1970 and 1990 and followed up for a median of 10 years, 5 of 6 patients with tumors ≥ 5 cm experienced recurrences while only 6 of 30 recurred when the tumor was <5 cm [19]. Similar were the results of another study by De Vile et al. [23], which showed that large tumor size, young age, and severe hydrocephalus were predictors of tumor recurrence in a cohort of 75 children treated for CP.

Tumor size ≥ 5 cm was also found to be an independent risk factor for CP recurrence in a more recent retrospective analysis of 86 children younger than 21 years of age [15]. In another study by Gupta et al. [26], 116 pediatric craniopharyngiomas (68 boys and 48 girls; age range 1.6–18 years) were reviewed and showed that tumor size > 4 cm was strongly associated with tumor recurrence. Similar were the results of two more recent studies [50,51]. The association of larger tumors with increased recurrence risk seems to be multifactorial. Larger tumors occupy larger intracranial compartments and invade surrounding anatomical structures and are, therefore, more difficult to remove completely [23,28]. For example, in a study of 309 patients with CP from China, in which the tumor size was 2–9 cm in diameter, patients with larger tumors showed a higher recurrence rate due to partial or subtotal resection [41]. Further, larger tumors increase the possibility of even a small tumor remaining after surgical excision, which increases the regrowth–recurrence risk [18,28] and possibly in a relatively short time after the first surgical intervention [15]. In addition, larger tumors present more frequently with severe hydrocephalus, which also precludes a total resection, thus increasing the recurrence risk.

Tumor location is another factor that has been associated with increased CP recurrence risk. Several investigators have observed that certain CP locations are more prone to recur, possibly due to difficulty in total resection due to attachment to and/or infiltration of the hypothalamus, attachment to important vascular structures, or involvement of the third ventricle [18,28,29,52]. Kim et al., for example [14], investigated retrospectively 36 children (age range 1–15 years) that had undergone radical excision without RT for a mean follow-up period of 52 months. They found that tumor location was the single most significant clinical predictor of recurrence since the 5-year recurrence-free survival rate was 39% for those who had an intrasellar tumor component and 81% for those who did not ($p < 0.05$). Anatomical structures adjacent to the tumor, such as the optic chiasm, the hypothalamus, and the pituitary stalk, were the most common sites for adhesion, and residual tumor in the optic apparatus was more likely to relapse [14]. Moreover, intracranial sites with intracellular compartments, especially in the vicinity of the pituitary fossa, were also associated with a high probability of relapse [14]. Several authors consider CP location relative to the hypothalamus so important as to support the need for a hypothalamus-referenced classification of CP [53–55].

A third morphological characteristic of CP that has been associated with an increased risk of recurrence is the degree of tumor adherence to surrounding vascular or neural structures. Although difficult to define precisely, tumor adherence refers to the neurosurgeon's ability to find a clear plan for adequate tumor resection [56]. Three factors define the type of adherence, namely, to which intracranial structures the tumor is attached, its adherence morphology, and its strength [56]. Several studies have shown a relationship between these factors and the success of tumor removal. The strongest and most extensive adhesions in the hypothalamus that preclude any attempt to perform a safe total removal are observed in CPs arising from the suprasellar cistern and secondarily invade the third ventricle, and in those with subpial growth at the third ventricle floor [1,18,28,29,41,55,57,58]. Indeed, in the series of children with CP by Tomita et al. [29], only 33% of CPs associated with the third ventricle were completely removed, in contrast to nearly 70% of extraventricular tumors. Similarly, Fahlbusch et al. [28] reported a much lower rate of total removal of intraventricular CPs compared to the general rate (21% vs. 50%, respectively). Indirect evidence of the role of tumor adherence in CP recurrence comes from the observation that the usual location of CP recurrences is frequently the anatomic areas where the primary tumor presented the tighter adherence [14,41]. The importance of tumor adherence regarding the surgical risk of hypothalamic injury, surgical removal extent, and, thus, the risk of tumor recurrence has led some authors to develop a comprehensive descriptive model based on the location, morphology, and strength of tumor attachment. This model is divided into five hierarchical levels of increasing severity, namely, mild, moderate, serious, severe, and critical, and can be used to anticipate the surgical risk of hypothalamic injury and to plan the degree of removal accordingly [56,59].

Finally, tumor consistency, meaning cystic, solid, or mixed cystic/solid tumor, has been associated with the risk of CP recurrence. A few studies in both adults and children have shown that the removal of cystic CPs is associated with a higher recurrence rate compared to the removal of predominantly solid CPs [16,26,60]. A possible explanation for this is the difficulty in removing an intact cystic tumor capsule during surgical removal.

Table 1. Categorized risk factors that have been studied in childhood-onset CP recurrence. Each factor is colored according to the following: dark blue for factors strongly protective against recurrence; light blue for factors that most probably have no association with recurrence; dark red as strongly heightened risk; light red as weakly heightened risk; grey for factors with inconclusive data.

Category	Risk Factor	Association Found	Study
Epidemiological features	Younger age	Increases the risk	Rajan et al. [25], De Vile et al. [23] Fisher et al. [40], Gautier et al. [24], Šteňo et al. [46], Drimtzias et al. [47]
		No association	Duff et al. [32], Lena et al. [48], Al Shail et al. [49]
	Male sex	Increases the risk	Gautier et al. [24], Mortini et al. [22]
		No association	Kim et al. [14], Lena et al. [48], Tena-Suck et al. [30], Tomita et al. [29], Al Shail et al. [49]
Morphological features	Large size	Increases the risk	Hetelekidis et al. [19], de Vile et al. [23], Elliot et al. [15] Gupta et al. [26], Shi et al. [41], Weiner et al. [27], Yosef et al. [50], Kobayashi et al. [51]
	Tumor location [e.g., third ventricle involvement]	Increases the risk	Kim et al. [14], Fahlbusch et al. [28], Tomita et al. [29], Van Effenterre et al. [18], Kim et al. [14]
	Tumor adherence to surrounding tissues	Increases the risk	Fahlbusch et al. [28], Tomita et al. [29], Karavitaki et al. [1], Pan et al. [57], Pascual et al. [55], Pascual et al. [58], Shi et al. [41], Effenterre et al. [18]
	Cystic tumor consistency	Increases the risk	Gupta et al. [26], Lee et al. [60], Prieto et al. [16]

Table 1. Cont.

Category	Risk Factor	Association Found	Study
Clinical presentation	Hydrocephalus (increased ICP)	Increases the risk	Prieto et al. [16], DeVile et al. [23], Gautier et al. [24]
		Some association	Kim et al. [14], Tomita et al. [29], Gupta et al. [26], Al Shail et al. [49], Poretti et al. [9], Liubinas et al. [61], Fahlbusch et al. [28]
		No association	Duff et al. [32], Karavitaki et al. [1], Kim et al. [14], Puget et al. [44]
	Visual disturbances at presentation	Increases the risk	Duff et al. [32], Lee et al. [62]
		No association	Shail et al. [49], Tena-Suck et al. [30], Drimtzias et al. [47]
	Hypothalamic involvement	Some association	Vinchon et al. [33], De Vile et al. [23], Poretti et al. [9]
		Decreases the risk	Gautier et al. [24]
	Hormonal-related symptoms	Increases the risk	Tena-suck et al. [30], Rogers et al. [63], Erfurth et al. [64]
		Better outcome	Gautier et al. [24]
Histological features	Adamantinomatous vs. papillary CP	Adamantinomatous increases recurrence risk	Adamson et al. [65], Szeifert et al. [66], Crotty et al. [67], Tavangar et al. [68]
		No difference between the two types	Duff et al. [32], Eldevik et al. [69], Gupta et al. [26], Kim et al. [14], Minamida et al. [70], Tena-Suck et al. [30], Weiner et al. [27], Prieto et al. [16], Agozzino et al. [35], Zygourakis et al. [71]
	Presence of finger-like epithelial protrusions	Increases the risk	Adamson et al. [65], Weiner et al. [27]
		No association	Duff et al. [32], Gupta et al. [26], Tena-Suck et al. [30]
	Presence of whorl-like arrays	Increases the risk	Stache et al. [31], Tena-Suck et al. [30],
	Intense reactive peritumoral gliosis	Possible risk increase	Pascual et al. [58], Qi et al. [57], Weiner et al. [27], Bartlett [72]
		Possible positive effect on number of recurrences	Vile et al. [23], Minamida et al. [70], Tomita et al. [29], Weiner et al. [27], Adamson et al. [65], Prieto et al. [16]
Molecular features	High Ki-67 expression	Increases the risk	Nishi et al. [73], Rodriguez et al. [34], Prieto et al. [16], Raghavan et al. [74], Izumoto et al. [75], Anegawa et al. [76], Guadagno et al. [77], Xu et al. [78]
		No association	Agozzino et al. [35], Kim et al. [14], Park et al. [79], Losa et al. [80], Duo et al. [81], Raghavan et al. [74], Yalçın et al. [82], Moszczyńska et al. [83]
	p53 gene loss of function	Increases the risk	Tena-Suck et al. [30]
		Possible association	Ishida et al. [36], Lefranc et al. [39], Prieto et al. [16], Ujifuku et al. [84]
		No association	Momota et al. [85], Yalcin et al. [82]
	Vascular endothelial growth factor (VEGF)	Increases the risk	Liu et al. [86], Sun et al. [87], Agozzino et al. [35], Xia et al. [88], Elmaci et al. [37]
		No association	Xu et al. [89]
	Expression of RAR isotypes and cathepsins	RARγ increases the risk	Lubansu et al. [38], Lefranc et al. [39]
	Hormones and their receptors	Possible association	Hofmann et al. [90], Li et al. [91]
		No association	Martínez-Ortega et al. [92]

Table 1. Cont.

Category	Risk Factor	Association Found	Study
Therapeutic approach	Presence of tumor remnants after excision	Increases the risk	Amendola et al. [93], Baskin et al. [94], Cabezudo et al. [95], Carmel et al. [96], Crotty et al. [67], De Vile et al. [23], Duff et al. [32], Elliot et al. [15], Fahlbusch et al. [28], Eldevik et al. [69], Gautier et al. [24], Gupta et al. [26], Hetelekidis et al. [19], Hoffman et al. [13], Karavitaki et al. [1], Khafaga et al. [97], Lena et al. [48], Mortini et al. [22], Puget et al. [44], Schoenfeld et al. [20], Shi et al. [41], Tena-Suck et al. [30], Thompson et al. [98], Tomita et al. [29], Van Effenterre et al. [18], Weiner et al. [27], Yasargil et al. [99], Zuccaro et al. [100]
	Neurosurgical team expertise	Affects the recurrence rate	Mortini et al. [101], Bao et al. [102], Yosef et al. [50], Zygourakis et al. [71], Prieto et al. [16], Tavangar et al. [68]
	Use of radiotherapy after subtotal surgical removal	Decreases the risk	Baskin et al. [94], Cabezudo et al. [95], Carmel et al. [96], Crotty et al. [67], De Vile et al. [23], Duff et al. [32], Eldevik et al. [69], Fisher et al. [40], Hetelekidis et al. [19], Karavitaki et al. [1], Khafaga et al. [97], Mortini et al. [22], Richmond et al. [103], Schoenfeld et al. [20], Stahnke et al. [104], Thompson et al. [98], Tomita et al. [29], Thomsett et al. [105], Weiss et al. [106], Wen et al. [107], Amendola et al. [93], Enayet et al. [108], Stripp et al. [109]
	Presence of calcifications	Increases the risk	Fahlbusch et al. [28], Fisher et al. [40], Zhang et al. 2008 [110], Cheng et al. [111]
		No association	Elliott et al. [42], Drimtzias et al. [47]
	Use of GH replacement therapy	Increases the risk	Taguchi et al. [112], Niu et al. [113]
		No association	Arslanian et al. [114], Olsson et al. [115], Kanev et al. [116], Moshang [43], Karavitaki et al. [117], Rohrer et al. [118], Boekhoff et al. [119], Boguszewski et al. [120], Puget et al. [44], Kim et al. [14], Elliott et al. [15], Clayton et al. [121], Child et al. [122], Darendeliler et al. [45], Moshang et al. [123], Price et al. [124], Smith et al. [125]
		Decreases the risk	Alotaibi et al. [126]

4.3. Clinical Presentation at Initial Diagnosis and Recurrence

Clinical manifestations of CP are suggestive of tumor invasion and damage to adjacent tissues. Typical initial CP manifestations include headache and vomiting in 60–80% of cases, hydrocephalus (all as a result of raised ICP), as well as visual deficits, hypothalamic damage, and hormonal-related manifestations (as a result of local invasion to adjacent structures). Of all clinical manifestations of CP, mostly hydrocephalus and visual symptoms have been associated with an increased risk of tumor recurrence (Table 1). Specifically, in a systematic review, it was reported that hydrocephalus at presentation was the unique symptom associated with tumor recurrence; however, this association was characterized as inconclusive as its role remains controversial [16]. In two studies, hydrocephalus at presentation was significantly associated with higher risk of tumor recurrence in children and mixed-age patients, respectively (DeVile et al.: Mann–Whitney U-test: $z = -3.15$, $p < 0.002$; Gautier et al.: HR: 2.12 95% CI [1.21–3.71], $p < 0.01$) [23,24]. In four other studies, the role of hydrocephalus and raised ICP as risk factors for recurrence were investigated, and both were associated with tumor recurrence since >30% of patients in the recurrence groups had hydrocephalus and intracranial hypertension at presentation (Gupta et al.: 33%; Al Shail et al.: 71.4%). However, no significant association was noted after statistical analysis (Kim et al.: $p = 0.1408$; Tomita et al.: $p = 0.41915$; Gupta et al.: $p = 0.32$; Al Shail et al.: $p = 0.122$) [14,26,29,49]. Other studies have also reported some association between hydrocephalus and tumor recurrence risk but without a detailed statistical analysis [9,15,28,61], and still others did not prove a consistent relationship [1,14,32,44].

Concerning visual deficits, almost half of the juvenile patients are referred to with such symptoms at the time of presentation, most usually as difficulty seeing at school and blurring of vision due to bitemporal hemianopia from optic chiasm compression [127,128]. Several studies have pointed out a possible association between visual symptoms and the risk of CP recurrence. For example, in the study by Duff et al. [32], pediatric patients with visual symptoms at presentation exhibited a higher rate of tumor recurrence (15.1% at 1 year) compared with those without visual symptoms (9.1%, $p = 0.024$). Within the gross total resection group, there was a significant increase in the recurrence rate among patients who presented with visual symptoms compared with those who did not (7.8% at 1 year vs. 3.6%, $p = 0.009$). This association was further reinforced by another study that showed that visual abnormalities at presentation were significantly associated with CP recurrence in children ($p < 0.001$), possibly due to tumor adhesion to the optic nerve or chiasm [62]. On the contrary, other studies performed in pediatric and adult patients showed no statistical significance between visual symptoms, such as chiasmatic syndrome and CP recurrence ($p = 0.682$), or between sixth cranial nerve palsy and recurrence ($p = 0.09$) [47,49], regardless of the higher recurrence rate that was observed in these patients (80% vs. 50%) [30]. These data come in contrast with the study by Duff et al. [32], which demonstrated a significant association between 6th cranial nerve palsy at presentation and CP recurrence ($p = 0.0337$).

Since the hypothalamic–pituitary axis is compromised or compressed by the tumor, symptoms, such as growth failure (75%), delayed puberty (60%), and diabetes insipidus (10–20%), are often reported, while most CP patients suffer from pituitary insufficiency or even panhypopituitarism (75–95%) [127]. When obstructive hydrocephalus is present, symptoms of functional decline manifest, such as psychomotor deficits or school performance decrease, due to frontal lobe compression [127,128]. While hypothalamic disturbance and hormonal-related manifestations have been indicated as risk factors for CP recurrence, very few studies have further investigated the significance of their association. One study in children reported that hypothalamic involvement was significantly associated with tumor recurrence in survival analysis ($p = 0.01$), but no significance was observed when logistic regression was performed ($p = 0.07$) [33]. Other researchers have reported that patients with hypothalamic damage, either by infiltration or compression at presentation, demonstrated more frequent recurrences; however, no further association was made [9,23].

Hormonal-related symptoms are typical manifestations of CP, and their potential role as prognostic factors of tumor recurrence has also been examined, albeit with contradictory results so far. Panhypopituitarism has been documented as a common symptom at presentation and associated with possible recurrence; however, either no statistical significance occurred (Tena-Suck et al.: $p = 0.191$, Rogers et al.: $p = 1.000$) [30,63] or no further analysis was performed [64]. It should be noted, however, that Gautier et al. [24] indicated that the isolated presence of hormonal-related manifestations is associated with a better outcome (OR: 0.38, 95%CI: [0.14–1.03]), while symptoms of raised ICP with a worse one.

4.4. Histological Features of the Tumor and Recurrence

Early studies have shown that the adamantinomatous CP tends to be more invasive [27,67] and to form villous elongations into the surrounding brain and particularly in the hypothalamus [39]. Histopathological examination of resected CPs frequently reveals isolated nests of tumor cells extending into, apparently, invading the surrounding gliotic brain tissue [26]. These features make gross-total resection of adamantinomatous CP more difficult. Since partial tumor resection has been linked with higher recurrence rates, it was assumed that these features render adamantinomatous CP a more aggressive and recurrent type [65,66]. However, several recent studies found no significant difference in recurrence rate between the two histological types of CP, and this lack of difference persisted independent of resection status [14,16,26,27,30,32,69,70]. In addition, several recent studies have challenged the claim that finger-like epithelial protrusions are associated with an increased risk of recurrence [26,32].

Since neither the histological type (adamantinomatous vs. papillary) nor the presence of finger-like protrusions seem to increase the tumor's recurrence risk, other histological features have been investigated as risk factors (Table 1). Among them, the presence of whorl-like arrays has recently been correlated with CP recurrence [30]. The structures are morule-like tumor cell nests that can be identified in histological sections of adamantinomatous CPs. They are thought to be caused by mutations in the β-catenin gene (*CTNNB1*), which are found almost exclusively in adamantinomatous CPs, as shown in a study by Brastianos et al. [129]. Such mutations are important in the Wnt signaling pathway [129,130], which has been shown to act as a promoter of epithelial migration through the regulation of fascin's gene expression, a protein implicated in filopodia formation [131]. Histologically, clusters of catenin-rich cells have been identified in the tumor–brain border and the tumor's cyst wall, suggesting a possible role of *CTNNB1* mutations in the aggressive expansion of some adamantinomatous CPs [31,132]. Similarly, a recent study by Guadagno et al. [77] reported that immunohistochemical expression of β-catenin in tumor tissue was strongly associated [$p = 0.0039$] with an increased CP recurrence risk.

Another feature that has been examined relative to the CP's recurrence risk is the presence of peritumoral gliosis. Reactive gliosis is the proliferation and hypertrophy of glial cells in response to brain tissue damage [133]. More than fifty years ago, Bartlett et al. described that rapidly growing CPs are characterized by a prominent gliotic reaction [72]. Subsequent studies have suggested that the presence of a thick layer of reactive gliosis at the tumor–brain interface may highlight a more aggressive tumor invading the adjacent tissues, with only one showing an increased recurrence risk [27,58,72,134]. On the contrary, a prominent peritumoral gliotic layer has been used as a non-functional dissection plane that facilitates a more extensive dissection of lesions. Indeed, in a study by Weiner et al. [27], 68% of totally removed CPs had a macroscopically visible layer of gliosis around the tumor, compared to 48% of the partially removed tumors. Likewise, several authors have identified the lack of peritumoral gliosis as a major risk factor for multiple subsequent operations [16,23,27,29,65,70].

4.5. Molecular Features of the Tumor and Recurrence

Several molecular features of CP have been studied as potential markers of their recurrence (Table 1). It is known that Ki-67 is a protein expressed in mammalian nucleated cells and directly associated with cell proliferation [135]. Extensive literature supports its use as a prognostic marker for tumor staging, assessment of cancer relapse, and prognosis in various tumor types in children and adults [136,137]. Increased Ki-67 expression has been noted in malignant CPs [34]. In addition, studies have examined this molecular index in relation to CP recurrence rate, albeit with conflicting results [16,138]. Nishi et al. [73] and Rodriguez et al. [34], for example, reported a significant correlation between high Ki-67 expression and CP recurrence. Other authors have reported a markedly increased Ki-67 expression in recurrent CP tumors [74–76,78], while several others failed to establish such a relationship [14,35,74,79–83]. The wide range of Ki-67 expression in recurrent CPs (0.1–49%) observed in various studies could be partly attributed to the fact that Ki-67 positive nuclei do not show a uniform distribution in each tissue sample [74,81], and on the other, Ki-67 expression may not be constant throughout tumor progression [139]. Prieto et al. [16], in a large systematic analysis of 298 patients from 12 studies, concluded that high Ki-67 expression was among the most reliable tumor markers for predicting an increased risk of recurrence and rapid tumor growth, as long as it was combined with pathological and therapeutic factors, particularly tumor topography and the degree of tumor removal [138].

Protein p53, a regulatory protein of the cell cycle with tumor suppressor properties, has been implicated in the pathogenesis of almost half of all cancers [140]. There are a few studies examining the possible role of altered p53 expression in the aggressivity and relapse of CP with conflicting results. Tena-Suck et al. [30], for example, found that altered immunoreactivity for p53 was significantly ($p = 0.022$) correlated with tumor recurrence or regrowth but without being associated with a specific histopathological subtype. The possible correlation between p53 expression and CP aggressiveness is further supported by the higher expression of p53 in malignant CPs compared to benign CPs [84] and the higher expression of p53 found in recurrent tumor specimens compared to primary CPs [16,36,39]. Nevertheless, there are studies that failed to demonstrate a correlation between p53 immunopositivity and CP histogenesis or recurrence rate, such as the ones by Momota et al. [85] and by Yalçın et al. [82], respectively.

Another molecular marker that, although not predictive of CP recurrence, appears to be of interest is the BRAF gene mutations. A particular mutation, namely, the BRAF p.Val600Glu mutation, has been described as a genetic hallmark of papillary CPs, as it is present in >95% of squamous papillary CPs and, surprisingly, in none of the adamantinomatous CPs [78,129]. This association suggests that activation of the MAPK/ERK pathway leading to suppression of apoptosis is probably the main oncogenic driver of papillary CP [141]. Indeed, BRAF-targeted chemotherapy in patients with papillary CP resulted in a dramatic reduction in tumor volume and cessation of tumor recurrences [142–145].

The main role of VEGF is the regulation of angiogenesis in both physiologic and pathologic [e.g., tumorigenesis] conditions [146]. Hypoxia-inducible factor 1α (HIF1α) is a transcription factor that regulates the cellular response to hypoxia and seems to be dysregulated in cancer cells [147]. Both of these factors have been examined as potential markers of increased risk of CP recurrence. In a study by Liu et al. [86], for example, CP recurrence was associated with higher VEGF and HIF1α expression, regardless of histopathological subtype, as the relative expression of VEGF and HIF1α in recurrent compared to non-recurrent CPs was 1.07 to 0.32 ($p = 0.001$) and 3.09 to 0.75 ($p = 0.001$), respectively. Similarly, previous studies have shown increased expression of both VEGF and its cellular receptor in recurrent or metastatic CPs, indicating a possible role of VEGF in neo-angiogenesis and tumor regrowth [35,37,87,88]. In another study by Vidal et al. [148], CPs with higher microvessel density were found to regrow more frequently compared to those with lower microvessel density, suggesting that the extent of angiogenesis and, thus, VEGF levels have prognostic value in CP patients. Despite the above data, a study by Xu et al. [89] examined 32 patients with adamantinomatous and 31 patients with papillary CP and found no difference in VEGF expression between the recurrent and non-recurrent CPs ($p > 0.05$).

Another possible marker of increased risk of recurrence is the RARs, which are nuclear receptors involved in epithelial maturation and differentiation. RARs family consists of three different isotypes, namely, alpha (RARα), beta (RARβ), and gamma (RARγ), and the corresponding retinoid X receptor with three subtypes, alpha, beta, and gamma. Two studies have shown a potential correlation between the levels of RARs and the risk of CP recurrence [38,39] since they showed higher expression of RARγ in CPs that recurred within two years of surgical resection. Interestingly, these tumors had lower expression of RARβ. A possible explanation for this discrepancy is the different expression of cathepsins, which are proteinases involved in the potential for local invasion. The different expression of cathepsins, specifically cathepsin D and cathepsin K, seems to contribute to the ability of RARs to influence CP recurrence.

Establishing a link between hormones and CP recurrence remains quite challenging. The most important hormonal mediator in the development and progression of CP seems to be the GH receptor. Indeed, in a study by Hofmann et al. [90], it was observed that CPs with high GH receptor expression had a higher proliferative potential than CPs with low

GH receptor expression. Accordingly, the insulin-like growth factor-1 (IGF-1) receptor was shown to be more abundantly expressed in adamantinomatous than in the papillary type of CP, an observation that possibly implicates the IGF-1 receptor in the recurrence of this type of tumor [91]. Other hormones, such as sex steroid hormones and their receptors, as well as leptin and insulin, have not been implicated in increasing the risk of CP recurrence, although results are somewhat conflicting regarding estrogen receptors [90,92].

4.6. Therapeutic Approach and Tumor Recurrence

Even though knowledge of the cellular and molecular mechanisms involved in tumor recurrence is limited, several clinical studies have found a significant association between the presence of residual tumor and the risk of CP recurrence in both children and adults [1,13,15,18–20,22–24,26–30,32,41,44,48,67,69,93–97,99,100] (Table 1). Therefore, a complete tumor resection, which includes resection of the outer tumor capsule adjacent to healthy tissues, is considered to be the best approach in order to minimize the possibility of tumor recurrence [7,149]. In a systematic review by Prieto et al. [16], for example, the mean recurrence rate after a total removal was 23% compared to 63% after a partial removal. The mean time between the first surgery and CP recurrence was also different between the two groups of patients (24 months for total and 45 months for subtotal surgical excision). In recent years, improvements in surgical techniques have increased the frequency with which a complete tumor resection can be achieved without excessive morbidity or mortality [15,41,150]. However, complete CP resection is still only achieved in a percentage of CP cases [41,70,100], and even then, the recurrence risk is high, reaching a 10-year rate of 95% [22]. In addition, an aggressive total resection is usually accompanied by endocrine dysfunction and hypothalamic damage, thus leading to increased morbidity for patients [149]. For these reasons, many authors advocate a less aggressive surgical treatment followed by RT, and in recent years, there has been an increasing tendency toward subtotal resection of complex craniopharyngiomas followed by adjuvant RT to maximize the quality of life while achieving tumor control [1,22]. Studies have shown that tumor control rates after subtotal resection and RT are similar to the ones reported after gross-tumor resection but with lower morbidity [20,100]. Even more controversial is the best approach for a child with recurrent CP. A study by Elliott et al. [15], including 86 children with primary and recurrent CP, showed that gross-total resection was more difficult to achieve in recurrent tumors, especially those with increasing size and after prior RT. Nevertheless, radical resection was still possible in patients with recurrent CPs with morbidity similar to that of primary tumors. Another factor strongly influencing the risk of tumor recurrence, independently of histopathology, both for primary and recurrent tumors, is the ability of the neurosurgeon and their team to achieve gross total resection in candidate patients [16,50,68,71,101,102]. Therefore, an experienced neurosurgical team should be in charge of dealing with these patients.

The use of adjuvant RT is another factor that has been shown in several patient series to significantly reduce the risk of recurrence after subtotal tumor removal [1,19,20,22,23,29,32,40,67,69,93–98,103–109]. In many of these studies that included pediatric patients with CP, the mean recurrence rate of patients treated with RT after subtotal removal was similar and sometimes superior [20] to the one observed in patients after total removal. In a meta-analysis including 442 patients who underwent tumor resection, Yang et al. showed that the 2- and 5-year progression-free survival rates for the gross-total resection group versus the subtotal resection followed by adjuvant RT group were 88 vs. 91%, and 67 vs. 69%, respectively [151]. Similar were the results of another systematic review of a cohort of 531 pediatric CP patients from a total of 109 studies showing similar rates of tumor control with both approaches [21]. These data suggest that subtotal resection followed by adjuvant RT may be equally efficient with gross-total resection without the morbidity associated with aggressive surgical procedures. In addition, contemporary RT techniques permit greater treatment precision and conformity. These approaches decrease but do not eliminate long-term toxicity by limiting the exposure of surrounding normal tissues to ionizing radiation [152]. In addition, there is still no consensus regarding the best irradiation technique, the most appropriate time to administer RT, and at what exact dosage. In addition, some studies have shown that once the pediatric CP recurs, it is exceedingly difficult to treat after prior irradiation since newer RT techniques decrease but do not eliminate long-term toxicity due to the exposure of surrounding normal tissues to ionizing radiation. Therefore, some authors suggest that gross-total resection may need to be the surgical goal at the time of first recurrence, if possible [153]. In total, it is of utmost importance to carefully evaluate each pediatric CP patient to reach the perfect balance between quality of life and the best tumor control approach.

Another factor that has been implicated in the risk of CP recurrence is the absence or presence of tumor calcifications. Elliott et al. [42] showed that minimal residual calcification does not have an impact on the risk of recurrence after gross-total removal in pediatric CPs. Given the potentially harmful effects of RT in the pediatric population, the authors suggest that RT should be withheld in patients after CP gross-total removal and only minimal residual calcification on MR or CT imaging CT, albeit with a close follow-up. In contrast, several authors found that the presence of calcifications in children with CP is an independent risk factor for unsuccessful complete tumor removal and, therefore, for an increased risk of tumor recurrence [28,40,108,110,111]. For example, Fahlbusch et al. [28], in 148 patients with CP who underwent initial (primary) surgery, found that the main reasons for incomplete removal were attachment to and/or infiltration of the hypothalamus, major calcifications, and attachment to vascular structures. Patients with total removal had a recurrence-free survival of 86.9% at 5 years vs. only 48.8% for those with subtotal removal and 41.5% for those with partial removal, implicating the initial presence of calcifications in a higher recurrence rate and lower survival. Similarly, in another cohort of children with CP that were operated on, the absence of calcification on diagnostic neuroimaging (n = 8/30) was significantly associated with improved 5-year progression-free survival (100% vs. 42.9% [SE = 14.7%], $p = 0.02$), even when adjusted for the extent of resection ($p = 0.03$). [40] In a more recent retrospective analysis of the clinical data of 92 children with CP who underwent surgical treatment, the authors found a statistically significant difference ($p < 0.05$) between the degree of tumor calcification and the recurrence rate after the operation and the mortality rate [111]. It, therefore, seems possible that, despite the conventional assumption that residual calcifications do not correspond to viable tumor tissue, their presence is frequently associated with higher rates of partial tumor excision, resulting in residual tumors, which increase the risk of tumor recurrence.

Selection of the right type of surgical approach is also crucial and must ensure complete tumor resection with the least possible damage to the adjacent important neuronal structures [22,41]. To achieve wide exposure of the chiasmatic region, a combination of subfrontal and pterional approaches is usually preferred, performing a frontotemporal method from the nondominant side, extending frontally near the midline [18,100]. The transsphenoidal approach has been used in patients in whom the lesion was exclusively intrasellar or in cases of intrasellar and suprasellar tumor extension with symmetrical and homogeneous intrasellar and suprasellar growth [154,155]. The transcranial approach was selected when the tumor was exclusively suprasellar or in cases of intrasellar and suprasellar extension with asymmetrical and larger suprasellar development [22]. In selected cases, by using the transsphenoidal approach, even tumors with large suprasellar expansion can be managed. The main disadvantage of endoscopic, endonasal, and transsphenoidal surgery, mainly with huge suprasellar expansion, is the increased risk of cerebrospinal fluid leakage [156,157]. Nevertheless, it seems that this approach may give excellent results with minor risks when used in appropriately located craniopharyngiomas and by neurosurgeons with extensive experience in pituitary surgery [158,159]. Recurrence rates associated with the various approaches vary among studies. For example, in a study by Minamida et al. [70], who compared different surgical approaches in 37 consecutive patients with CPs, the recurrence rates were as follows: 20% in patients treated with the basal interhemispheric approach; 25% in those treated with the pterional approach; and 60% in those treated with the transsphenoidal approach.

Safety concerns related to GH treatment and CP recurrence or regrowth come from in vitro studies that have demonstrated the growth of CP cells cultured in the presence of exogenous GH [91], from the identification of GH receptors on CP cells [90], and from the observation that increased GH receptors expression may indicate higher tumor aggressiveness [160]. In addition, there are a few case reports describing a rapid CP enlargement after GH therapy initiation [112,113]. On the contrary, robust data come from carefully conducted case-control studies in pediatric or mixed pediatric–adult populations, most of which have failed to demonstrate any evidence of CP recurrence or regrowth with GH therapy [14,15,43,44,114–121]. Similarly, in adults, a recent well-conducted, retrospective analysis of 89 patients with adult-onset craniopharyngioma with a median follow-up of >7 years demonstrated no increased risk of CP recurrence after surgical excision in those treated with GH [161]. Furthermore, a recent meta-analysis comparing 3436 patients who received GH with 51 who did not [126] demonstrated a protective effect of GH treatment on CP recurrence (overall CP recurrence rate 10.9%, 95%CI: 9.80% vs. 35.2%, 95%CI: 23.1%, for patients with or without GH treatment, respectively; $p < 0.01$). These results, however, may reflect a selection bias in the included studies favoring GH treatment in patients with less aggressive CP. In addition, safety data of GH treatment come from post-marketing surveillance studies sponsored by the pharmaceutical industry, with equally reassuring results [45,122–125].

5. Conclusions

Despite the extensive research conducted over the past four decades on the mechanisms of CP recurrence in children and adolescents, many aspects of this intriguing process remain elusive. Data from large case series and cohort studies are quite often conflicting, mainly due to the heterogeneity of the specific characteristics of each CP in terms of topography, size, adhesiveness, histology, molecular characteristics, long-term behavior, and so forth. Subtotal surgical removal not followed by RT is the predictor of CP recurrence. Further, a younger age, large cystic tumors, tight adherence to surrounding structures, specific clinical findings at diagnosis, presence of histological whorl-like arrays, and some specific molecular features may all be associated with a higher rate of CP recurrence.

Systematic reviews and meta-analyses of each of the individual factors examined, but mostly, well-designed multicenter prospective studies with large numbers of CP patients, will shed further light on the pathomechanisms involved. This will not only assist in identifying prognostic factors for the risk of CP recurrence for each individual patient, thus helping in the best treatment therapeutic strategy already at the time of initial diagnosis. It will also guide the development of new targeted adjunct therapies that, together with tumor resection and local RT, will increase recurrence-free survival rates and improve the quality of life of these patients in the long run.

Author Contributions: Conceptualization, A.S. and A.G.-T.; methodology, A.S., V.R.T., A.P., S.G., E.P.K. and A.G.-T.; validation, V.R.T., A.P., S.K., E.I.S., K.M., E.L. and S.N.; investigation, A.S., V.R.T., A.P., S.K., E.I.S., K.M., E.L., S.N., S.G. and E.P.K.; data curation, A.S., V.R.T., A.P., S.K., E.I.S., K.M., E.L., S.N., S.G. and E.P.K.; writing—original draft preparation, A.S., V.R.T., A.P., S.K., E.I.S., K.M., E.L., S.N. and S.G.; writing—review and editing, A.S., S.G., E.P.K. and A.G.-T.; visualization, A.S., S.G. and E.P.K.; supervision, A.G.-T. All authors have read and agreed to the published version of the manuscript.

Funding: This research received no external funding.

Institutional Review Board Statement: Not applicable.

Informed Consent Statement: Not applicable.

Data Availability Statement: Not applicable.

Conflicts of Interest: The authors declare no conflict of interest.

References

1. Karavitaki, N.; Brufani, C.; Warner, J.T.; Adams, C.B.T.; Richards, P.; Ansorge, O.; Shine, B.; Turner, H.E.; Wass, J.A.H. Craniopharyngiomas in children and adults: Systematic analysis of 121 cases with long-term follow-up. *Clin. Endocrinol.* 2005, *62*, 397–409. [CrossRef] [PubMed]
2. Larkin, S.; Karavitaki, N. Recent advances in molecular pathology of craniopharyngioma. *F1000Research* 2017, *6*, 1202. [CrossRef]
3. Louis, D.N.; Ohgaki, H.; Wiestler, O.D.; Cavenee, W.K.; Burger, P.C.; Jouvet, A.; Scheithauer, B.W.; Kleihues, P. The 2007 WHO Classification of Tumours of the Central Nervous System. *Acta Neuropathol.* 2007, *114*, 97–109. [CrossRef] [PubMed]
4. Karavitaki, N.; Wass, J.A.H. Craniopharyngiomas. *Endocrinol. Metab. Clin. N. Am.* 2008, *37*, 173–193. [CrossRef]
5. Marszałek, A.; Szylberg, L.; Wiśniewski, S. Pathologic aspects of skull base tumors. *Rep. Pract. Oncol. Radiother.* 2016, *21*, 288–303. [CrossRef]
6. Gong, J.; Zhang, H.; Xing, S.; Li, C.; Ma, Z.; Jia, G.; Hu, W. High expression levels of CXCL12 and CXCR4 predict recurrence of adamanti-nomatous craniopharyngiomas in children. *Cancer Biomark.* 2014, *14*, 241–251. [CrossRef] [PubMed]
7. Müller, H.L.; Merchant, T.E.; Warmuth-Metz, M.; Martinez-Barbera, J.P.; Puget, S. Craniopharyngioma. *Nat. Rev. Dis. Primers* 2019, *5*, 75–94. [CrossRef] [PubMed]
8. Sughrue, M.E.; Yang, I.; Kane, A.J.; Fang, S.; Clark, A.J.; Aranda, D.; Barani, I.J.; Parsa, A.T. Endocrinologic, neurologic, and visual morbidity after treatment for craniopharyngioma. *J. Neuro-Oncol.* 2010, *101*, 463–476. [CrossRef]
9. Poretti, A.; Grotzer, M.A.; Ribi, K.; Schönle, E.; Boltshauser, E. Outcome of craniopharyngioma in children: Long-term complications and quality of life. *Dev. Med. Child Neurol.* 2004, *6*, 220–229.
10. Yuen, K.C.J.; Mattsson, A.F.; Burman, P.; Erfurth, E.-M.; Camacho-Hubner, C.; Fox, J.L.; Verhelst, J.; Geffner, M.E.; Abs, R. Relative Risks of Contributing Factors to Morbidity and Mortality in Adults with Craniopharyngioma on Growth Hormone Replacement. *J. Clin. Endocrinol. Metab.* 2018, *103*, 768–777. [CrossRef]
11. Wijnen, M.; Olsson, D.S.; Van Den Heuvel-Eibrink, M.M.; Hammarstrand, C.; Janssen, J.A.M.J.L.; van der Lely, A.J.; Johannsson, G.; Neggers, S.J.C.M.M. Excess morbidity and mortality in patients with craniopharyngioma: A hospital-based retrospective cohort study. *Eur. J. Endocrinol.* 2018, *178*, 93–102. [CrossRef]
12. Cohen, M.; Guger, S.; Hamilton, J. Long Term Sequelae of Pediatric Craniopharyngioma—Literature Review and 20 Years of Experience. *Front. Endocrinol.* 2011, *2*, 81. [CrossRef]
13. Hoffman, H.J.; De Silva, M.; Humphreys, R.P.; Drake, J.M.; Smith, M.L.; Blaser, S.I. Aggressive surgical management of craniopharyngiomas in children. *J. Neurosurg.* 1992, *76*, 47–52. [CrossRef]
14. Kim, S.-K.; Wang, K.-C.; Shin, S.-H.; Choe, G.; Chi, J.G.; Cho, B.-K. Radical excision of pediatric craniopharyngioma: Recurrence pattern and prognostic factors. *Child's Nerv. Syst.* 2001, *17*, 531–536. [CrossRef]
15. Elliott, R.E.; Hsieh, K.; Hochman, T.; Belitskaya-Levy, I.; Wisoff, J.; Wisoff, J.H. Efficacy and safety of radical resection of primary and recurrent craniopharyngiomas in 86 children. *J. Neurosurg. Pediatr.* 2010, *5*, 30–48. [CrossRef] [PubMed]
16. Prieto, R.; Pascual, J.M.; Subhi-Issa, I.; Jorquera, M.; Yus, M.; Martínez, R. Predictive Factors for Craniopharyngioma Recurrence: A Systematic Review and Illustrative Case Report of a Rapid Recurrence. *World Neurosurg.* 2013, *79*, 733–749. [CrossRef] [PubMed]
17. Coury, J.R.; Davis, B.N.; Koumas, C.P.; Manzano, G.S.; Dehdashti, A.R. Histopathological and molecular predictors of growth patterns and recurrence in craniopharyngiomas: A systematic review. *Neurosurg. Rev.* 2020, *43*, 41–48. [CrossRef]
18. Van Effenterre, R.; Boch, A.-L. Craniopharyngioma in adults and children: A study of 122 surgical cases. *J. Neurosurg.* 2002, *97*, 3–11. [CrossRef]
19. Hetelekidis, S.; Barnes, P.D.; Tao, M.L.; Fischer, E.G.; Schneider, L.; Scott, R.; Tarbell, N.J. 20-Year experience in childhood craniopharyngioma. *Int. J. Radiat. Oncol. Biol. Phys.* 1993, *27*, 189–195. [CrossRef] [PubMed]
20. Schoenfeld, A.; Pekmezci, M.; Barnes, M.J.; Tihan, T.; Gupta, N.; Lamborn, K.R.; Banerjee, A.; Mueller, S.; Chang, S.; Berger, M.S.; et al. The superiority of conservative resection and adjuvant radiation for craniopharyngiomas. *J. Neuro-Oncol.* 2012, *108*, 133–139. [CrossRef]
21. Clark, A.J.; Cage, T.A.; Aranda, D.; Parsa, A.T.; Sun, P.P.; Auguste, K.I.; Gupta, N. A systematic review of the results of surgery and radiotherapy on tumor control for pediatric craniopharyngioma. *Child's Nerv. Syst.* 2012, *29*, 231–238. [CrossRef] [PubMed]
22. Mortini, P.; Losa, M.; Pozzobon, G.; Barzaghi, R.; Riva, M.; Acerno, S.; Angius, D.; Weber, G.; Chiumello, G.; Giovanelli, M.; et al. Neurosurgical treatment of craniopharyngioma in adults and children: Early and long-term results in a large case series. *J. Neurosurg.* 2011, *114*, 1350–1359. [CrossRef]
23. De Vile, C.J.; Grant, D.B.; Kendall, B.E.; Neville, B.G.R.; Stanhope, R.; Watkins, K.E.; Hayward, R.D. Management of childhood craniopharyngioma: Can the morbidity of radical surgery be predicted? *J. Neurosurg.* 1996, *85*, 73–81. [CrossRef]
24. Gautier, A.; Godbout, A.; Grosheny, C.; Tejedor, I.; Coudert, M.; Courtillot, C.; Jublanc, C.; De Kerdanet, M.; Poirier, J.-Y.; Riffaud, L.; et al. Markers of Recurrence and Long-Term Morbidity in Craniopharyngioma: A Systematic Analysis of 171 Patients. *J. Clin. Endocrinol. Metab.* 2012, *97*, 1258–1267. [CrossRef]
25. Rajan, B.; Ashley, S.; Gorman, C.; Jose, C.; Horwich, A.; Bloom, H.; Marsh, H.; Brada, M. Craniopharyngioma—A long-term results following limited surgery and radiotherapy. *Radiother. Oncol.* 1993, *26*, 1–10. [CrossRef]
26. Gupta, D.K.; Ojha, B.K.; Sarkar, C.; Mahapatra, A.K.; Sharma, B.S.; Mehta, V.S. Recurrence in pediatric craniopharyngiomas: Analysis of clinical and histological features. *Child's Nerv. Syst.* 2006, *22*, 50–55. [CrossRef]

27. Weiner, H.L.; Wisoff, J.H.; Rosenberg, M.E.; Kupersmith, M.J.; Cohen, H.; Zagzag, D.; Shiminski-Maher, T.; Flamm, E.S.; Epstein, F.J.; Miller, D.C. Craniopharyngiomas: A clinicopathological analysis of factors predictive of recurrence and functional outcome. *Neurosurgery* **1994**, *35*, 1001–1011. [CrossRef]
28. Fahlbusch, R.; Honegger, J.; Paulus, W.; Huk, W.; Buchfelder, M. Surgical treatment of craniopharyngiomas: Experience with 168 patients. *J. Neurosurg.* **1999**, *90*, 237–250. [CrossRef]
29. Tomita, T.; Bowman, R.M. Craniopharyngiomas in children: Surgical experience at Children's Memorial Hospital. *Child's Nerv. Syst.* **2005**, *21*, 729–746. [CrossRef] [PubMed]
30. Tena-Suck, M.L.; Salinas-Lara, C.; Arce-Arellano, R.I.; Rembao-Bojórquez, D.; Morales-Espinosa, D.; Sotelo, J.; Arrieta, O. Clinicopathological and immunohistochemical characteristics associated to recurrence/regrowth of craniopharyngiomas. *Clin. Neurol. Neurosurg.* **2006**, *108*, 661–669. [CrossRef] [PubMed]
31. Stache, C.; Hölsken, A.; Schlaffer, S.-M.; Hess, A.; Metzler, M.; Frey, B.; Fahlbusch, R.; Flitsch, J.; Buchfelder, M.; Buslei, R. Insights into the Infiltrative Behavior of Adamantinomatous Craniopharyngioma in a New Xenotransplant Mouse Model. *Brain Pathol.* **2015**, *25*, 1–10. [CrossRef]
32. Duff, J.M.; Meyer, F.B.; Ilstrup, D.M.; Laws, E.R.; Schleck, C.D.; Scheithauer, B.W. Long-term Outcomes for Surgically Resected Craniopharyngiomas. *Neurosurgery* **2000**, *46*, 291–305. [CrossRef]
33. Vinchon, M.; Dhellemmes, P. Craniopharyngiomas in children: Recurrence, reoperation and outcome. *Child's Nerv. Syst.* **2008**, *24*, 211–217. [CrossRef]
34. Rodriguez, F.J.; Scheithauer, B.W.; Tsunoda, S.; Kovacs, K.; Vidal, S.; Piepgras, D.G. The Spectrum of Malignancy in Craniopharyngioma. *Am. J. Surg. Pathol.* **2007**, *31*, 1020–1028. [CrossRef] [PubMed]
35. Agozzino, L.; Ferraraccio, F.; Accardo, M.; Esposito, S.; Agozzino, M.; Cuccurullo, L. Morphological and Ultrastructural Findings of Prognostic Impact in Craniopharyngiomas. *Ultrastruct. Pathol.* **2006**, *30*, 143–150. [CrossRef] [PubMed]
36. Ishida, M.; Hotta, M.; Tsukamura, A.; Taga, T.; Kato, H.; Ohta, S.; Takeuchi, Y.; Nakasu, S.; Okabe, H. Malignant transformation in craniopharyngioma after radiation therapy: A case report and review of the literature. *Clin. Neuropathol.* **2010**, *29*, 2–8. [CrossRef] [PubMed]
37. Elmaci, L.; Kurtkaya-Yapicier, O.; Ekinci, G.; Sav, A.; Pamir, M.N.; Vidal, S.; Kovacs, K.; Scheithauer, B.W. Metastatic papillary craniopharyngioma: Case study and study of tumor angiogenesis. *Neuro-Oncology* **2002**, *4*, 123–128. [CrossRef]
38. Lubansu, A.; Ruchoux, M.-M.; Brotchi, J.; Salmon, I.; Kiss, R.; Lefranc, F. Cathepsin B, D and K expression in adamantinomatous craniopharyngiomas relates to their levels of differentiation as determined by the patterns of retinoic acid receptor expression. *Histopathology* **2003**, *43*, 563–572. [CrossRef]
39. Lefranc, F.; Mijatovic, T.; Decaestecker, C.; Kaltner, H.; André, S.; Brotchi, J.; Salmon, I.; Gabius, H.-J.; Kiss, R. Monitoring the Expression Profiles of Integrins and Adhesion/Growth-regulatory Galectins in Adamantinomatous Craniopharyngiomas: Their Ability to Regulate Tumor Adhesiveness to Surrounding Tissue and Their Contribution to Prognosis. *Neurosurgery* **2005**, *56*, 763–775. [CrossRef]
40. Fisher, P.G.; Jenab, J.; Goldthwaite, P.T.; Tihan, T.; Wharam, M.D.; Foer, D.R.; Burger, P.C. Outcomes and failure patterns in childhood craniopharyngiomas. *Child's Nerv. Syst.* **1998**, *14*, 558–563. [CrossRef]
41. Shi, X.-E.; Wu, B.; Fan, T.; Zhou, Z.-Q.; Zhang, Y.-L. Craniopharyngioma: Surgical experience of 309 cases in China. *Clin. Neurol. Neurosurg.* **2008**, *110*, 151–159. [CrossRef] [PubMed]
42. Elliott, R.E.; Moshel, Y.A.; Wisoff, J.H. Minimal residual calcification and recurrence after gross-total resection of craniopharyngioma in children. *J. Neurosurg. Pediatr.* **2009**, *3*, 276–283. [CrossRef] [PubMed]
43. Moshang, T. Is brain tumor recurrence increased following growth hormone treatment? *Trends Endocrinol. Metab.* **1995**, *6*, 205–209. [CrossRef] [PubMed]
44. Puget, S.; Garnett, M.; Wray, A.; Grill, J.; Habrand, J.-L.; Bodaert, N.; Zerah, M.; Bezerra, M.; Renier, D.; Pierre-Kahn, A.; et al. Pediatric craniopharyngiomas: Classification and treatment according to the degree of hypothalamic involvement. *J. Neurosurg. Pediatr.* **2007**, *106*, 3–12. [CrossRef] [PubMed]
45. Darendeliler, F.; Karagiannis, G.; Wilton, P.; Ranke, M.B.; Albertsson-Wikland, K.; Price, D.A. Recurrence of brain tumours in patients treated with growth hormone: Analysis of KIGS [Pfizer International Growth Database]. *Acta Paediatr.* **2006**, *95*, 1284–1290. [CrossRef]
46. teňo, J.; Bízik, I.; Šteňo, A.; Matejčík, V. Recurrent craniopharyngiomas in children and adults: Long-term recurrence rate and management. *Acta Neurochir. [Wien.]* **2014**, *156*, 113–122.
47. Drimtzias, E.; Falzon, K.; Picton, S.; Jeeva, I.; Guy, D.; Nelson, O.; Simmons, I. The ophthalmic natural history of paediatric craniopharyngioma: A long-term review. *J. Neuro-Oncol.* **2014**, *120*, 651–656. [CrossRef]
48. Lena, G.; Paredes, A.P.; Scavarda, D.; Giusiano, B. Craniopharyngioma in children: Marseille experience. *Child's Nerv. Syst.* **2005**, *21*, 778–784. [CrossRef]
49. Al Shail, E.; Al-Shenkiti, A.; Alotaibi, M.T.; Siddiqui, K.; Al-Kofide, A. Excision of pediatric craniopharyngioma: Pattern of recurrence in 35 patients at a tertiary care hospital in Saudi Arabia. *Child's Nerv. Syst.* **2020**, *36*, 297–304. [CrossRef]
50. Yosef, L.; Ekkehard, K.M.; Shalom, M. Giant craniopharyngiomas in children: Short- and long-term implications. *Child's Nerv. Syst.* **2016**, *32*, 79–88. [CrossRef]
51. Kobayashi, T.; Tsugawa, T.; Hatano, M.; Hashizume, C.; Mori, Y.; Shibamoto, Y. Gamma knife radiosurgery of craniopharyngioma: Results of 30 cases treated at Nagoya Radiosurgery Center. *Nagoya J. Med. Sci.* **2015**, *77*, 447–454. [PubMed]

52. Pascual, J.M.; Prieto, R. Craniopharyngioma and the Third Ventricle: This Inescapable Topographical Relationship. *Front. Oncol.* **2022**, *12*, 872689. [CrossRef]
53. Müller, H.L.; Gebhardt, U.; Teske, C.; Faldum, A.; Zwiener, I.; Warmuth-Metz, M.; Pietsch, T.; Pohl, F.; Sörensen, N.; Calaminus, G. Post-operative hypothalamic lesions and obesity in childhood craniopharyngioma: Results of the multinational prospective trial KRANIOPHARYNGEOM 2000 after 3-year follow-up. *Eur. J. Endocrinol.* **2011**, *165*, 17–24. [CrossRef]
54. Müller, H.L.; Gebhardt, U.; Faldum, A.; Warmuth-Metz, M.; Pietsch, T.; Pohl, F.; Calaminus, G.; Sörensen, N.; Kraniopharyngeom 2000 Study Committee. Xanthogranuloma, Rathke's cyst, and childhood craniopharyngioma: Results of prospective multinational studies of children and adolescents with rare sellar malformations. *J. Clin. Endocrinol. Metab.* **2012**, *97*, 3935–3943. [CrossRef]
55. Pascual, J.M.; Prieto, R.; Carrasco, R. Infundibulo-tuberal or not strictly intraventricular craniopharyngioma: Evidence for a major topographical category. *Acta Neurochir.* **2011**, *153*, 2403–2425. [CrossRef]
56. Prieto, R.; Pascual, J.M.; Hofecker, V.; Winter, E.; Castro-Dufourny, I.; Carrasco, R.; Barrios, L. Craniopharyngioma adherence: A reappraisal of the evidence. *Neurosurg. Rev.* **2020**, *43*, 453–472. [CrossRef]
57. Pan, J.; Qi, S.; Lu, Y.; Fan, J.; Zhang, X.; Zhou, J.; Peng, J. Intraventricular craniopharyngioma: Morphological analysis and outcome evaluation of 17 cases. *Acta Neurochir.* **2011**, *153*, 773–784. [CrossRef]
58. Pascual, J.M.; González-Llanos, F.; Barrios, L.; Roda, J.M. Intraventricular craniopharyngiomas: Topographical classification and surgical approach selection based on an extensive overview. *Acta Neurochir.* **2004**, *146*, 785–800. [CrossRef]
59. Prieto, R.; Pascual, J.M.; Rosdolsky, M.; Castro-Dufourny, I.; Carrasco, R.; Strauss, S.; Barrios, L. Craniopharyngioma adherence: A comprehensive topographical categorization and outcome-related risk stratification model based on the methodical examination of 500 tumors. *Neurosurg. Focus* **2016**, *41*, E13. [CrossRef]
60. Lee, E.J.; Cho, Y.H.; Hong, S.H.; Kim, J.H.; Kim, C.J. Is the Complete Resection of Craniopharyngiomas in Adults Feasible Considering Both the Oncologic and Functional Outcomes? *J. Korean Neurosurg. Soc.* **2015**, *58*, 432–441. [CrossRef]
61. Liubinas, S.V.; Munshey, A.S.; Kaye, A.H. Management of recurrent craniopharyngioma. *J. Clin. Neurosci.* **2011**, *18*, 451–457. [CrossRef]
62. Lee, M.J.; Hwang, J.M. Initial visual field as a predictor of recurrence and postoperative visual outcome in children with craniopharyngioma. *J. Pediatr. Ophthalmol. Strabismus* **2012**, *49*, 38–42. [CrossRef]
63. Rogers, M.; Davies, D.-M.; Halliday, J.; Pal, A.; Marland, A.; Foord, T.; Jafar-Mohammadi, B. Characterisation of paediatric craniopharyngiomas in a single centre study—Analysis of factors affecting recurrence rates. *Endocr. Abstr.* **2018**, *59*, 133. [CrossRef]
64. Erfurth, E.M. Endocrine aspects and sequel in patients with craniopharyngioma. *J. Pediatr. Endocrinol. Metab.* **2015**, *28*, 19–26. [CrossRef]
65. Adamson, T.E.; Wiestler, O.D.; Kleihues, P.; Yaşargil, M.G. Correlation of clinical and pathological features in surgically treated craniopharyngiomas. *J. Neurosurg.* **1990**, *73*, 12–17. [CrossRef] [PubMed]
66. Szeifert, G.T.; Sipos, L.; Horváth, M.; Sarker, M.H.; Major, O.; Salomváry, B.; Czirják, S.; Bálint, K.; Slowik, F.; Kolonics, L. Pathological characteristics of surgically removed craniopharyngiomas: Analysis of 131 cases. *Acta Neurochir.* **1993**, *124*, 139–143.
67. Crotty, T.B.; Scheithauer, B.W.; Young, W.F.; Davis, D.H.; Shaw, E.G.; Miller, G.M.; Burger, P.C. Papillary craniopharyngioma: A clinicopathological study of 48 cases. *J. Neurosurg.* **1995**, *83*, 206–214. [CrossRef]
68. Tavangar, S.M.; Larijani, B.; Mahta, A.; Hosseini, S.M.A.; Mehrazine, M.; Bandarian, F. Craniopharyngioma: A Clinicopathological Study of 141 Cases. *Endocr. Pathol.* **2004**, *15*, 339–344. [CrossRef]
69. Eldevik, O.P.; Blaivas, M.; Gabrielsen, T.O.; Hald, J.K.; Chandler, W.F. Craniopharyngioma: Radiologic and histologic findings and recurrence. *Am. J. Neuroradiol.* **1996**, *17*, 1427–1439. [PubMed]
70. Minamida, Y.; Mikami, T.; Hashi, K.; Houkin, K. Surgical management of the recurrence and regrowth of craniopharyngiomas. *J. Neurosurg.* **2005**, *103*, 224–232. [CrossRef]
71. Zygourakis, C.C.; Kaur, G.; Kunwar, S.; McDermott, M.W.; Madden, M.; Oh, T.; Parsa, A.T. Modern treatment of 84 newly diagnosed craniopharyngiomas. *J. Clin. Neurosci.* **2014**, *21*, 1558–1566. [CrossRef] [PubMed]
72. Bartlett, J.R. Craniopharyngiomas. An analysis of some aspects of symptomatology, radiology and histology. *Brain* **1971**, *94*, 725–732. [CrossRef] [PubMed]
73. Nishi, T.; Kuratsu, J.; Takeshima, H.; Saito, Y.; Kochi, M.; Ushio, Y. Prognostic significance of the MIB-1 labeling index for patient with craniopharyngioma. *Int. J. Mol. Med.* **1999**, *3*, 157–161. [CrossRef]
74. Raghavan, R.; Dickey, W.T.; Margraf, L.R.; White, C.L.; Coimbra, C.; Hynan, L.S.; Rushing, E.J. Proliferative activity in craniopharyngiomas: Clinicopathological correlations in adults and children. *Surg. Neurol.* **2000**, *54*, 241–248. [CrossRef]
75. Izumoto, S.; Suzuki, T.; Kinoshita, M.; Hashiba, T.; Kagawa, N.; Wada, K.; Fujimoto, Y.; Hashimoto, N.; Saitoh, Y.; Maruno, M.; et al. Immunohistochemical detection of female sex hormone receptors in craniopharyngiomas: Correlation with clinical and histologic features. *Surg. Neurol.* **2005**, *63*, 520–525. [CrossRef]
76. Anegawa, S.; Hayashi, T.; Nakagawa, S.; Furukawa, Y.; Tomokiyo, M. Craniopharyngioma with rapid regrowth–role of MIB-1 labeling index. *No Shinkei Geka* **2001**, *29*, 727–733.
77. Guadagno, E.; De Divitiis, O.; Solari, D.; Borrelli, G.; Bracale, U.M.; Di Somma, A.; Cappabianca, P.; Caro, M.D.B.D. Can recurrences be predicted in craniopharyngiomas? β-catenin coexisting with stem cells markers and p-ATM in a clinicopathologic study of 45 cases. *J. Exp. Clin. Cancer Res.* **2017**, *36*, 95–106. [CrossRef]

78. Xu, C.; Ge, S.; Cheng, J.; Gao, H.; Zhang, F.; Han, A. Pathological and Prognostic Characterization of Craniopharyngioma Based on the Expression of TrkA, β-Catenin, Cell Cycle Markers, and BRAF V600E Mutation. *Front. Endocrinol.* **2022**, *13*, 859381. [CrossRef]
79. Park, H.J.; Dho, Y.S.; Kim, J.H.; Kim, J.W.; Park, C.K.; Kim, Y.H. Recurrence Rate and Prognostic Factors for the Adult Craniopharyngiomas in Long-Term Follow-Up. *World Neurosurg.* **2020**, *133*, e211–e217. [CrossRef]
80. Losa, M.; Vimercati, A.; Acerno, S.; Barzaghi, R.L.; Mortini, P.; Mangili, F.; Terreni, M.R.; Santambrogio, G.; Giovanelli, M. Correlation between clinical characteristics and proliferative activity in patients with craniopharyngioma. *J. Neurol. Neurosurg. Psychiatry* **2004**, *75*, 889–892. [CrossRef]
81. Duò, D.; Gasverde, S.; Benech, F.; Zenga, F.; Giordana, M.T. MIB-1 immunoreactivity in craniopharyngiomas: A clinicopathological analysis. *Clin. Neuropathol.* **2003**, *22*, 229–234. [PubMed]
82. Yalcin, N.; Akbulut, M.; Sedat, C.; Bir, F.; Demirtaş, E. Prognostic significance of the Ki-67 labeling index and p53 protein expression for patient with craniopharyngioma. *J. Neurol. Sci.* **2009**, *26*, 286–291.
83. Moszczyńska, E.; Prokop-Piotrkowska, M.; Bogusz-Wójcik, A.; Grajkowska, W.; Szymańska, S.; Szalecki, M. Ki67 as a prognostic factor of craniopharyngioma's recurrence in paediatric population. *Child's Nerv. Syst.* **2020**, *36*, 1461–1469. [CrossRef]
84. Ujifuku, K.; Matsuo, T.; Takeshita, T.; Hayashi, Y.; Hayashi, K.; Kitagawa, N.; Hayashi, T.; Suyama, K.; Nagata, I. Malignant Transformation of Craniopharyngioma Associated with Moyamoya Syndrome. *Neurol. Med. Chir.* **2010**, *50*, 599–603. [CrossRef]
85. Momota, H.; Ichimiya, S.; Ikeda, T.; Yamaki, T.; Kikuchi, T.; Houkin, K.; Sato, N. Immunohistochemical analysis of the p53 family members in human craniopharyngioma. *Brain Tumor Pathol.* **2003**, *20*, 73–77. [CrossRef]
86. Liu, H.; Liu, Z.; Li, J.; Li, Q.; You, C.; Xu, J. Relative quantitative expression of hypoxia-inducible factor 1α messenger ribonucleic acid in recurrent craniopharyngiomas. *Neurol. India* **2014**, *62*, 53–56.
87. Sun, H.I.; Akgun, E.; Bicer, A.; Ozkan, A.; Bozkurt, S.U.; Kurtkaya, O.; Koc, D.Y.; Pamir, M.N.; Kilic, T. Expression of angiogenic factors in craniopharyngiomas: Implications for tumor recurrence. *Neurosurgery* **2010**, *66*, 744–750. [CrossRef]
88. Xia, Z.; Liu, W.; Li, S.; Jia, G.; Zhang, Y.; Li, C.; Ma, Z.; Tian, J.; Gong, J. Expression of Matrix Metalloproteinase-9, Type IV Collagen and Vascular Endothelial Growth Factor in Adamantinous Craniopharyngioma. *Neurochem. Res.* **2011**, *36*, 2346–2351. [CrossRef]
89. Xu, J.; Zhang, S.; You, C.; Wang, X.; Zhou, Q. Microvascular density and vascular endothelial growth factor have little correlation with prognosis of craniopharyngioma. *Surg. Neurol.* **2006**, *66*, S30–S34. [CrossRef]
90. Hofmann, B.M.; Hoelsken, A.; Fahlbusch, R.; Blümcke, I.; Buslei, R. Hormone receptor expression in craniopharyngiomas: A clinicopathological correlation. *Neurosurgery* **2010**, *67*, 617–625. [CrossRef]
91. Li, Q.; You, C.; Liu, L.; Rao, Z.; Sima, X.; Zhou, L.; Xu, J. Craniopharyngioma cell growth is promoted by growth hormone [GH] and is inhibited by tamoxifen: Involvement of growth hormone receptor [GHR] and IGF-1 receptor [IGF-1R]. *J. Clin. Neurosci.* **2013**, *20*, 153–157. [CrossRef]
92. Martínez-Ortega, A.; Flores-Martinez, Á.; Venegas-Moreno, E.; Dios, E.; Del Can, G.; Rivas, E.; Kaen, A.; Ruiz-Valdepeñas, E.C.; Fajardo, E.; Roldán, F.; et al. Sex Hormone Receptor Expression in Craniopharyngiomas and Association with Tumor Aggressiveness Characteristics. *J. Clin. Med.* **2022**, *11*, 281–290. [CrossRef] [PubMed]
93. Amendola, B.E.; Gebarski, S.S.; Bermudez, A.G. Analysis of treatment results in craniopharyngioma. *J. Clin. Oncol.* **1985**, *3*, 252–258. [CrossRef]
94. Baskin, D.S.; Wilson, C.B. Surgical management of craniopharyngiomas. A review of 74 cases. *J. Neurosurg.* **1986**, *65*, 22–27. [CrossRef]
95. Cabezudo, J.M.; Vaquero, J.; Areitio, E.; Martinez, R.; de Sola, R.G.; Bravo, G. Craniopharyngiomas: A critical approach to treatment. *J. Neurosurg.* **1981**, *55*, 371–375. [CrossRef]
96. Carmel, P.W.; Antunes, J.L.; Chang, C.H. Craniopharyngiomas in children. *Neurosurgery* **1982**, *11*, 382–389. [CrossRef]
97. Khafaga, Y.; Jenkin, D.; Kanaan, I.; Hassounah, M.; Al Shabanah, M.; Gray, A. Craniopharyngioma in children. *Int. J. Radiat. Oncol. Biol. Phys.* **1998**, *42*, 601–606. [CrossRef]
98. Thompson, D.; Phipps, K.; Hayward, R. Craniopharyngioma in childhood: Our evidence-based approach to management. *Child's Nerv. Syst.* **2005**, *21*, 660–668. [CrossRef]
99. Yaşargil, M.G.; Curcic, M.; Kis, M.; Siegenthaler, G.; Teddy, P.J.; Roth, P. Total removal of craniopharyngiomas. Approaches and long-term results in 144 patients. *J. Neurosurg.* **1990**, *73*, 355–357. [CrossRef]
100. Zuccaro, G. Radical resection of craniopharyngioma. *Child's Nerv. Syst.* **2005**, *21*, 679–690. [CrossRef]
101. Mortini, P.; Gagliardi, F.; Boari, N.; Losa, M. Surgical strategies and modern therapeutic options in the treatment of craniopharyngiomas. *Crit. Rev. Oncol.* **2013**, *88*, 514–529. [CrossRef] [PubMed]
102. Bao, Y.; Qiu, B.; Qi, S.; Pan, J.; Lu, Y.; Peng, J. Influence of previous treatments on repeat surgery for recurrent craniopharyngiomas in children. *Child's Nerv. Syst.* **2016**, *32*, 485–491. [CrossRef]
103. Richmond, I.L.; Wara, W.M.; Wilson, C.B. Role of Radiation Therapy in the Management of Craniopharyngiomas in Children. *Neurosurgery* **1980**, *6*, 513–517. [CrossRef]
104. Stahnke, N.; Grubel, G.; Lagenstein, I.; Willig, R.P. Long-term follow-up of children with craniopharyngioma. *Eur. J. Pediatr.* **1984**, *142*, 179–185. [CrossRef] [PubMed]
105. Thomsett, M.; Conte, F.; Kaplan, S.; Grumbach, M. Endocrine and neurologic outcome in childhood craniopharyngioma: Review of effect of treatment in 42 patients. *J. Pediatr.* **1980**, *97*, 728–735. [CrossRef]

106. Weiss, M.; Sutton, L.; Marcial, V.; Fowble, B.; Packer, R.; Zimmerman, R.; Schut, L.; Bruce, D.; D'Angio, G. The role of radiation therapy in the management of childhood craniopharyngioma. *Int. J. Radiat. Oncol. Biol. Phys.* **1989**, *17*, 1313–1321. [CrossRef]
107. Wen, B.-C.; Hussey, D.H.; Staples, J.; Hitchon, P.W.; Jani, S.K.; Vigliotti, A.P.; Doornbos, J. A comparison of the roles of surgery and radiation therapy in the management of craniopharyngiomas. *Int. J. Radiat. Oncol. Biol. Phys.* **1989**, *16*, 17–24. [CrossRef]
108. Enayet, A.E.R.; Atteya, M.M.E.; Taha, H.; Zaghloul, M.S.; Refaat, A.; Maher, E.; Abdelaziz, A.; El Beltagy, M.A. Management of pediatric craniopharyngioma: 10-year experience from high-flow center. *Child's Nerv. Syst.* **2021**, *37*, 391–401. [CrossRef]
109. Stripp, D.C.; Maity, A.; Janss, A.J.; Belasco, J.B.; Tochner, Z.A.; Goldwein, J.W.; Moshang, T.; Rorke, L.B.; Phillips, P.C.; Sutton, L.N.; et al. Surgery with or without radiation therapy in the management of craniopharyngiomas in children and young adults. *Int. J. Radiat. Oncol. Biol Phys.* **2004**, *58*, 714–720. [CrossRef]
110. Zhang, Y.Q.; Ma, Z.Y.; Wu, Z.B.; Luo, S.Q.; Wang, Z.C. Radical Resection of 202 Pediatric Craniopharyngiomas with Special Reference to the Surgical Approaches and Hypothalamic Protection. *Pediatr. Neurosurg.* **2008**, *44*, 435–443. [CrossRef]
111. Cheng, J.; Shao, Q.; Pan, Z.; You, J. Analysis and Long-Term Follow-Up of the Surgical Treatment of Children With Craniopharyngioma. *J. Craniofacial Surg.* **2016**, *27*, e763–e766. [CrossRef] [PubMed]
112. Taguchi, T.; Takao, T.; Iwasaki, Y.; Pooh, K.; Okazaki, M.; Hashimoto, K.; Terada, Y. Rapid recurrence of craniopharyngioma following recombinant human growth hormone replacement. *J. Neuro-Oncol.* **2010**, *100*, 321–322. [CrossRef]
113. Niu, D.-M.; Guo, W.-Y.; Pan, H.-C.; Wong, T.-T. Rapid enlargement of a residual craniopharyngioma during short-term growth hormone replacement. *Child's Nerv. Syst.* **2002**, *18*, 164–165. [CrossRef] [PubMed]
114. Arslanian, S.A.; Becker, D.J.; Lee, P.A.; Drash, A.L.; Foley, T.P. Growth Hormone Therapy and Tumor Recurrence: Findings in Children With Brain Neoplasms and Hypopituitarism. *Am. J. Dis. Children* **1985**, *139*, 347–350. [CrossRef]
115. Olsson, D.S.; Buchfelder, M.; Wiendieck, K.; Kremenevskaja, N.; Bengtsson, B.Å.; Jakobsson, K.-E.; Jarfelt, M.; Johannsson, G.; Nilsson, A.G. Tumour recurrence and enlargement in patients with craniopharyngioma with and without GH replacement therapy during more than 10 years of follow-up. *Eur. J. Endocrinol.* **2012**, *166*, 1061–1068. [CrossRef]
116. Kanev, P.M.; Lefebvre, J.F.; Mauseth, R.S.; Berger, M.S.; Alotaibi, N.M.; Noormohamed, N.; Cote, D.J.; Alharthi, S.; Doucette, J.; Zaidi, H.A.; et al. Growth hormone deficiency following radiation therapy of primary brain tumors in children. *J. Neurosurg.* **1991**, *74*, 743–748. [CrossRef]
117. Karavitaki, N.; Warner, J.T.; Marland, A.; Shine, B.; Ryan, F.; Arnold, J.; Turner, H.E.; Wass, J.A.H. GH replacement does not increase the risk of recurrence in patients with craniopharyngioma. *Clin. Endocrinol.* **2006**, *64*, 556–560. [CrossRef]
118. Rohrer, T.R.; Langer, T.; Grabenbauer, G.G.; Buchfelder, M.; Glowatzki, M.; Dörr, H.G. Growth Hormone Therapy and the Risk of Tumor Recurrence after Brain Tumor Treatment in Children. *J. Pediatr. Endocrinol. Metab.* **2010**, *23*, 935–942. [CrossRef]
119. Boekhoff, S.; Bogusz, A.; Sterkenburg, A.S.; Eveslage, M.; Müller, H.L. Long-term effects of growth hormone replacement therapy in childhood-onset craniopharyngioma: Results of the German Craniopharyngioma Registry [HIT-Endo]. *Eur. J. Endocrinol.* **2018**, *179*, 331–341. [CrossRef]
120. Boguszewski, M.C.S.; Cardoso-Demartini, A.A.; Boguszewski, C.L.; Chemaitilly, W.; Higham, C.E.; Johannsson, G.; Yuen, K.C.J. Safety of growth hormone [GH] treatment in GH deficient children and adults treated for cancer and non-malignant intracranial tumors—A review of research and clinical practice. *Pituitary* **2021**, *24*, 810–827. [CrossRef]
121. Clayton, P.E.; Price, D.A.; Shalet, S.M.; Gattemaneni, H.R. Craniopharyngioma Recurrence and Growth Hormone Therapy. *Lancet* **1988**, *331*, 642. [CrossRef] [PubMed]
122. Child, C.J.; Conroy, D.; Zimmermann, A.G.; Woodmansee, W.W.; Erfurth, E.M.; Robison, L.L. Incidence of primary cancers and intracranial tumour recurrences in GH-treated and untreated adult hypopituitary patients: Analyses from the Hypopituitary Control and Complications Study. *Eur. J. Endocrinol.* **2015**, *172*, 779–790. [CrossRef]
123. Moshang, T.; Rundle, A.C.; Graves, D.A.; Nickas, J.; Johanson, A.; Meadows, A. Brain tumor recurrence in children treated with growth hormone: The National Cooperative Growth Study experience. *J. Pediatr.* **1996**, *128*, S4–S7. [CrossRef]
124. Price, D.; Wilton, P.; Jönsson, P.; Albertsson-Wikland, K.; Chatelain, P.; Cutfield, W.; Ranke, M. Efficacy and Safety of Growth Hormone Treatment in Children with Prior Craniopharyngioma: An Analysis of the Pharmacia and Upjohn International Growth Database [KIGS] from 1988 to 1996. *Horm. Res. Paediatr.* **1998**, *49*, 91–97. [CrossRef]
125. Smith, T.R.; Cote, D.J.; Jane, J.A.; Laws, E.R. Physiological growth hormone replacement and rate of recurrence of craniopharyngioma: The Genentech National Cooperative Growth Study. *J. Neurosurg. Pediatr.* **2016**, *18*, 408–412. [CrossRef]
126. Alotaibi, N.M.; Noormohamed, N.; Cote, D.J.; Alharthi, S.; Doucette, J.; Zaidi, H.A.; Mekary, R.A.; Smith, T.R. Physiologic Growth Hormone—Replacement Therapy and Craniopharyngioma Recurrence in Pediatric Patients: A Meta-Analysis. *World Neurosurg.* **2018**, *109*, 487–496. [CrossRef]
127. Drapeau, A.; Walz, P.C.; Eide, J.G.; Rugino, A.J.; Shaikhouni, A.; Mohyeldin, A.; Carrau, R.L.; Prevedello, D.M. Pediatric craniopharyngioma. *Child's Nerv. Syst.* **2019**, *35*, 2133–2145. [CrossRef]
128. Steinbok, P. Craniopharyngioma in Children: Long-term Outcomes. *Neurol. Med. Chir.* **2015**, *55*, 722–726. [CrossRef]
129. Brastianos, P.K.; Taylor-Weiner, A.; Manley, P.E.; Jones, R.T.; Dias-Santagata, D.; Thorner, A.R.; Lawrence, M.S.; Rodriguez, F.J.; A Bernardo, J.; Schubert, L.; et al. Exome sequencing identifies BRAF mutations in papillary craniopharyngiomas. *Nat. Genet.* **2014**, *46*, 161–165. [CrossRef]
130. Buslei, R.; Hölsken, A.; Hofmann, M.; Kreutzer, J.; Siebzehnrubl, F.; Hans, V.; Oppel, F.; Buchfelder, M.; Fahlbusch, R.; Blümcke, I. Nuclear beta-catenin accumulation associates with epithelial morphogenesis in craniopharyngiomas. *Acta Neuropathol.* **2007**, *113*, 585–590. [CrossRef]

131. Hölsken, A.; Stache, C.; Schlaffer, S.M.; Flitsch, J.; Fahlbusch, R.; Buchfelder, M.; Oppel, F.; Buchfelder, M.; Fahlbusch, R.; Blümcke, I. Adamantinomatous craniopharyngiomas express tumor stem cell markers in cells with activated Wnt signaling: Further evidence for the existence of a tumor stem cell niche? *Pituitary* **2014**, *17*, 546–556. [CrossRef] [PubMed]
132. Zhao, C.; Wang, Y.; Liu, H.; Qi, X.; Zhou, Z.; Wang, X.; Lin, Z. Molecular biological features of cyst wall of adamantinomatous craniopharyngioma. *Sci. Rep.* **2023**, *13*, 3049. [CrossRef] [PubMed]
133. Khakh, B.S.; Sofroniew, M.V. Diversity of astrocyte functions and phenotypes in neural circuits. *Nat. Neurosci.* **2015**, *18*, 942–952. [CrossRef]
134. Qi, S.; Lu, Y.; Pan, J.; Zhang, X.; Long, H.; Fan, J. Anatomic relations of the arachnoidea around the pituitary stalk: Relevance for surgical removal of craniopharyngiomas. *Acta Neurochir.* **2011**, *153*, 785–796. [CrossRef]
135. Scholzen, T.; Gerdes, J. The Ki-67 protein: From the known and the unknown. *J. Cell. Physiol.* **2000**, *182*, 311–322. [CrossRef]
136. Mrouj, K.; Andrés-Sánchez, N.; Dubra, G.; Singh, P.; Sobecki, M.; Chahar, D.; Al Ghoul, E.; Aznar, A.B.; Prieto, S.; Pirot, N.; et al. Ki-67 regulates global gene expression and promotes sequential stages of carcinogenesis. *Proc. Natl. Acad. Sci. USA* **2021**, *118*, e2026507118. [CrossRef]
137. Sengupta, S.; Chatterjee, U.; Banerjee, U.; Ghosh, S.; Chatterjee, S.; Ghosh, A.K. A study of histopathological spectrum and expression of Ki-67, TP53 in primary brain tumors of pediatric age group. *Indian J. Med. Paediatr. Oncol.* **2012**, *33*, 25–31. [CrossRef]
138. Prieto, R.; Pascual, J.M. Can tissue biomarkers reliably predict the biological behavior of craniopharyngiomas? A comprehensive overview. *Pituitary* **2018**, *21*, 431–442. [CrossRef]
139. Broggi, G.; Franzini, A.; Cajola, L.; Pluchino, F. Cell Kinetic Investigations in Craniopharyngioma: Preliminary Results and Considerations. *Pediatr. Neurosurg.* **1994**, *21*, 21–23. [CrossRef]
140. Kim, S.; An, S.S.A. Role of p53 isoforms and aggregations in cancer. *Medicine* **2016**, *95*, e3993. [CrossRef]
141. Brastianos, P.K.; Santagata, S. Endocrine Tumors: BRAF V600E mutations in papillary craniopharyngioma. *Eur. J. Endocrinol.* **2016**, *174*, R139–R144. [CrossRef]
142. Rao, M.; Bhattacharjee, M.; Shepard, S.; Hsu, S. Newly diagnosed papillary craniopharyngioma with *BRAF V600E* mutation treated with single-agent selective BRAF inhibitor dabrafenib: A case report. *Oncotarget* **2019**, *10*, 6038–6042. [CrossRef] [PubMed]
143. Himes, B.T.; Ruff, M.W.; Van Gompel, J.J.; Park, S.S.; Galanis, E.; Kaufmann, T.J.; Uhm, J.H. Recurrent papillary craniopharyngioma with BRAF V600E mutation treated with dabrafenib: Case report. *J. Neurosurg.* **2018**, *130*, 1299–1303. [CrossRef]
144. Fasano, M.; Della Corte, C.M.; Caterino, M.; Pirozzi, M.; Rauso, R.; Troiani, T.; Martini, G.; Napolitano, S.; Morgillo, F.; Ciardiello, F. Dramatic Therapeutic Response to Dabrafenib Plus Trametinib in BRAF V600E Mutated Papillary Craniopharyngiomas: A Case Report and Literature Review. *Front. Med.* **2022**, *8*, 652005. [CrossRef]
145. Brastianos, P.K.; Shankar, G.M.; Gill, C.M.; Taylor-Weiner, A.; Nayyar, N.; Panka, D.J.; Sullivan, R.J.; Frederick, D.T.; Abedalthagafi, M.; Jones, P.S.; et al. Dramatic Response of BRAF V600E Mutant Papillary Craniopharyngioma to Targeted Therapy. *Gynecol. Oncol.* **2015**, *108*, djv310. [CrossRef]
146. Apte, R.S.; Chen, D.S.; Ferrara, N. VEGF in Signaling and Disease: Beyond Discovery and Development. *Cell* **2019**, *176*, 1248–1264. [CrossRef]
147. Jun, J.C.; Rathore, A.; Younas, H.; Gilkes, D.; Polotsky, V.Y. Hypoxia-Inducible Factors and Cancer. *Curr. Sleep Med. Rep.* **2017**, *3*, 1–10. [CrossRef]
148. Vidal, S.; Kovacs, K.; Lloyd, R.V.; Meyer, F.B.; Scheithauer, B.W. Angiogenesis in patients with craniopharyngiomas: Correlation with treatment and outcome. *Cancer* **2002**, *94*, 738–745. [CrossRef]
149. Flitsch, J.; Müller, H.L.; Burkhardt, T. Surgical Strategies in Childhood Craniopharyngioma. *Front. Endocrinol.* **2011**, *2*, 96. [CrossRef]
150. Yamada, S.; Fukuhara, N.; Yamaguchi-Okada, M.; Nishioka, H.; Takeshita, A.; Takeuchi, Y.; Inoshita, N.; Ito, J. Therapeutic outcomes of transsphenoidal surgery in pediatric patients with craniopharyngiomas: A single-center study. *J. Neurosurg. Pediatr.* **2018**, *21*, 549–562. [CrossRef]
151. Yang, I.; Sughrue, M.E.; Rutkowski, M.J.; Kaur, R.; Ivan, M.E.; Aranda, D.; Barani, I.J.; Parsa, A.T. Craniopharyngioma: A comparison of tumor control with various treatment strategies. *Neurosurg. Focus* **2010**, *28*, E5. [CrossRef] [PubMed]
152. Jalali, R.; Gupta, T.; Goda, J.S.; Goswami, S.; Shah, N.; Dutta, D.; Uday, K.; Jayita, D.; Padmavathy, M.; Sadhana, K.; et al. Efficacy of Stereotactic Conformal Radiotherapy vs Conventional Radiotherapy on Benign and Low-Grade Brain Tumors: A Randomized Clinical Trial. *JAMA Oncol.* **2017**, *3*, 1368–1376. [CrossRef]
153. Klimo, P.; Venable, G.T.; Boop, F.A.; Merchant, T.E. Recurrent craniopharyngioma after conformal radiation in children and the burden of treatment. *J. Neurosurg. Pediatr.* **2015**, *15*, 499–505. [CrossRef] [PubMed]
154. Matsuo, T.; Kamada, K.; Izumo, T.; Nagata, I. Indication and Limitations of Endoscopic Extended Transsphenoidal Surgery for Craniopharyngioma. *Neurol. Med. Chir.* **2014**, *54*, 974–982. [CrossRef] [PubMed]
155. de Divitiis, E.; Cappabianca, P.; Cavallo, L.M.; Esposito, F.; de Divitiis, O.; Messina, A. Extended Endoscopic Transsphenoidal Approach for Extrasellar Craniopharyngiomas. *Neurosurgery* **2007**, *61*, 219–228. [CrossRef]
156. Koutourousiou, M.; Fernandez-Miranda, J.C.; Wang, E.W.; Snyderman, C.H.; Gardner, P.A. The limits of transsellar/transtuberculum surgery for craniopharyngioma. *J. Neurosurg. Sci.* **2018**, *62*, 301–309. [CrossRef]
157. Taylor, D.G.; Jane, J.A. Editorial. Endoscopic endonasal surgery for pediatric craniopharyngiomas. *J. Neurosurg. Pediatr.* **2018**, *21*, 546–548. [CrossRef]

158. Maira, G.; Anile, C.; Albanese, A.; Cabezas, D.; Pardi, F.; Vignati, A. The role of transsphenoidal surgery in the treatment of craniopharyngiomas. *J. Neurosurg.* **2004**, *100*, 445–451. [CrossRef]
159. Komotar, R.J.; Starke, R.M.; Raper, D.M.M.; Anand, V.K.; Schwartz, T.H. Endoscopic Endonasal Compared with Microscopic Transsphenoidal and Open Transcranial Resection of Craniopharyngiomas. *World Neurosurg.* **2012**, *77*, 329–341. [CrossRef]
160. Ogawa, Y.; Kudo, M.; Watanabe, M.; Tominaga, T. Heterogeneity of Growth Hormone Receptor Expression in Craniopharyngioma—Implications for Surgical Strategy. *World Neurosurg.* **2020**, *138*, 89–92. [CrossRef]
161. Losa, M.; Castellino, L.; Pagnano, A.; Rossini, A.; Mortini, P.; Lanzi, R. Growth Hormone Therapy Does Not Increase the Risk of Craniopharyngioma and Nonfunctioning Pituitary Adenoma Recurrence. *J. Clin. Endocrinol. Metab.* **2020**, *105*, 1573–1580. [CrossRef]

Disclaimer/Publisher's Note: The statements, opinions and data contained in all publications are solely those of the individual author(s) and contributor(s) and not of MDPI and/or the editor(s). MDPI and/or the editor(s) disclaim responsibility for any injury to people or property resulting from any ideas, methods, instructions or products referred to in the content.

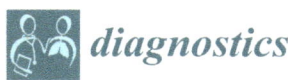

Review

Therapeutic Management and Prognostic Factors for Ovarian Malignant Tumours in Adolescents: A Comprehensive Review of Current Guidelines

Chrysoula Margioula-Siarkou [1], Stamatios Petousis [1,*], Georgia Margioula-Siarkou [1], George Mavromatidis [1], Fotios Chatzinikolaou [1], Emmanouel Hatzipantelis [2], Frédéric Guyon [3] and Konstantinos Dinas [1]

- [1] 2nd Department of Obstetrics and Gynaecology, Aristotle University of Thessaloniki, 541 24 Thessaloniki, Greece; margioulasiarkouc@gmail.com (C.M.-S.); gmargioulasiarkou@gmail.com (G.M.-S.)
- [2] Children's & Adolescent's Haematology–Oncology Unit, 2nd Department of Paediatrics, School of Medicine, Aristotle University of Thessaloniki, 541 24 Thessaloniki, Greece
- [3] Gynaecologic Oncology Unit, Institut Bergonié, 33000 Bordeaux, France
- * Correspondence: petousisstamatios@gmail.com; Tel.: +30-693-405-0763

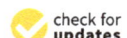

Citation: Margioula-Siarkou, C.; Petousis, S.; Margioula-Siarkou, G.; Mavromatidis, G.; Chatzinikolaou, F.; Hatzipantelis, E.; Guyon, F.; Dinas, K. Therapeutic Management and Prognostic Factors for Ovarian Malignant Tumours in Adolescents: A Comprehensive Review of Current Guidelines. *Diagnostics* **2023**, *13*, 1080. https://doi.org/10.3390/diagnostics13061080

Academic Editors: Edward J. Pavlik and Gustavo Baldassarre

Received: 28 December 2022
Revised: 27 February 2023
Accepted: 3 March 2023
Published: 13 March 2023

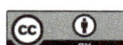

Copyright: © 2023 by the authors. Licensee MDPI, Basel, Switzerland. This article is an open access article distributed under the terms and conditions of the Creative Commons Attribution (CC BY) license (https://creativecommons.org/licenses/by/4.0/).

Abstract: Background: Ovarian malignant tumours are rarely diagnosed in adolescents but may have a significant impact on their survival, future fertility and quality of life. The management of such cases is rather complex and requires expertise and careful planning according to scarce existing evidence and recommendations. **Objective:** The aim of this study was to review and compare recommendations from published guidelines regarding the diagnosis, prognosis and treatment of malignant ovarian tumours in adolescents. **Evidence acquisition:** A comparative descriptive/narrative review of guidelines issued by L'Observatoire des Tumeurs Malignes Rares Gynécologiques, the British Society for Paediatric & Adolescent Gynaecology, the European Society for Medical Oncology, the European Society of Gynecological Oncology-European Society for Paediatric Oncology and the European Cooperative Study Group for Pediatric Rare Tumors was conducted. **Results:** All guidelines recommend a thorough diagnostic work-up, consisting of both imaging tests and serum tumour marker measurement, as well as the use of immunohistochemical methods to confirm the diagnosis and complete surgical staging prior to constructing the treatment plan. There is a lack of recommendations regarding the assessment of prognostic factors, with only one guideline providing detailed information. Treatment strategies, as suggested by the majority of guidelines and with only a few discrepancies between them, should include both surgery and adjuvant therapies, mainly chemotherapy, with great emphasis on fertility preservation when it is considered oncologically safe and on the significance of regular and long-term follow-up. **Conclusions:** There is a significant degree of agreement among recommendations of existing guidelines. The reported differences, although limited, highlight the need for the adoption of an international consensus in order to further improve the management of adolescent ovarian cancer.

Keywords: ovarian cancer; adolescents; diagnosis; prognosis; treatment; therapy; guidelines

1. Introduction

Ovarian tumours are the most common neoplasms affecting the reproductive system in adolescents [1,2]. They are rarely diagnosed in childhood and adolescence, with an estimated incidence of 2.6 cases per 100,000 girls per year. Approximately 10–30% of all ovarian masses detected in girls up to 17 years are malignant, accounting for 1% of all childhood malignancies and 8% of all abdominal tumours in children [3–5]. As expected, due to the particularities of the pediatric population, there are substantial differences between adults and adolescents regarding the incidence, histologic distribution, clinical manifestations, diagnostic evaluation and therapeutic management of ovarian cancer [6,7]. Although epithelial ovarian cancer is the most predominant pathological subtype in adults, ovarian tumours in children and adolescents originate mainly from non-epithelial tissues and cells that are specific to the ovary. Specifically, about 85% of all preadolescent malignant ovarian masses are germ cell tumours (GCTs), 8% are epithelial cell carcinomas, 5% are sex cord stromal tumours (SCSTs) and steroid cell tumours, while less than 1% of them are small cell carcinomas of the ovary [4,8,9]. Germ cell tumours are the most common ovarian neoplasms in pediatric patients, with dysgerminomas and yolk sac tumours being accordingly the most prominent seminomatous and nonseminomatous GCTs in this population [10–12]. Regarding sex cord stromal tumours and steroid cell tumours, adolescents are mostly diagnosed with juvenile granulosa cell tumours, Sertoli cell tumours and Sertoli–Leydig cell tumours, rather than granulosa cell tumours and thecomas, which mostly affect peri- and postmenopausal women [9]. The current WHO classification of GCTs and SCSTs are presented in Table 1 [13,14].

Table 1. WHO (World Health Organisation) 2020 classification of germ cell tumours (GCTs) and sex cord-stromal tumours (SCSTs).

SEX CORD-STROMAL TUMOURS	GERM CELL TUMOURS
Pure stromal tumours	Teratoma, benign
Fibroma, NOS	Immature teratoma, NOS
Cellular fibroma	Extra-gonadal teratoma
Thecoma	Post-pubertal type teratoma
Luteinised thecoma associated with sclerosing peritonitis	Dysgerminoma
Sclerosing stromal tumour	Yolk sac tumour
Microcystic stromal tumour	Embryonal carcinoma
Signet ring stromal tumour	Choriocarcinoma, NOS
Leydig cell tumour	Fetus in fetu
Steroid cell tumour	Mixed germ cell tumour
Malignant steroid cell tumour	Monodermal teratomas and somatic type tumours arising from a dermoid cyst
Fibrosarcoma	Struma ovarii, NOS
Pure sex cord tumours	Struma ovarii, malignant
Adult granulosa cell tumour	Struma carcinoid
Juvenile granulosa cell tumour	Teratoma with malignant transformation
Sertoli cell tumour, NOS	Cystic teratoma, NOS
Sex cord tumour with annular tubules	Germ cell sex cord stromal tumours
Mixed sex cord stromal tumours	Gonadoblastoma
Sertoli–Leydig cell tumour	Dissecting gonadoblastoma
Well differentiated	Undifferentiated gonadal tissue
Moderately differentiated	Mixed germ cell-sec cord stromal tumour, unclassified
Poorly differentiated	
Retiform	
Sex cord stromal tumour, NOS	
Gynandroblastoma	
Other	
Papillary cystadenoma	

The diagnosis of ovarian cancer in the adolescent population can pose challenges in clinical practice, considering the low suspicion of the disease due to young age, the heterogenous and often subtle clinical presentation and the potential limitations in diagnostic imaging in an effort to reduce radiation exposure [15,16]. Ovarian-mass related symptoms are usually non-specific, such as diffuse subacute abdominal and pelvic pain, feeling of pelvic pressure, distended abdomen, rapid increase in abdominal volume, urinary or bowel transit disorders, nausea, vomiting and, much rarer in early puberty, vaginal bleeding and menstrual irregularities [17,18]. Therefore, they can be easily attributed at first in conditions related to other systems rather than the reproductive and, in the majority of cases, the mass is already large at the time of the initial diagnosis [4,19,20]. Moreover, the therapeutic management of ovarian tumours is rather demanding, requiring expertise and precise design, tailored to the specific needs of non-adult patients [21]. Suggested treatment should simultaneously be curative and oncologically safe, ovarian function and fertility-sparing if possible, minimally invasive and sensitive to the psycho–emotional impact on this vulnerable population [1,22,23]. The rarity of ovarian cancer in adolescents further complicates the management of the disease, since the majority of information available to clinicians handling such cases can mostly be obtained by case reports and case series, while only a small number of official guidelines relevant to this topic have been issued. Considering all the above, an effort to combine and concisely summarise all existing guidelines referring to the management of ovarian malignancies in the adolescent population could be very useful to pediatricians, gynecologists and all related specialties involved in such complex cases and it could further facilitate the establishment of evidence-based and generally accepted principals of clinical practice.

The aim of this descriptive review is to compare and synthesise recommendations from published international guidelines regarding the diagnosis, prognosis and treatment of malignant ovarian tumours in adolescents.

2. Methods

The main objective of the present narrative review was to identify existing guidelines or recommendations issued by official medical organisations, colleges, associations, societies, committees and study groups regarding the management of ovarian malignant tumours in pediatric and adolescent populations. A search of the literature was conducted in September 2022 through PubMed, Scopus and Web of Science databases. The literature search was performed regarding the period 1990–2022. Electronic search was conducted by using combinations of terms "ovarian cancer" [tiab] OR "ovarian mass"[tiab] AND "adolescent" [tiab] OR "children" [tiab] OR "pediatric" OR "paediatric" [tiab] AND "guidelines" [tiab] OR "recommendations" [tiab]. Additionally, the websites of internationally recognised medical organisations and societies with scientific interest on gynecologic and pediatric oncology were also searched in order to identify official published guidelines relevant to the objective of the present review. Namely, American College of Obstetricians and Gynaecology (ACOG), American Academy of Pediatrics (AAP), American Pediatric Surgical Association (APSA), Society of Obstetricians and Gynaecologists of Canada (SOGC), International Federation of Gynecology and Obstetrics (FIGO), Royal College of Obstetricians and Gynaecologists (RCOG), British Society for Paediatric and Adolescent Gynaecology (BritSPAG), National Institute for Health and Care Excellence (NICE), French Society of Gynaecologic Oncology (SFOG), L'observatoire des tumeurs rares malignes gynécologiques (IMAGYN), European Society of Gynaecologic Oncology (ESGO), European Society of Paediatric Oncology (SIOPE), European Society of Medical Oncology (ESMO), Paediatric Rare Tumours Network-European Registry (PARTNER), Royal Australian and New Zealand College of Obstetricians and Gynaecologists (RANZCOG) and Chinese Society of Obstetrics and Gynaecology (CSOG) were reviewed.

Exclusion criteria included all other types of studies, except for official guidelines and recommendations, as well as guidelines written in any language except for English and French. The main outcomes of interest to identify in the included guidelines/recommendations were the most common types of ovarian cancer in non-adult population, staging and therapeutic management of each type of ovarian cancer in adolescents, as well as suggested follow-up.

Systematic search revealed 96 items with potential for inclusion in our narrative review, of which 12 were duplicated and another 74 were excluded based on title/abstract. There were finally twelve items reviewed as potentially eligible for our review, of which three were excluded because of not reporting guidelines/recommendations, two items were excluded because of not reporting guidelines for paediatric/adolescent population, one item was excluded for reporting only on population with hereditary cancer and one item was excluded because of reporting on population with cancer in pregnancy.

There were finally five published guidelines/official recommendations regarding the management of ovarian tumours in children and adolescents that were retrieved and included in the present descriptive/narrative review. In particular, two national guidelines were identified, issued by L'Observatoire des Tumeurs Malignes Rares Gynécologiques (Centres Experts TMRG, 2022) [24] and by the British Society for Paediatric & Adolescent Gynaecology (BritSPAG 2018) [25], as well as two international guidelines, issued by the European Society for Medical Oncology (ESMO 2018) [9], by the European Society of Gynecological Oncology and the European Society for Paediatric Oncology (ESGO-SIOPE 2020) [26] and by the European Cooperative Study Group for Pediatric Rare Tumors as part of the Paediatric Rare Tumours Network-European Registry (EXPeRT/PARTNER 2021) [27,28]. The flowchart of study selection is presented in Figure 1. An overview of recommendations of all five guidelines is presented in Table 2.

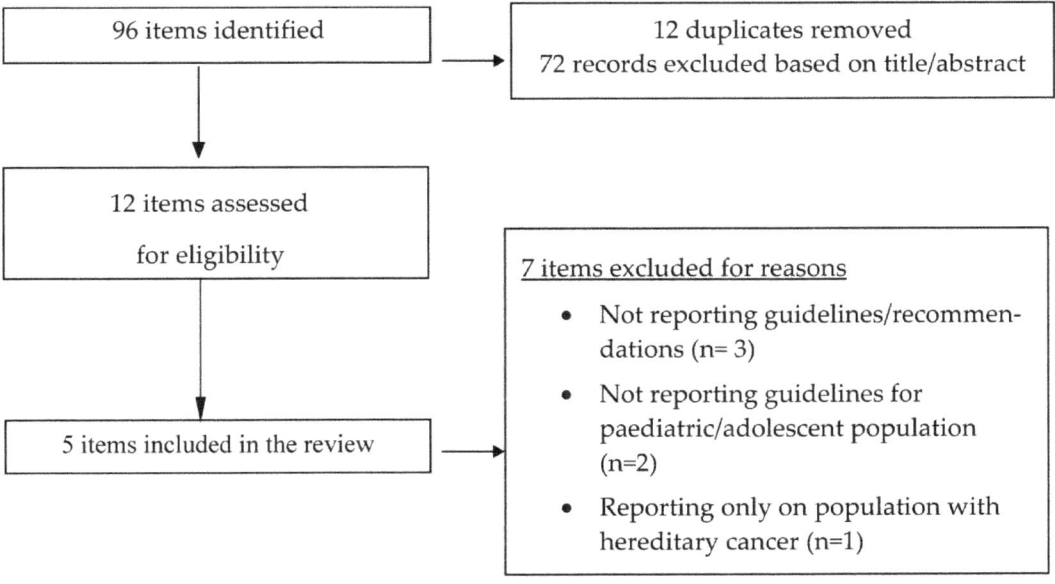

Figure 1. Flowchart of study selection.

Table 2. Summary of recommendations.

	L'Observatoire des Tumeurs Malignes Rares Gynécologiques (Centres Experts TRMG)	ESGO-SIOPE	ESMO	BritSPAG	EXPeRT/ PARTNER Consensus
Country	France	International/European	International/European	United Kingdom	International/European
Issued	2022	2020	2018	2018	2021
Title	Les tumeurs malignes rares gynécologiques—Référentiels	Non-epithelial ovarian cancers in adolescents and young adults	Non-epithelial ovarian cancer: ESMO Clinical Practice Guidelines for diagnosis, treatment and follow-up	Guideline for the management of ovarian cysts in children and adolescents	Consensus recommendations from the EXPeRT/PARTNER groups for the diagnosis and therapy of sex cord stromal tumours in children and adolescents
Diagnostic evaluation					
Reference to specialised centre with multidisciplinary board	Not discussed	Recommended	Not discussed	Recommended	Not discussed
Abdominal–pelvic ultrasound	Recommended as initial imaging	Not discussed	Recommended	Recommended as initial imaging	Recommended
Evaluation of endometrial thickness	Recommended for suspected hormone-producing tumours	Recommended for suspected hormone-producing tumours	Endometrial curettage recommended for adults	Not discussed	Not discussed
Chest X-ray	Not discussed	Not discussed	Recommended	Not discussed	Recommended
CT scan	Not discussed	Recommended thoracic CT scan	Recommended abdominal–pelvic CT scan	Not discussed	Low-dose chest CT as an alternative to chest X-ray
Abdominal–pelvic MRI	Recommended for suspected GCTs	Recommended	Not discussed	Not discussed	Recommended
PET scan	Recommended in selected cases	Not recommended	Recommended in selected cases	Not discussed	Not discussed
Serum tumour markers (basic panel: β-hCG, AFP, LDH, CA125)	Recommended, pre- and post-operative measurement	Recommended, pre- and post-operative measurement	Recommended, pre- and post-operative measurement	Recommended	Recommended
Hormonal profile	Not discussed	Recommended if signs of hormonal production/precocious puberty	Not discussed	Recommended if signs of hormonal production/precocious puberty	Recommended
Post-operative imaging if omitted preoperatively	Not discussed	Recommended	Not discussed	Recommended	Not discussed
Pathology and molecular biology					
Preoperative biopsy	Not discussed	Recommended if extraovarian spread, avoided if cystic component	Not discussed	Not discussed	Ovarian biopsy strongly discouraged at diagnosis
Opinion of expert pathologist	Not discussed	Recommended	Recommended	Not discussed	Recommended
Use of immunohistochemical markers	Recommended	Recommended	Recommended	Not discussed	Recommended, FOXL2 for granulosa cell tumours to distinguish adult and juvenile types
Karyotyping	Recommended for suspected gonadoblastoma	Recommended for suspected gonadoblastoma	Recommended for suspected gonadoblastoma	Not discussed	Not discussed
Mutational analysis	Recommended, DICER1 mutations for suspect SCSTs, SMARCA4 mutations for SCCOHT	Recommended, DICER1 mutations for suspect SCCOHT, Germline mutation analysis for bilateral GCTs, unilateral GCTs with pubertal retardation, Sertoli–Leydig cell tumours and SCCOHT	Recommended, DICER1 mutations for suspect SCSTs, SMARCA4 mutations for SCCOHT	Not discussed	Recommended, DICER1 mutations for suspected SLCTs or gynadroblastoma

Table 2. Cont.

	L'Observatoire des Tumeurs Malignes Rares Gynécologiques (Centres Experts TRMG)	ESGO-SIOPE	ESMO	BritSPAG	EXPeRT/PARTNER Consensus
Assessment of prognostic factors					
GCTs	Not discussed	Recommended, based on age at diagnosis, FIGO stage, tumour histology, residual disease after surgical resection	Not discussed	Not discussed	Not discussed
SCSTs	Not discussed	Recommended, based on FIGO stage, size of tumour, intraoperative tumour rupture	Not discussed	Not discussed	Not discussed
SCCOHT	Not discussed	Recommended based on FIGO stage, size of tumour, preoperative calcium levels, presence of large cells, residual disease after surgical resection	Not discussed	Not discussed	Not discussed
Surgical staging					
Surgical approach	Not discussed	Open route recommended	Not discussed	Not discussed	Open route recommended
Complete surgical staging (peritoneal fluid cytology, complete examination of peritoneal cavity, biopsies of diaphragmatic–paracolic–pelvic peritoneum and abnormal areas, biopsy of omentum, inspection of pelvic–paraaortic lymph nodes and excision of enlarged ones)	Recommended	Recommended	Recommended	Not discussed	Recommended
Biopsy of contralateral ovary	Not discussed	Not recommended if macroscopically normal	Not recommended if macroscopically normal	Not discussed	Not recommended if unsuspicious in palpation and by ultrasound
Systematic pelvic–paraaortic lymphadenectomy	Not discussed	Not routinely recommended	Not routinely recommended, highly indicated for SCCOHT	Not discussed	Not routinely recommended
General principles of therapeutic management					
Surgical approach	Not discussed	Median laparotomy recommended when high suspicion of malignancy	Open route recommended	Not discussed	Median laparotomy recommended, sub-umbilical transverse Incision or pfannenstiel laparotomy can be accepted
Tumour resection	Not discussed	Oophorectomy recommended, tumourectomy–cystectomy to be avoided	Unilateral salpingo-oophorectomy recommended	Not discussed	Oophorectomy or adnexectomy is recommended
Fertility-sparing surgery	Not discussed	Recommended if oncologically safe	Recommended if oncologically safe	Recommended if oncologically safe	Recommended for FIGO stage IA SCSTs
Fertility preservation	Ovarian stimulation recommended for GCTs and stage IA granulosa SCSTs	Oncofertility counselling recommended	Oocyte cryopreservation with ovarian stimulation recommended	Not discussed	Not discussed
Hormone replacement therapy	Recommended for GCTs and SCCOHT, to be discussed for IA and IB granulosa SCSTs, not recommended for other SCSTs	Not discussed	Recommended for GCTs and SCCOHT, not recommended for SCSTs	Not discussed	Not discussed

Table 2. Cont.

	L'Observatoire des Tumeurs Malignes Rares Gynécologiques (Centres Experts TRMG)	ESGO-SIOPE	ESMO	BritSPAG	EXPeRT/PARTNER Consensus
Hormonal contraception (if desired)	Recommended for GCTs, recommended for SCSTs with oestrogen-free products	Not discussed	Recommended for GCTs	Not discussed	Not discussed
Follow-up	Recommended with serum tumour markers, tailored depending on histological type of tumour	Recommended with serum tumour markers, tailored depending on histological type of tumour	Recommended with serum tumour markers, ultrasound and CT scan of abdomen, pelvis ± chest, tailored depending on histological type of tumour	Not discussed	Recommended with serum tumour markers, ultrasound, chest X-ray and abdominal MRI in case of equivocal findings and poor visibility on ultrasound
Supportive care and psycho-oncological support	Not discussed	Recommended	Not discussed	Not discussed	Not discussed
Treatment of GCTs					
Early stage				Not discussed	
- Surgery	Unilateral oophorectomy recommended. For bilateral disease, recommendation for preservation of ovarian tissue if possible	Open unilateral oophorectomy recommended. For bilateral disease, recommendation for genetic analysis and preservation of ovarian tissue if possible (bilateral salpingo-oophorectomy recommended if gonadoblastoma or dysgerminoma). Lymphadenectomy only if preoperative/intraoperative evidence of nodal involvement. Not recommended for stage IA GCTs with complete surgical resection (only active surveillance needed). Potentially recommended for stage IB GCTs—to be discussed. For stage IC1 GCTs, either ChT or active surveillance recommended. For stage IC2-IC3 GCTs, ChT is recommended	Unilateral salpingo-oophorectomy recommended		
- Adjuvant chemotherapy (ChT)	BEP is most used regimen		BEP is most used regimen		
- Dysgerminomas	Stage IA+IB: active surveillance recommended. Stage IC: active surveillance (if complete surgical resection) or ChT recommended	Stage IA: active surveillance recommended. Stage IB+IC: active surveillance (if complete surgical resection) or ChT recommended	Stage IA: active surveillance recommended. Stage IB+IC: active surveillance (if complete surgical resection) or ChT recommended		

Table 2. Cont.

	L'Observatoire des Tumeurs Malignes Rares Gynécologiques (Centres Experts TRMG)	ESGO-SIOPE	ESMO	BritSPAG	EXPeRT/PARTNER Consensus
- Immature teratomas	Stage IA-IC2 grade 1–2: active surveillance recommended. Stage IA-IC2 grade 3: active surveillance (if complete surgical resection) or ChT recommended. Stage IC3 grade 1: active surveillance recommended. Stage IC3 grade 2–3: active surveillance (if complete surgical resection) or ChT recommended.	Not discussed	Stage IA: active surveillance recommended. Stage IB+IC: active surveillance (if complete surgical resection) or ChT recommended.		
- Yolk sac tumours	Stage IA: active surveillance (if complete surgical resection) or ChT recommended. Stage IB+ IC: ChT recommended.	Stage IA: active surveillance (if complete surgical resection) or ChT recommended. Stage IB+ IC: ChT recommended.	Stage IA+IB: active surveillance (if complete surgical resection) or ChT recommended. Stage IC: ChT recommended.		
Advanced stage					
- Surgery	Fertility sparing surgery to be considered. Second surgery recommended in case of residual disease, immature teratomas, embryonal carcinomas, non-secreting mixed germ-cell tumours with post-chemotherapy residual lesions	Fertility sparing surgery to be considered. Second surgery recommended in case of residual disease and immature teratomas (exception: immature teratoma and gliomatosis peritonei, where large biopsies can instead be taken).	Fertility sparing surgery to be considered. Second surgery recommended in case of residual disease and immature teratomas.		
- Adjuvant chemotherapy (ChT)	BEP regimen is recommended.	BEP regimen for three–four cycles (bleomycin omitted after cycle three) is recommended. Alternative regimens: cisplatine-etoposide-ifosfamide, cisplatin-etoposide-dose-reduced bleomycin, carboplatin-etoposide-bleomycin. Role of surgery unclear, mostly treated with chemotherapy.	BEP regimen for three–four cycles (bleomycin omitted after cycle three) is recommended. Platinum-sensitive relapse: use of combinations with platinum to be considered.		
Refractory or recurrent disease	Role of surgery unclear, mostly treated with chemotherapy. Prior administration of ChT: BEP (three–four cycles) are recommended. No prior administration of ChT: VeIP (vinblastine, ifosfamide, cisplatin) or TIP (paclitaxel, ifosfamide, platine) for three–four cycles to be considered.	Prior administration of ChT: previous regimens and the time interval between initial diagnosis and relapse to be considered.	Not discussed		

Table 2. Cont.

	L'Observatoire des Tumeurs Malignes Rares Gynécologiques (Centres Experts TRMG)	ESGO-SIOPE	ESMO	BritSPAG	EXPeRT/PARTNER Consensus
	Intensified chemotherapy ± stem cell support to be considered in case of incomplete response.	Intensified chemotherapy ± stem cell support to be considered in case of incomplete response. Growing teratoma syndrome with only mature tissues in histology: extensive surgical resection is recommended. Recurrent pure dysgerminoma: radiotherapy to be discussed.			
Treatment of SCSTs				Not discussed	
Early stage					
- Surgery	Complete surgical staging (±endometrial curettage) recommended. Total hysterectomy as part only recommended in stage II+. Lymphadenectomy only if preoperative or intraoperative evidence of nodal involvement. Stage IA: only surgery is recommended, fertility preservation acceptable if macroscopic lesions are excised.	Complete surgical staging is recommended. Lymphadenectomy only if preoperative or intraoperative evidence of nodal involvement. Stage IA: only surgery is recommended. Stage IA+: chemotherapy to be considered.	Stage IA: only surgery is recommended.		Complete surgical staging is recommended. If adhesions to the omentum, omentectomy is recommended; routine omentectomy not required if unsuspicious. Routine retroperitoneal lymph node dissection is not recommended if unsuspicious. Stage IA: only surgery is recommended, fertility preservation is acceptable. Stage IA/IB tumours do not require adjuvant ChT if histology shows good to intermediate differentiation.
- Adjuvant chemotherapy (ChT)	BEP (three–four cycles) is recommended, carboplatin–paclitaxel is alternative option.	BEP (three–four cycles) is recommended, carboplatin–paclitaxel is alternative option.	BEP (three–four cycles) is recommended, carboplatin–paclitaxel is alternative option.		ChT protocols include cisplatin-based regimen (e.g., bleomycin–etoposide–cisplatin or etoposide–ifosfamide–cisplatin). In stage IC tumours, three–four cycles of ChT are recommended.
- Juvenile granulosa cell tumours	Stage IA-IC1: ChT may be avoided if complete surgical resection. Stage IC2-IC3: ChT is recommended.	Stage IA-IC1: ChT may be avoided if complete surgical resection. Stage IC2-IC3: ChT is recommended.	Stage IC: ChT is recommended.		Stage IC: ChT is certainly recommended if preoperative spontaneous tumour rupture and/or malignant ascites
- Adult granulosa cell tumours	Stage IA-IC2: may be avoided if complete surgical resection. Stage IC3: ChT is recommended.		Stage IC2-IC3: ChT is recommended.		Stage IC: adjuvant ChT is recommended, irrespective of the time of the tumour rupture
- Sertoli–Leydig cells tumours	Stage IA-IC2 well or moderately differentiated Sertoli–Leydig cell tumours: omission of chemotherapy is acceptable.	Stage IC: ChT is recommended.	Stage IA poorly differentiated tumours or with heterologous elements/retiform patterns and Stage >IA: ChT is recommended.		

Table 2. Cont.

	L'Observatoire des Tumeurs Malignes Rares Gynécologiques (Centres Experts TRMG)	ESGO-SIOPE	ESMO	BritSPAG	ExPeRT/PARTNER Consensus
Advanced stage					
- Surgery	Debulking surgery: recommended for advanced stages.	Stage III with incomplete initial macroscopic resection and residual disease after chemotherapy: second surgery to be discussed.	Debulking surgery: recommended for advanced stage granulosa cell tumours.		There is no role for debulking surgery (apart from palliative surgery)—inoperable tumours should be biopsied and upfront ChT should be initiated followed by delayed tumour resection.
- Adjuvant chemotherapy (ChT)	Recommended.	Recommended.	Recommended.		In stages II–IV tumours, four cycles of ChT are recommended, with second-look surgery if initial macroscopic incomplete resection or residual disease. Adjuvant ChT is recommended in all tumours with locoregional spread, distant metastases or unresectable tumours.
	BEP regimen for three-four cycles (alternative option: carboplatine-paclitaxel for six cycles).	BEP regimen for at least four cycles (alternative options: cisplatin-etoposide-ifosfamide for at least four cycles or carboplatine-paclitaxel).	BEP regimen for three cycles (alternative option: carboplatine-paclitaxel for six cycles).		
Refractory/recurrent disease	Platinum-based chemotherapy is recommended.	Treatment plan to be discussed in multidisciplinary board. Cytoreductive surgery recommended treatment of choice for relapsed patients. Additional treatment options to be considered.	Platinum-based chemotherapy is recommended. Additional treatment options to be considered.		Additional treatment options to be considered.
Treatment of SCCOHT					
Early stage					
- Surgery	Fertility-sparing surgery is not recommended. Radical surgery is recommended (including total abdominal hysterectomy, bilateral salpingo-oophorectomy, full pelvic and para-aortic lympadenectomy)	Fertility-sparing surgery is not recommended. Radical surgery is recommended (including total abdominal hysterectomy, bilateral salpingo-oophorectomy, full pelvic and para-aortic lympadenectomy). ChT with platinum and etoposide combinations is recommended. Complete remission after initial chemotherapy: dose-intensive chemotherapy with stem cell support to be discussed.	Fertility-sparing surgery is not recommended. Radical surgery is recommended (including total abdominal hysterectomy, bilateral salpingo-oophorectomy, full pelvic and para-aortic lympadenectomy) ChT with platinum and etoposide (and potentially paclitaxel) combinations is recommended.	Not discussed	Not discussed
- Adjuvant chemotherapy (ChT)	ChT is recommended.				
	Pelvic radiotherapy to be discussed.	Pelvic radiotherapy to be discussed.	Pelvic radiotherapy to be discussed.		

Table 2. Cont.

	L'Observatoire des Tumeurs Malignes Rares Gynécologiques (Centres Experts TRMG)	ESGO-SIOPE	ESMO	BritSPAG	EXPeRT/ PARTNER Consensus
Advanced stage					
- Surgery	Debulking surgery, either initial or interval after three–six cycles of chemotherapy (including systematic pelvic and para-aortic lymphadenectomy) is recommended.	Debulking surgery, either initial or interval after three–six cycles of chemotherapy (including systematic pelvic and para-aortic lymphadenectomy) is recommended.	Debulking surgery, either initial or interval after three–six cycles of chemotherapy (including systematic pelvic and para-aortic lymphadenectomy) is recommended.		
- Adjuvant chemotherapy (ChT)	ChT is recommended.	ChT with platinum and etoposide combinations is recommended. Complete remission after initial surgery and ChT: dose-intensive regimen, followed by high-dose chemotherapy with stem cell support and pelvic radiotherapy to be considered.	ChT with platinum and etoposide combinations is recommended.		
Refractory/recurrent disease	Not discussed	No suggested treatment.	Not discussed		

AFP: Alpha Fetoprotein; BEP: Bleomycin/Etoposide/Cisplatin; β-hCG: β human chorionic gonadotropin; BritSPAG: British Society for Paediatric & Adolescent Gynaecology; CA125: cancer antigen 125; ChT: Chemotherapy; CT scan: Computerised Tomography scan; ESGO: European Society of Gynecological Oncology; ESMO: European Society for Medical Oncology; EXPeRT: European Cooperative Study Group for Paediatric Rare Tumors; FIGO: International Federation of Gynecology and Obstetrics; GCTs: Germ Cell Tumors; LDH: Lactate Dehydrogenase; MRI: Magnetic Resonance Imaging; PARTNER: Paediatric Rare Tumours Network-European Registry; PET scan: Positron Emission Tomography scan; SCCOHT: Small Cell Carcinomas of the Ovary Hypercalcemic Type; SCSTs: Sex Cord Stromal Tumours; SLCs: Sertoli–Leydig cell tumours; SIOPE: European Society for Paediatric Oncology; TIP: Paclitaxel/Ifosfamide/Platine; TRMG: Tumeurs Malignes Rares Gynécologiques; VeIP: Vinblastine/Ifosfamide/Cisplatin.

3. Diagnostic Evaluation

In order to ensure optimal management and due to the rarity of these cases, paediatric and adolescent patients with suspected ovarian malignancies should be referred to a specialised center with a multidisciplinary team composed of trained gynaecological and paediatric oncologists with experience in such cases (ESGO-SIOPE 2020, BritSPAG 2018) [25,26,29,30]. The involvement of a gynaecologist with specialist knowledge of pediatric and adolescent gynaecology is considered necessary, both pre-operatively and post-operatively, even in patients treated for ovarian cysts with low suspicion of malignancy, in terms of supervising the diagnostic and therapeutic management and providing correct counselling about potential future fertility issues (BritSPAG 2018) [25,31].

The preoperative diagnostic work-up should include a combination of tests and modalities, performed to further evaluate suspicious ovarian masses and confirm the diagnosis of ovarian cancer, as well as for staging purposes and the assessment of prognostic factors (ESGO-SIOPE 2020, ESMO 2018, EXPeRT/PARTNER 2021) [9,26,27]. Abdominal and pelvic ultrasound is the initial imaging of choice when investigating ovarian tumours in non-adult patients and it should be performed, if possible, by a gynaecologist or radiologist experienced in paediatric population imaging (Centres Experts TRMG 2022, BritSPAG 2018, EXPeRT/PARTNER 2021) [24,25,27,32]. Transvaginal route of scanning is preferred when the patient is sexually active, while transabdominal scanning is reserved for patients with no sexual relations (BritSPAG 2018) [25], focusing on the pelvis, ovaries, para-aortic lymph nodes (in case of right ovarian tumour) and renal lymph nodes (in case of left ovarian tumour) (EXPeRT/PARTNER 2021) [27]. Evaluation of endometrial thickness should be additionally performed via ultrasound in patients with suspected hormone-producing ovarian tumours, especially SCSTs (ESGO-SIOPE 2020, Centres Experts TMRG 2022) [24,26]. Additional imaging is required, but the recommended imaging tests differ among guidelines; ESGO-SIOPE guidelines suggest that thoracic computed tomography (CT) scan and abdomino–pelvic magnetic resonance imaging (MRI) are necessary, with the latter considered notably useful in assessing bilateral ovarian masses and guiding the choice of surgical approach without exposing the patient to radiation (ESGO-SIOPE 2020, EXPeRT/PARTNER 2021) [26,27,33,34]. On the other hand, an abdomino–pelvic computed tomography (CT) scan and chest X-ray are suggested by ESMO guidelines as additional preoperative imaging tests [9], while guidelines by EXPeRT/PARTNER 2021 recommend chest X-rays for the identification of distant metastases, with the alternative of a low-dose chest CT scan [27]. The use of a positron emission tomography (PET) scan is also debatable, with guidelines by ESMO and L'Observatoire des Tumeurs malignes Rares Gynécologiques underlining that it should be performed in selected patients with suspected germ-cell tumours [9,24], while ESGO-SIOPE guidelines do not support its use due to its low negative predictive value [26]. Preoperative imaging may be omitted in acute settings in favor of immediate surgery (e.g., in clinically suspected ovarian torsion). In that case, the recommended imaging tests should be performed as soon as possible after surgery (ESGO-SIOPE 2020, BritSPAG 2018) [25,26].

There is a consensus among all guidelines that serum tumour markers, especially β-human chorionic gonadotropin (β-hCG), alpha-fetoprotein (AFP), lactate dehydrogenase (LDH) and cancer antigen 125 (CA125), should be measured in all ovarian masses with suspicious features (ESGO-SIOPE 2020, ESMO 2018, BritSPAG 2018, Centres Experts TRMG 2022, EXPeRT/PARTNER 2021) [9,24–27,35]. A hormonal profile, including oestrogen, testosterone, dehydroepiandrosterone, dehydroepiandrosterone sulfate, luteinising hormone and follicle stimulating hormone levels, is also essential when signs of hormonal production and precocious puberty are identified (BritSPAG 2018, ESGO-SIOPE 2020, EXPeRT/PARTNER 2021) [25–27]. Other biomarkers can also be useful; serum calcium, chromogranin A and neuron specific enolase levels can be elevated in small cell carcinoma of the ovary of hypercalcemic type (ESGO-SIOPE 2020, EXPeRT/PARTNER 2021) [26,27], whereas anti-Mullerian hormone (AMH) and inhibin B may indicate the presence of granulosa cell tumours (ESMO 2018, Centres Experts TRMG 2022, EXPeRT/PARTNER 2021) [9,24,27].

Preoperative measurements of tumour markers can provide both diagnostic and prognostic information. In case they are preoperatively elevated, repeated measurements should be performed postoperatively and before the start of adjuvant treatment (for patients receiving adjuvant chemotherapy, new measurements should be obtained before each cycle of treatment) (Centres Experts TRMG 2022, ESGO-SIOPE 2020, ESMO 2018) [9,24,26].

4. Pathology and Molecular Biology

A preoperative diagnostic biopsy can definitively provide a histological confirmation of ovarian malignancy, but it should be avoided if a cystic component is identified within the suspicious mass and it is formally indicated only in the case of extraovarian spread of the disease (ESGO-SIOPE 2020, EXPeRT/PARTNER 2021) [26,27]. Tissues retrieved through biopsy and surgical specimens should be examined by an experienced specialist gynaecological or paediatric pathologist, considering that the risk of misdiagnosis is significant due to the rarity of ovarian malignant neoplasms in non-adult patients (ESGO-SIOPE 2020, ESMO 2018, EXPeRT/PARTNER 2021) [9,26,27,36]. The use of immunohistochemistry and molecular tests, if available, is strongly recommended in order to resolve potential diagnostic dilemmas and confirm diagnosis (ESGO-SIOPE 2020) [26]. In suspected germ-cell tumours (GTCs), a panel of immunohistochemical markers including Sall4, OCT3/4, PLAP, NANOG, D2-40, SCFR, a-fetoprotein, glypican-3, SOX2 and SOX10 as well as chromosome 12p fluorescent in situ hybridisation (FISH) for the identification of isochromosome 12 can facilitate the diagnosis in difficult cases. Karyotyping may also be useful, especially in premenarche girls with suspected gonadoblastoma, considering that this type of tumour usually arises in dysgenetic gonads (ESMO 2018, ESGO-SIOPE 2020, Centres Experts TRMG 2022) [9,24,26]. Inhibin A, calretinin, NCAM-1, MART-1, CD99, antigen-like protein 2, steroidogenic factor 1, Forkhead box protein L2, Wilms tumour protein and FOXL2 may be expressed and can be of value in diagnosing sex cord–stromal tumours (SCSTs), especially when they are evaluated in combination, while DICER1 mutations should also be investigated in suspected SCSTs and gynandroblastomas (ESMO 2018, ESGO-SIOPE 2020, Centres Experts TRMG 2022, EXPeRT/PARTNER 2021) [9,24,26,27,37]. Small cell carcinomas of the ovary hypercalcemic type (SCCOHTs) are characterised by the presence of mutations in the SMARCA4 gene, a SWItch/Sucrose Non-Fermentable (SWI/SNF) chromatin-remodelling gene that encodes BRG1 protein. The identification of these mutations, which leads to the loss of BRG1 protein expression, can confirm the diagnosis of SCCOHTs with high sensitivity and specificity (ESMO 2018, ESGO-SIOPE 2020, Centres Experts TRMG 2022) [9,24,26,38–40]. Germline mutation analysis and genetic counselling should generally be considered in cases of bilateral GCTs, unilateral GCTs with streak gonad or pubertal retardation, Sertoli–Leydig cell tumour and SCCOHT since these types of tumours can occur as part of a familial tumour syndrome (ESGO-SIOPE 2020) [26].

5. Assessment of Prognostic Factors

Although different factors define the prognosis among the various histological types of ovarian cancer in adolescents, the treatment of patients in large specified cancer centers is considered a favourable prognostic factor that applies to all cases (ESMO 2018) [9]. For patients with GCTs, the age of diagnosis can significantly affect the prognosis; premenarche girls may face a worse prognosis than post-adolescent females due to differences in tumour biology. Stage > I, incomplete surgical resection and yolk sac tumour histology are additional adverse prognostic factors for GCTs (ESMO 2018) [9,41,42]. Patients with SCSTs generally have a better prognosis, with 20% of them relapsing or dying from metastatic cancer. Advanced FIGO stage is also recognised as a factor associated with poor outcome for SCSTs along with intraperitoneal tumour rupture and size of tumour > 5 cm (ESMO 2018) [9,35]. On the other hand, prognosis of SCCOHT is poor, given that the percentage of long-time survivors is estimated at 30–40%. The most significant favourable prognostic factors for patients with SCCOHT are stage IA, normal preoperative calcium level, tumour size < 10 cm, absence of large cells and complete surgical resection including bilateral oophorectomy (ESMO 2018) [9,43].

6. Surgical Staging

Patients should be staged according to the FIGO 2014 staging system (ESGO-SIOPE 2020, EXPeRT/PARTNER 2021) [26,27]. Surgical staging is of utmost importance to correctly determine the stage of the disease and consequently to further decide on the extent of surgery and the need for postoperative treatment. Regarding a surgical approach, the open route is usually preferred in order to avoid tumour rupture, but a laparoscopic or robotic approach is also acceptable in selected cases (ESMO 2018) [9]. Complete surgical staging includes the sampling of peritoneal fluid before manipulating the tumour or peritoneal washings when no free fluid is detected, careful examination of the abdominal cavity and peritoneal surfaces, biopsy of the diaphragmatic peritoneum, paracolic gutters, pelvic peritoneum, inspection, palpation and large biopsy of the omentum if normal, infracolic omentectomy if omentum is macroscopically abnormal, examination and palpation of pelvic and para-aortic lymph nodes and excision of enlarged ones, inspection of contralateral ovary and biopsy of abnormal appearing areas (ESMO 2018, ESGO-SIOPE 2020, Centres Experts TMRG 2022, EXPeRT/PARTNER 2021) [9,24,26,27]. In case macroscopic disease is detected on other pelvic or abdominal organs, precise description and biopsies of the lesions are also required (ESGO-SIOPE 2020) [26]. For patients with GCTs, systematic ovarian biopsy should be avoided when the non-affected ovary is macroscopically normal. However, in cases with macroscopic bilateral involvement, preservation of a healthy part of one ovary and the uterus should be attempted without compromising oncological safety (ESMO 2018) [9,44]. The role of systematic lymphadenectomy in GCTs in not well-established and should be reserved for cases with nodal abnormalities or residual disease after chemotherapy, considering that nodal recurrence in patients who did not receive initial surgical nodal assessment can be effectively cured with adjuvant chemotherapy (ESMO 2018) [9,45,46]. Early-stage SCSTs rarely produce retroperitoneal or nodal metastases; thus, retroperitoneal evaluation and lymphadenectomy are not mandatory in these cases (ESMO 2018, EXPeRT/PARTNER 2021) [9,27]. On the contrary, extensive peritoneal and nodal surgical staging is indicated in patients with SCCOHT because of the high incidence of extra-ovarian spread (ESMO 2018) [9,47,48].

7. General Principles of Therapeutic Management

Although the therapeutic management of ovarian malignances in adolescents is tailored according to the histological type, the stage of the disease and the individual characteristics and needs of each patient, there are some general principles that apply in all cases. Adolescents with non-epithelial ovarian cancer should preferably be treated, when feasible, in the setting of clinical trials (ESGO-SIOPE 2020) [26]. The choice of the surgical approach should be guided by the findings of preoperative imaging and on the basis of avoiding intraoperative tumour rupture. In cases with high suspicion of malignancy, median laparotomy is indicated (ESGO-SIOPE 2020) [26], but in children, a sub-umbilical transverse incision or a Pfannenstiel laparotomy can also be accepted (depending on size of the tumour and the initial tumour spread) (EXPeRT/PARTNER 2021) [27]. On the other hand, a minimally invasive approach is considered an acceptable alternative only if the surgeon is experienced and properly trained in laparoscopic oncological surgery and able to perform a full exploration of the peritoneal cavity and excision of the tumour with no morcellation or accidental rupture (ESGO-SIOPE 2020, EXPeRT/PARTNER 2021) [26,27]. Regarding the radicality of surgical approach, oophorectomy should be, in general, preferred compared to cystectomy or tumourectomy (ESGO-SIOPE 2020, ESMO 2018, EXPeRT/PARTNER 2021) [9,26,27]. However, all efforts should be made to perform, if it is oncologically safe and technically feasible, a fertility sparing surgery at first, with preservation of the uterus and at least a part of one adnexa, considering that saving healthy ovarian tissue is critical both for pubertal development and future fertility (BritSPAG 2018, ESMO 2018, ESGO-SIOPE 2020,

EXPeRT/PARTNER 2021) [9,25–27,49,50]. A more radical second surgery might be required after the definitive pathological results. In the event of an incidental discovery of a suspicious ovarian tumour during surgery performed by a non-gynaecology specialty for other medical conditions, a gynaecologist should be consulted before attempting surgical manipulations near or on the tumour (BritSPAG 2018) [25].

Oncofertility counselling should be provided to all adolescent patients with ovarian cancer before receiving treatment (ESGO-SIOPE 2020) [26]. Even if ovarian tissue can be preserved during surgery, without compromising the oncological management, there is a significant risk of gonadal dysfunction in patients receiving chemotherapy. The likelihood of chemotherapy-induced amenorrhea depends on the type of administrated drugs, their cumulative dose and the duration of the treatment. Apart from these factors, the age of the patient at the time of chemotherapy also has great impact on the return of menstruation and ovulation, with more favorable results being reported in younger patients (ESMO 2018) [9,51,52]. Taking all the above into consideration, it is evident that oocyte cryopreservation is an option that should be offered to all patients scheduled to receive chemotherapy, either by ovulation induction and oocyte aspiration prior to the beginning of treatment or by controlled ovarian hyperstimulation followed by oocyte cryopreservation 12 months after the end of chemotherapy (ESMO 2018) [9,53,54]. While ovarian stimulation is a safe choice for patients with GCTs, it is permitted only for stage IA granulosa-type SCSTs and after discussion in a multidisciplinary board, while it is contraindicated for stages > IA, in which other fertility preservation techniques that do not require ovarian stimulation should be applied (Centres Experts TMRG 2022) [24]. Fertility and gonadal function preservation is extremely difficult to achieve in patients with SCCOHT, even if one ovary is preserved, due to high-dose combined chemotherapy and radiotherapy that usually follows after surgery (ESMO 2018) [9]. In this setting, it is also crucial to address other acute or delayed side effects of chemotherapy and offer supportive care to minimise adverse symptoms and improve the quality of life of the patients (ESGO-SIOPE 2020) [26].

Young premenopausal patients with GCTs or SCSTs treated with chemotherapy are also eligible for hormone replacement therapy (HRT) in order to relieve the symptoms of potential oestrogen deficiency and iatrogenic menopause, which are often more pronounced compared to those following naturally occurring menopause. HRT can be safely administered to patients with GCTs and SCCOHT, but it should generally be avoided in cases of SCSTs, with the exception of stage IA and IB granulosa-type tumours, where it might be considered upon approval of a multidisciplinary board (ESMO 2018, Centres Experts TMRG 2022) [9,24]. For patients receiving fertility-sparing treatment but wish to postpone pregnancies, hormonal contraception is permitted both in case of a GCT or a SCST, but for the latter, contraceptive products containing oestrogens are contraindicated (ESMO 2018, Centres Experts TMRG 2022) [9,24].

Regular, targeted and long-term follow-up is essential to monitor the response to treatment and to early diagnose a potential recurrence. As already mentioned, the postoperative measurement of serum tumour markers (βhCG, AFP, LDH, CA125, inhibin B) is used to assess tumour response during chemotherapy, in addition to imaging by pelvic ultrasound and CT scan of the abdomen, pelvis and chest, when lung metastases are suspected, while an abdominal MRI could also be useful in case of equivocal findings and patients with poor visibility on ultrasound (ESMO 2018, ESGO-SIOPE 2020, EXPeRT/PARTNER 2021) [9,26,27]. Routine post-treatment monitoring for patients that received fertility-sparing surgery usually includes a pelvic ultrasound every 6 months, whereas a CT scan of the abdomen and pelvis is performed only upon clinical indication. PET scan is not recommended as a tool for follow-up evaluation or tumour response monitoring (ESMO 2018) [9]. The time intervals between each follow-up appointment can vary depending on the histological type of tumour, while discrepancies are also detected between existing guidelines. Apart from clinical care, it is important to continuously offer psycho–oncological support to all patients and their families throughout treatment and follow-up (ESGO-SIOPE 2020) [26].

Specific recommendations for the therapeutic management of germ-cell tumours, sex cord stromal tumours and small cell carcinomas of the ovary will be presented in the following respective sections of the article.

8. Germ Cell Tumours (GCTs)

8.1. Early Stages

Preoperative MRI is necessary in patients with suspected malignant GTCs with a solid or partially solid mass on ultrasound and if a solid component is also present on MRI; then, surgery is the suggested initial treatment (ESGO-SIOPE 2020) [26]. When planning the surgical approach, it is crucial to assess the likelihood of malignancy according to preoperative imaging. Laparotomy is preferable for the excision of a GCT with imaging findings suggestive of malignancy because it enables complete surgical staging without increasing the risk of intraperitoneal spillage. During staging, the biopsy of contralateral ovary is not encouraged if it appears to be macroscopically normal (ESGO-SIOPE 2020) [26]. Fertility-sparing surgery should always be offered in adolescent patients with malignant GCTs when it does not jeopardise oncological safety (ESMO 2018, ESGO-SIOPE 2020, Centres Experts TMRG 2022) [9,24,26]. For solid unilateral tumours, total en bloc oophorectomy is recommended, while cystectomy should be avoided in case of a cystic tumour (ESMO 2018, ESGO-SIOPE 2020, Centres Experts TMRG 2022) [9,24,26]. When both ovaries are macroscopically involved, bilateral salpingo-oophorectomy should always be avoided if possible, and maximal effort to preserve at least a part of one ovary and the uterus is encouraged even in stage IB tumours, except when genetic analysis is suggestive of dysgenetic gonads (ESGO-SIOPE 2020, Centres Experts TMRG 2022) [24,26]. Genetic analysis and counselling should be offered to all patients with bilateral ovarian tumours to identify potential sex chromosomal aberrations accompanied by dysgenetic gonads. In that case, bilateral salpingo-oophorectomy is indicated due to the high risk of gonadoblastoma or dysgerminoma (ESGO-SIOPE 2020) [26]. Comprehensive surgical staging with lymphadenectomy should be avoided and reserved only for cases with preoperative or intraoperative evidence of nodal involvement (ESGO-SIOPE 2020) [26].

The need for adjuvant chemotherapy in patients with early-stage GCTs is determined according to the histological type and the stage of the disease. The most used combination is the 5-day bleomycin/etoposide/cisplatin (BEP) regimen (ESMO 2018, Centres Experts TMRG 2022) [9,24]. In stage IA neoplasms where complete surgical resection is achieved, along with normalising or negative post-operative serum tumour markers, active surveillance without adjuvant chemotherapy is usually the approach of choice (ESGO-SIOPE 2020) [26]. Active surveillance involves regular clinical assessment; radiological imaging, including abdominal–pelvic ultrasound CT scan of the abdomen and pelvis, chest X-ray and/or CT scan; and close monitoring of serum tumour marker levels over a period of 10 years, with a gradual increase of intervals between clinical appointments (ESMO 2018, ESGO-SIOPE 2020, Centres Experts TMRG 2022) [9,24,26]. The management of stage IB GCTs is usually more complex and is tailored according to the histotype of the tumours. For stage IC1 GCTs, ESGO-SIOPE guidelines suggest either active surveillance or adjuvant chemotherapy (maximum two cycles), with the latter being the only recommended option for stage IC2-IC3 tumours of any histological type (maximum three cycles) [26], as opposed to the other guidelines which still suggest, as it will be presented below, active surveillance for some IC2-IC3 GCTs. It is worth mentioning that ESGO-SIOPE guidelines [26] are the only official recommendations suggesting two cycles of chemotherapy for stage IC GCTs compared to the guidelines by L'Observatoire des Tumeurs malignes Rares Gynécologiques [24], which recommend two–three cycles of BEP and the guidelines of ESMO [9], which suggest the standard three cycles of chemotherapy, in case the alternative option of close active surveillance (recommended by all three aforementioned guidelines as an acceptable option) is not preferred. The decision both for the administration of chemotherapy instead of surveillance and the duration of the chemotherapy should be carefully made by the multidisciplinary team treating the patient, and the chemotherapy regimen should be tailored individually according to the specific needs of each patient, after taking into consideration the biological behavior and the molecular characteristics of the tumour, since there are slight disparities among guidelines regarding the duration of the regimen.

Active surveillance can be applied for stage IA (and IB, as per guideline by L'Observatoire des Tumeurs malignes Rares Gynécologiques) [24] pure dysgerminomas (ESGO-SIOPE 2020, ESMO 2018) [9,26]. It remains an option for stage IB-IC dysgerminomas with complete surgical resection, with the alternative of adjuvant chemotherapy (ESMO 2018, Centres Experts TMRG 2022) [9,24]. For immature teratomas, active surveillance is recommended for stage IA-IC3 grade 1 tumours (ESMO 2018) [9], whereas it can also be acceptable for IA-IC2 grade 2 tumours (Centres Experts TMRG 2022) [24], for which adjuvant chemotherapy can be alternatively applied (ESMO 2018) [9]. For IA-IC2 grade 3 and IC3 grade 2–3 immature teratomas, adjuvant chemotherapy is usually preferred compared to active surveillance (ESMO 2018, Centres Experts TMRG 2022) [9,24]. Regarding yolk sac tumours, properly staged patients with stage IA (and potentially IB, as suggested by ESMO guidelines) [9] and negative postoperative tumour markers may be monitored with active surveillance instead of receiving adjuvant chemotherapy, which is the sole option for stage IB and IC tumours (ESGO-SIOPE 2020, Centres Experts TMRG 2022) [24,26].

8.2. Advanced Stages

Fertility-sparing surgery should be considered even in patients with advanced-stage disease due to the high chemosensitivity of malignant GCTs. For the same reason and given the fact that adjuvant chemotherapy is indicated for all patients with advanced stage GTCs, extensive cytoreductive surgery, which may pose delays in the commencement of postoperative chemotherapy and significantly increase long-term morbidity, should be avoided during initial surgical management (ESMO 2018, ESGO-SIOPE 2020, Centres Experts TMRG 2022) [9,24,26].

Platinum-based chemotherapy agents, mainly the 5-day BEP regimen, remain the treatment of choice for adolescent as well as adult patients. In general, the regimen is administered for three cycles in patients with complete surgical resection and for four cycles in case of macroscopical residual disease, with bleomycin omitted after cycle three to reduce the risk of lung toxicity (ESMO 2018, ESGO-SIOPE 2020) [9,26]. Other regimens that can be used in adolescent population are cisplatine-etoposide-ifosfamide, cisplatin-etoposide-dose-reduced bleomycin or carboplatin-etoposide-bleomycin, all administered for three–four cycles. Patients with elevated serum tumour markers at initial diagnosis who do not have negative markers after cycle four are classified as non-responders to chemotherapy, while if the reduction of marker levels is not the expected, according to their half-life, after cycle two, the patients are identified as high-risk cases in need of potential intensification of the therapy (ESGO-SIOPE 2020) [26]. Moreover, patients already treated with platinum who are diagnosed with a platinum-sensitive relapse (defined as evidence of progression at 4–6 weeks after completion of chemotherapy), the use of combinations with platinum should be considered (ESMO 2018) [9].

A second surgical resection is not always necessary after the completion of chemotherapy. It is recommended in all patients with residual disease (in peritoneum, remaining ovary or lymph nodes) and normal serum cancer markers after chemotherapy, as well as in cases of embryonal carcinomas or non-secreting mixed germ-cell tumours with post-chemotherapy residual lesions. The same applies for immature teratomas, in order to avoid the growing teratoma syndrome (ESMO 2018, ESGO-SIOPE 2020, Centres Experts TMRG 2022) [9,24,26]. However, in patients with immature teratoma and extraovarian spread that comprises gliomatosis peritonei (morphologically benign glial tissue with no immature elements), large and multiple biopsies can be taken instead of complete surgical resection of all lesions (ESGO-SIOPE 2020) [26].

8.3. Refractory or Recurrent Disease

When a recurrence of the disease is suspected, a biopsy is necessary to obtain histological confirmation before deciding on additional treatment. It is important to thoroughly examine retrieved specimens in order to identify or rule out the presence of immature tissues. In patients with recurrent disease, normal serum cancer markers and histopathology indicative of an immature teratoma or a mixed tumour with a component of immature teratoma, growing teratoma syndrome should always be included in differential diagnosis. If confirmed, it should be exclusively treated with surgical resection, on the condition of the absence of immature tissues on histological examination (ESGO-SIOPE 2020) [26]. The role of salvage surgery in recurrent disease is not yet established; it is almost exclusively treated with chemotherapy, although there are no well-defined treatment strategies (ESGO-SIOPE 2020, Centres Experts TMRG 2022) [24,26]. Suggested regimens and the duration of therapy depend on the prior administration of chemotherapy. For patients not previously treated with chemotherapy, three or four cycles of BEP (bleomycin, etoposide, cisplatin) should be offered (Centres Experts TMRG 2022) [24]. In patients who have already received chemotherapy, the previous lines of therapy and the time interval between initial diagnosis and relapse should be considered (ESGO-SIOPE 2020) [26]. If BEP regimen was previously administered, patients may benefit from four cycles of either VelP (vinblastine, ifosfamide, cisplatin) or TIP (paclitaxel, ifosfamide, platine) (Centres Experts TMRG 2022) [24]. Intensified chemotherapy with or without stem cell support can be considered when complete response is not achieved (ESGO-SIOPE 2020, Centres Experts TMRG 2022) [24,26]. Finally, for patients with recurrent pure dysgerminoma, the option of radiotherapy could also be discussed (ESGO-SIOPE 2020) [26].

9. Sex Cord Stromal Tumours (SCSTs)

9.1. Early Stages

Complete surgical staging is imperative in patients with SCSTs, including peritoneal fluid sampling or peritoneal washings, unilateral adnexectomy, examination of contralateral ovary, large omental biopsy or infracolic omentectomy, endometrial curettage for older patients, random blind peritoneal sampling and resection of any suspicious lesions (ESGO-SIOPE 2020, Centres Experts TRMG 2022, EXPeRT/PARTNER 2021) [24,26,27]. Total hysterectomy as part of initial surgery should only be performed in patients with stage II+ disease (Centres Experts TRMG 2022) [24], while omentectomy is recommended only in cases of adhesions to the omentum and not as a routine procedure (EXPeRT/PARTNER 2021) [27]. Systematic lymphadenectomy is not recommended, but the excision of lymph nodes with suspicious preoperative or intraoperative findings is encouraged (ESGO-SIOPE 2020, Centres Experts TRMG 2022, EXPeRT/PARTNER 2021) [24,26,27]. Patients with confirmed Stage IA disease should be treated only with surgery (ESMO 2018, ESGO-SIOPE 2020, Centres Experts TRMG 2022, EXPeRT/PARTNER 2021) [9,24,26,27], during which fertility preservation is feasible as long as all macroscopic lesions are excised (Centres Experts TRMG 2022, EXPeRT/PARTNER 2021) [24,27]. Tumours staged higher than IA (or higher than IB, according to guidelines by EXPeRT/PARTNER) [27] may require chemotherapy (ESGO-SIOPE 2020) [26], which usually consists of three or four cycles of cisplatin-based regimens, mainly BEP, while carboplatin-paclitaxel is also an acceptable option (ESMO 2018, ESGO-SIOPE 2020, Centres Experts TRMG 2022, EXPeRT/PARTNER 2021) [9,24,26,27].

Regarding juvenile granulosa cell tumours, patients with stage IA-IC1 disease and complete surgical resection may avoid chemotherapy, which is otherwise required for stages IC2-IC3 (and potentially for IC1, according to ESMO guidelines (ESMO 2018, ESGO-SIOPE 2020, Centres Experts TRMG 2022 EXPeRT/PARTNER 2021) [9,24,26,27]. For adult granulosa cell tumours, adjuvant chemotherapy is recommended for patients staged as IC3 after complete surgery (and potentially for IC2, as per ESMO guidelines), while it is considered safe to omit it for stage IA-IC2 patients (ESMO 2018, ESGO-SIOPE 2020, Centres Experts TRMG 2022) [9,24,26]. Finally, in completely surgically staged patients with stage IA-IC2 well or moderately differentiated Sertoli–Leydig cell tumours, the omission of chemotherapy is acceptable (Centres Experts TRMG 2022) [24], but it is necessary for poorly differentiated tumours or when heterologous elements/retiform patterns are recognised, even for stage IA cases (ESMO 2018, ESGO-SIOPE 2020) [9,26]. However, guidelines by EXPeRT/PARTNER suggest that adjuvant chemotherapy is recommended in all stage IC Sertoli–Leydig cell tumours, irrespectively of the time of tumour rupture [27].

9.2. Advanced Stages

Debulking surgery is considered the most effective course of treatment for advanced stage granulosa cell tumours (ESMO 2018, Centres Experts TRMG 2022) [9,24], although it is considered to have no role in SCSTs except for palliative management, according to EXPeRT/PARTNER guidelines [27]. Adjuvant chemotherapy is generally recommended for patients with advanced-stage SCSTs, preferably with platinum-based combinations. BEP regimen for at least three–four cycles is mainly administered, whereas cisplatin-etoposide-ifosfamide for at least four cycles or carboplatine-paclitaxel for six cycles are alternative options (ESMO 2018, ESGO-SIOPE 2020, Centres Experts TRMG 2022, EXPeRT/PARTNER 2021) [9,24,26,27]. Especially for stage III disease with incomplete initial macroscopic resection and residual disease after chemotherapy, a delayed second surgery after neoadjuvant chemotherapy should be discussed (ESGO-SIOPE 2020, EXPeRT/PARTNER 2021) [26,27].

9.3. Refractory or Recurrent Disease

The treatment plan for patients with recurrent SCSTs should be discussed in a multidisciplinary board setting and tailored according to the site of recurrence, histological subtype, dissemination, tumour-free interval and previous therapeutic management. Cytoreductive surgery is the treatment of choice for relapsed patients (ESGO-SIOPE 2020) [26], followed by additional platinum-based chemotherapy (ESMO 2018, Centres Experts TRMG 2022) [9,24]. For patients treated in the setting of a clinical trial, other treatment options may also be available, such as hormone therapy (GnRH agonists, tamoxifen, progestin, aromatase inhibitors) and antiangiogenic and targeted drugs (ESMO 2018, ESGO-SIOPE 2020) [9,26], while the addition of bevacizumab, HIPEC (hyperthermic intraperitoneal chemotherapy with cytoreductive surgery) and regional deep hyperthermia in combination with platinum-based chemotherapy, high-dose chemotherapy with autologous hematopoietic stem cell transplantation and even radiotherapy could be considered on an individual basis for patients with tumour progression and recurrence not responding to other therapeutic options (EXPeRT/PARTNER 2021) [27].

10. Small Cell Carcinoma of the Ovary Hypercalcemic Type (SCCOHT)

10.1. Early Stages

Confirmation of diagnosis by an expert pathologist and discussion of therapeutic management in a specialised tumour board is suggested due to the rarity of these tumours (ESMO 2018) [9]. Considering treatment strategies, a multimodal approach combining radical surgery, chemotherapy and radiotherapy is recommended. Surgery is always required, including total abdominal hysterectomy, bilateral salpingo-oophorectomy, full pelvic and para-aortic lympadenectomy and peritoneal cytology and peritoneal staging. Due to the aggressive nature of the tumour, a conservative fertility-sparing surgical approach is not oncologically safe. Adjuvant chemotherapy with regimens combining mainly cisplatin and etoposide and potentially paclitaxel is suggested (ESMO 2018, ESGO-SIOPE 2020, Centres Experts TRMG 2022) [9,24,26]. In the absence of evidence of disease after completion of initial chemotherapy, dose-intensive chemotherapy with stem cell support can be applied (ESGO-SIOPE 2020) [26]. The use of pelvic radiotherapy, usually following chemotherapy, may also benefit patients with SCCOHT (ESMO 2018, ESGO-SIOPE 2020, Centres Experts TRMG 2022) [9,24,26].

10.2. Advanced Stages

Debulking surgery, either initially or after an interval of three–six cycles of chemotherapy, including omentectomy, systematic pelvic and para-aortic lymph node dissection and complete removal of peritoneal disease is the optional treatment for advanced stage SCCOHT (ESMO 2018, ESGO-SIOPE 2020, Centres experts TRMG 2022) [9,24,26]. Chemotherapy is also indicated with an administration of regimens including platinum and etoposide. When patients achieve complete remission after initial surgery and chemotherapy, they may subsequently be treated with a dose-intensive regimen, followed by high-dose chemotherapy with stem cell support and pelvic radiotherapy (ESGO-SIOPE 2020) [26].

10.3. Refractory or Recurrent Disease

Currently, there are no official guidelines about the treatment of patients with recurrent SCCOHT. However, close follow-up is recommended due to the aggressive course and rapid progression of the disease (ESGO-SIOPE 2020) [26].

11. Conclusions

Ovarian cancer is rarely diagnosed in children and adolescents, whose diagnostic and therapeutic management can pose great challenges and requires expertise and experience. There is a significant degree of agreement in the recommendations of the existing reviewed guidelines, which generally overlap or complement each other, with only a few areas of dispute. All guidelines suggest that diagnostic work should include both imaging tests (at least ultrasound of abdomen and pelvis) and the measurement of a basic panel of serum tumour markers, while there is debate around the necessity of MRI and the diagnostic value of PET scan. There is a consensus among guidelines about the significant role of molecular biology and immunohistochemistry in confirming the diagnosis, as well as about the procedures that a complete surgical staging should include. On the other hand, only ESMO guidelines provide suggestions about the prognostic factors that should be taken into consideration for adolescent patients with ovarian malignancies. Finally, considering basic therapeutic principles and treatment strategies, recommendations from existing guidelines are mostly identical, suggesting that a combination of fertility-preserving surgery (when it is oncologically safe) and adjuvant therapy is effective in most cases of ovarian cancer in adolescents, with a few discrepancies, mainly detected in proposed time intervals between follow-up appointments. The differences in the reviewed guidelines, although they are limited, highlight the need for the adoption of an international consensus in order to further improve the management of ovarian malignant tumours in the adolescent population.

Author Contributions: All authors contributed equally to the conception and design of the work, the search of the literature, the collection and analysis of data and the writing of the manuscript. The submitted manuscript has been read and approved for submission by all named authors. All authors have read and agreed to the published version of the manuscript.

Funding: This research received no external funding.

Institutional Review Board Statement: Not applicable.

Informed Consent Statement: Not applicable.

Conflicts of Interest: The authors declare no conflict of interest.

References

1. Liu, H.; Wang, X.; Lu, D.; Liu, Z.; Shi, G. Ovarian Masses in Children and Adolescents in China: Analysis of 203 Cases. *J. Ovarian Res.* **2013**, *6*, 47. [CrossRef] [PubMed]
2. Zhang, M.; Jiang, W.; Li, G.; Xu, C. Ovarian Masses in Children and Adolescents—An Analysis of 521 Clinical Cases. *J. Pediatr. Adolesc. Gynecol.* **2014**, *27*, e73–e77. [CrossRef] [PubMed]
3. Rathore, R.; Sharma, S.; Arora, D. Spectrum of Childhood and Adolescent Ovarian Tumors in India: 25 Years Experience at a Single Institution. *Open Access Maced. J. Med. Sci.* **2016**, *4*, 551. [CrossRef]
4. Mahadik, K.; Ghorpade, K. Childhood Ovarian Malignancy. *J. Obstet. Gynaecol. India* **2014**, *64*, 91. [CrossRef] [PubMed]

5. Banlı-Cesur, I.; Tanrıdan-Okcu, N.; Özçelik, Z. Ovarian Masses in Children and Adolescents: Analysis on 146 Patients. *J. Gynecol. Obstet. Hum. Reprod.* **2021**, *50*, 101901. [CrossRef] [PubMed]
6. Heo, S.H.; Kim, J.W.; Shin, S.S.; Jeong, S.I.; Lim, H.S.; Choi, Y.D.; Lee, K.H.; Kang, W.D.; Jeong, Y.Y.; Kang, H.K. Review of Ovarian Tumors in Children and Adolescents: Radiologic-Pathologic Correlation. *Radiographics* **2014**, *34*, 2039–2055. [CrossRef]
7. Shaaban, A.M.; Rezvani, M.; Elsayes, K.M.; Baskin, H.; Mourad, A.; Foster, B.R.; Jarboe, E.A.; Menias, C.O. Ovarian Malignant Germ Cell Tumors: Cellular Classification and Clinical and Imaging Features. *Radiographics* **2014**, *34*, 777–801. [CrossRef] [PubMed]
8. Grigore, M.; Murarasu, M.; Himiniuc, L.M.; Toma, B.F.; Duma, O.; Popovici, R. Large Ovarian Tumors in Adolescents, a Systematic Review of Reported Cases, Diagnostic Findings and Surgical Management. *Taiwan. J. Obstet. Gynecol.* **2021**, *60*, 602–608. [CrossRef]
9. Ray-Coquard, I.; Morice, P.; Lorusso, D.; Prat, J.; Oaknin, A.; Pautier, P.; Colombo, N. Non-Epithelial Ovarian Cancer: ESMO Clinical Practice Guidelines for Diagnosis, Treatment and Follow-Up. *Ann. Oncol.* **2018**, *29*, iv1–iv18. [CrossRef]
10. Fonseca, A.; Lindsay Frazier, A.; Shaikh, F. Germ Cell Tumors in Adolescents and Young Adults. *J. Oncol. Pract.* **2019**, *15*, 433–441. [CrossRef]
11. Pierce, J.L.; Frazier, A.L.; Amatruda, J.F. Pediatric Germ Cell Tumors: A Developmental Perspective. *Adv. Urol.* **2018**, *2018*, 9059382. [CrossRef] [PubMed]
12. Gupta, B.; Guleria, K.; Suneja, A.; Vaid, N.B.; Rajaram, S.; Wadhwa, N. Adolescent Ovarian Masses: A Retrospective Analysis. *J. Obstet. Gynaecol.* **2016**, *36*, 515–517. [CrossRef] [PubMed]
13. Herrington, C.S.; Editorial Board. WHO Classification of Tumours. Tumours of the Ovary (Chapter 1). In *WHO Classification of Tumours of Female Reproductive Organs*, 5th ed.; International Agency for Research on Cancer: Lyon, France, 2020; pp. 93–143.
14. Alaggio, R.; Hill, D.A.; Jacques, T.S.; Jarzembowski, J.A.; López-Terrada, D.H.; Pfister, S.M. *WHO Classification of Tumours: Pediatric Tumors*, 1st ed.; International Agency for Research on Cancer: Lyon, France, 2021.
15. Baert, T.; Storme, N.; Van Nieuwenhuysen, E.; Uyttebroeck, A.; Van Damme, N.; Vergote, I.; Coosemans, A. Ovarian Cancer in Children and Adolescents: A Rare Disease That Needs More Attention. *Maturitas* **2016**, *88*, 3–8. [CrossRef] [PubMed]
16. Tarca, E.; Trandafir, L.M.; Cojocaru, E.; Costea, C.F.; Rosu, S.T.; Butnariu, L.I.; Iordache, A.C.; Munteanu, V.; Luca, A.C. Diagnosis Difficulties and Minimally Invasive Treatment for Ovarian Masses in Adolescents. *Int. J. Women's Health* **2022**, *14*, 1047. [CrossRef]
17. Takayasu, H.; Masumoto, K.; Tanaka, N.; Aiyoshi, T.; Sasaki, T.; Ono, K.; Chiba, F.; Urita, Y.; Shinkai, T. A Clinical Review of Ovarian Tumors in Children and Adolescents. *Pediatr. Surg. Int.* **2020**, *36*, 701–709. [CrossRef]
18. Cartault, A.; Caula-Legriel, S.; Baunin, C.; Le Mandat, A.; Lemasson, F.; Galinier, P.; Pienkowski, C. Ovarian Masses in Adolescent Girls. *Endocr. Dev.* **2012**, *22*, 194–207. [CrossRef]
19. Zhang, B.; Zhang, L.; Meng, G. Clinical Analysis of 52 Adolescent Patients with Ovarian Masses ≥10 Cm in Diameter. *J. Int. Med. Res.* **2021**, *49*, 1–13. [CrossRef]
20. Marginean, C.O.; Marginean, C.; Chinceşan, M.; Marginean, M.O.; Melit, L.E.; Sasaran, V.; Marginean, C.D. Pediatric Ovarian Tumors, a Challenge for Pediatrician and Gynecologist: Three Case Reports (CARE Compliant). *Medicine* **2019**, *98*, e15242. [CrossRef]
21. Sadeghian, N.; Sadeghian, I.; Mirshemirani, A.; Tabari, A.K.; Ghoroubi, J.; Gorji, F.A.; Roushanzamir, F. Types and Frequency of Ovarian Masses in Children over a 10-Year Period. *Casp. J. Intern. Med.* **2015**, *6*, 220.
22. van Heerden, J.; Tjalma, W.A. The Multidisciplinary Approach to Ovarian Tumours in Children and Adolescents. *Eur. J. Obstet. Gynecol. Reprod. Biol.* **2019**, *243*, 103–110. [CrossRef]
23. AlDakhil, L.; Aljuhaimi, A.; AlKhattabi, M.; Alobaid, S.; Mattar, R.E.; Alobaid, A. Ovarian Neoplasia in Adolescence: A Retrospective Chart Review of Girls with Neoplastic Ovarian Tumors in Saudi Arabia. *J. Ovarian Res.* **2022**, *15*, 105. [CrossRef] [PubMed]
24. L'Observatoire des Tumeurs Malignes Rares Gynécologiques. Référentiels, Version Février 2022. Available online: https://www.ovaire-rare.org/ (accessed on 12 October 2022).
25. Ritchie, J.; O'Mahony, F.; Garden, A. Guideline for the Management of Ovarian Cysts in Children and Adolescents. *Br. Soc. Paediatr. Adolesc. Gynaecol.* **2018**, *11*, 2–11.
26. Sessa, C.; Schneider, D.T.; Planchamp, F.; Baust, K.; Braicu, E.I.; Concin, N.; Godzinski, J.; McCluggage, W.G.; Orbach, D.; Pautier, P.; et al. ESGO–SIOPE Guidelines for the Management of Adolescents and Young Adults with Non-Epithelial Ovarian Cancers. *Lancet Oncol.* **2020**, *21*, e360–e368. [CrossRef] [PubMed]
27. Schneider, D.T.; Orbach, D.; Ben-Ami, T.; Bien, E.; Bisogno, G.; Brecht, I.B.; Cecchetto, G.; Ferrari, A.; Godzinski, J.; Janic, D.; et al. Consensus recommendations from the EXPeRT/PARTNER groups for the diagnosis and therapy of sex cord stromal tumors in children and adolescents. *Pediatr Blood Cancer.* **2021**, *68* (Suppl. S4), e29017. [CrossRef]
28. de Faria, F.W.; Valera, E.T.; Macedo, C.R.P.D.; Azevedo, E.F.; Vieira, A.G.S.; Martins, G.E.; Júnior, A.G.D.C.; dos Reis, M.B.F.; Foulkes, W.D.; Lopes, L.F. Comment on: Consensus recommendations from the EXPeRT/PARTNER groups for the diagnosis and therapy of sex cord stromal tumors in children and adolescents. *Pediatr. Blood Cancer* **2022**, *69*, e29650. [CrossRef]
29. Lockley, M.; Stoneham, S.J.; Olson, T.A. Ovarian Cancer in Adolescents and Young Adults. *Pediatr. Blood Cancer* **2019**, *66*, e27512. [CrossRef]

30. Solheim, O.; Kærn, J.; Tropé, C.G.; Rokkones, E.; Dahl, A.A.; Nesland, J.M.; Fosså, S.D. Malignant Ovarian Germ Cell Tumors: Presentation, Survival and Second Cancer in a Population Based Norwegian Cohort (1953–2009). *Gynecol. Oncol.* **2013**, *131*, 330–335. [CrossRef]
31. Chaopotong, P.; Therasakvichya, S.; Leelapatanadit, C.; Jaishuen, A.; Kuljarusnont, S. Ovarian Cancer in Children and Adolescents: Treatment and Reproductive Outcomes. *Asian Pac. J. Cancer Prev.* **2015**, *16*, 4787–4790. [CrossRef]
32. Yeap, S.T.; Hsiao, C.C.; Hsieh, C.S.; Yu, H.R.; Chen, Y.C.; Chuang, J.H.; Sheen, J.M. Pediatric Malignant Ovarian Tumors: 15 Years of Experience at a Single Institution. *Pediatr. Neonatol.* **2011**, *52*, 140–144. [CrossRef]
33. Janssen, C.L.; Littooij, A.S.; Fiocco, M.; Huige, J.C.B.; de Krijger, R.R.; Hulsker, C.C.C.; Goverde, A.J.; Zsiros, J.; Mavinkurve-Groothuis, A.M.C. The Diagnostic Value of Magnetic Resonance Imaging in Differentiating Benign and Malignant Pediatric Ovarian Tumors. *Pediatr. Radiol.* **2021**, *51*, 427. [CrossRef]
34. van Nimwegen, L.W.E.; Mavinkurve-Groothuis, A.M.C.; de Krijger, R.R.; Hulsker, C.C.C.; Goverde, A.J.; Zsiros, J.; Littooij, A.S. MR Imaging in Discriminating between Benign and Malignant Paediatric Ovarian Masses: A Systematic Review. *Eur. Radiol.* **2020**, *30*, 1166. [CrossRef] [PubMed]
35. Gershenson, D.M. Current Advances in the Management of Malignant Germ Cell and Sex Cord-Stromal Tumors of the Ovary. *Gynecol. Oncol.* **2012**, *125*, 515–517. [CrossRef] [PubMed]
36. Akakpo, P.K.; Derkyi-Kwarteng, L.; Quayson, S.E.; Gyasi, R.K.; Anim, J.T. Ovarian Tumors in Children and Adolescents: A 10-Yr Histopathologic Review in Korle-Bu Teaching Hospital, Ghana. *Int. J. Gynecol. Pathol.* **2016**, *35*, 479–507. [CrossRef]
37. Al-Agha, O.M.; Huwait, H.F.; Chow, C.; Yang, W.; Senz, J.; Kalloger, S.E.; Huntsman, D.G.; Young, R.H.; Gilks, C.B. FOXL2 Is a Sensitive and Specific Marker for Sex Cord-Stromal Tumors of the Ovary. *Am. J. Surg. Pathol.* **2011**, *35*, 484–494. [CrossRef] [PubMed]
38. Ramos, P.; Karnezis, A.N.; Craig, D.W.; Sekulic, A.; Russell, M.L.; Hendricks, W.P.D.; Corneveaux, J.J.; Barrett, M.T.; Shumansky, K.; Yang, Y.; et al. Small Cell Carcinoma of the Ovary, Hypercalcemic Type, Displays Frequent Inactivating Germline and Somatic Mutations in SMARCA4. *Nat. Genet.* **2014**, *46*, 427–429. [CrossRef]
39. Karnezis, A.N.; Wang, Y.; Ramos, P.; Hendricks, W.P.D.; Oliva, E.; D'Angelo, E.; Prat, J.; Nucci, M.R.; Nielsen, T.O.; Chow, C.; et al. Dual Loss of the SWI/SNF Complex ATPases SMARCA4/BRG1 and SMARCA2/BRM Is Highly Sensitive and Specific for Small Cell Carcinoma of the Ovary, Hypercalcaemic Type. *J. Pathol.* **2016**, *238*, 389–400. [CrossRef]
40. Jelinic, P.; Mueller, J.J.; Olvera, N.; Dao, F.; Scott, S.N.; Shah, R.; Gao, J.; Schultz, N.; Gonen, M.; Soslow, R.A.; et al. Recurrent SMARCA4 Mutations in Small Cell Carcinoma of the Ovary. *Nat. Genet.* **2014**, *46*, 424–426. [CrossRef]
41. Mangili, G.; Sigismondi, C.; Gadducci, A.; Cormio, G.; Scollo, P.; Tateo, S.; Ferrandina, G.; Greggi, S.; Candiani, M.; Lorusso, D. Outcome and Risk Factors for Recurrence in Malignant Ovarian Germ Cell Tumors: A MITO-9 Retrospective Study. *Int. J. Gynecol. Cancer* **2011**, *21*, 1414–1421. [CrossRef]
42. de la Motte Rouge, T.; Pautier, P.; Genestie, C.; Rey, A.; Gouy, S.; Leary, A.; Haie-Meder, C.; Kerbrat, P.; Culine, S.; Fizazi, K.; et al. Prognostic Significance of an Early Decline in Serum Alpha-Fetoprotein during Chemotherapy for Ovarian Yolk Sac Tumors. *Gynecol. Oncol.* **2016**, *142*, 452–457. [CrossRef]
43. Reed, N.S.; Pautier, P.; Åvall-Lundqvist, E.; Choi, C.H.; Du Bois, A.; Friedlander, M.; Fyles, A.; Kichenadasse, G.; Provencher, D.M.; Ray-Coquard, I. Gynecologic Cancer InterGroup (GCIG) Consensus Review for Ovarian Small Cell Cancers. *Int. J. Gynecol. Cancer* **2014**, *24* (Suppl. S3), S30–S34. [CrossRef]
44. Brown, J.; Friedlander, M.; Backes, F.J.; Harter, P.; O'Connor, D.M.; De La Motte Rouge, T.; Lorusso, D.; Maenpaa, J.; Kim, J.W.; Tenney, M.E.; et al. Gynecologic Cancer Intergroup (GCIG) Consensus Review for Ovarian Germ Cell Tumors. *Int. J. Gynecol. Cancer* **2014**, *24* (Suppl. S3), S48–S54. [CrossRef]
45. Mangili, G.; Sigismondi, C.; Lorusso, D.; Cormio, G.; Candiani, M.; Scarfone, G.; Mascilini, F.; Gadducci, A.; Mosconi, A.M.; Scollo, P.; et al. The Role of Staging and Adjuvant Chemotherapy in Stage I Malignant Ovarian Germ Cell Tumors (MOGTs): The MITO-9 Study. *Ann. Oncol. Off. J. Eur. Soc. Med. Oncol.* **2017**, *28*, 333–338. [CrossRef]
46. Billmire, D.F.; Vinocur, C.; Rescorla, F.; Cushing, B.; London, W.; Schlatter, M.; Davis, M.; Giller, R.; Lauer, S.; Olson, T.; et al. Outcome and Staging Evaluation in Malignant Germ Cell Tumors of the Ovary in Children and Adolescents: An Intergroup Study. *J. Pediatr. Surg.* **2004**, *39*, 424–429. [CrossRef]
47. Young, R.H.; Oliva, E.; Scully, R.E. Small Cell Carcinoma of the Ovary, Hypercalcemic Type. A Clinicopathological Analysis of 150 Cases. *Am. J. Surg. Pathol.* **1994**, *18*, 1102–1116. [CrossRef]
48. Nasioudis, D.; Kanninen, T.T.; Holcomb, K.; Sisti, G.; Witkin, S.S. Prevalence of Lymph Node Metastasis and Prognostic Significance of Lymphadenectomy in Apparent Early-Stage Malignant Ovarian Sex Cord-Stromal Tumors. *Gynecol. Oncol.* **2017**, *145*, 243–247. [CrossRef]
49. Park, J.Y.; Kim, D.Y.; Suh, D.S.; Kim, J.H.; Kim, Y.M.; Kim, Y.T.; Nam, J.H. Outcomes of Pediatric and Adolescent Girls with Malignant Ovarian Germ Cell Tumors. *Gynecol. Oncol.* **2015**, *137*, 418–422. [CrossRef]
50. Braungart, S.; Craigie, R.J.; Farrelly, P.; Losty, P.D. Operative Management of Pediatric Ovarian Tumors and the Challenge of Fertility-Preservation: Results from the UK CCLG Surgeons Cancer Group Nationwide Study. *J. Pediatr. Surg.* **2020**, *55*, 2425–2429. [CrossRef]
51. Gershenson, D.M. Treatment of Ovarian Cancer in Young Women. *Clin. Obstet. Gynecol.* **2012**, *55*, 65–74. [CrossRef]
52. Tomao, F.; Peccatori, F.; del Pup, L.; Franchi, D.; Zanagnolo, V.; Panici, P.B.; Colombo, N. Special Issues in Fertility Preservation for Gynecologic Malignancies. *Crit. Rev. Oncol. Hematol.* **2016**, *97*, 206–219. [CrossRef]

53. Arapaki, A.; Christopoulos, P.; Kalampokas, E.; Triantafyllidou, O.; Matsas, A.; Vlahos, N.F. Ovarian Tissue Cryopreservation in Children and Adolescents. *Children* **2022**, *9*, 1256. [CrossRef]
54. McKenzie, N.D.; Kennard, J.A.; Ahmad, S. Fertility Preserving Options for Gynecologic Malignancies: A Review of Current Understanding and Future Directions. *Crit. Rev. Oncol. Hematol.* **2018**, *132*, 116–124. [CrossRef] [PubMed]

Disclaimer/Publisher's Note: The statements, opinions and data contained in all publications are solely those of the individual author(s) and contributor(s) and not of MDPI and/or the editor(s). MDPI and/or the editor(s) disclaim responsibility for any injury to people or property resulting from any ideas, methods, instructions or products referred to in the content.

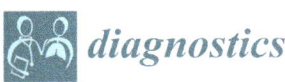

Review

Clinical, Histological, and Molecular Prognostic Factors in Childhood Medulloblastoma: Where Do We Stand?

Charikleia Ntenti [1,†], Konstantinos Lallas [2,†] and Georgios Papazisis [3,*]

1. First Department of Pharmacology, School of Medicine, Aristotle University of Thessaloniki, 54621 Thessaloniki, Greece
2. Department of Medical Oncology, School of Medicine, Aristotle University of Thessaloniki, 54621 Thessaloniki, Greece
3. Clinical Research Unit, Special Unit for Biomedical Research and Education (BRESU), School of Medicine, Aristotle University of Thessaloniki, 54621 Thessaloniki, Greece
* Correspondence: papazisg@auth.gr
† These authors contributed equally to this work.

Abstract: Medulloblastomas, highly aggressive neoplasms of the central nervous system (CNS) that present significant heterogeneity in clinical presentation, disease course, and treatment outcomes, are common in childhood. Moreover, patients who survive may be diagnosed with subsequent malignancies during their life or could develop treatment-related medical conditions. Genetic and transcriptomic studies have classified MBs into four subgroups: wingless type (WNT), Sonic Hedgehog (SHH), Group 3, and Group 4, with distinct histological and molecular profiles. However, recent molecular findings resulted in the WHO updating their guidelines and stratifying medulloblastomas into further molecular subgroups, changing the clinical stratification and treatment management. In this review, we discuss most of the histological, clinical, and molecular prognostic factors, as well the feasibility of their application, for better characterization, prognostication, and treatment of medulloblastomas.

Keywords: medulloblastoma; tumor; histologic; pediatrics; micro-RNAs; non-coding RNAs; prognosis; molecular subgroup; stratification

1. Introduction

Medulloblastomas (MBs) are highly aggressive neoplasms of the central nervous system (CNS) and are considered the most common malignant brain tumor in childhood [1,2]. First described by Cushing and Bailey in 1925, these tumors derive from discrete neuronal lineages based on molecularly defined subgroups, as shown by recent studies. For example, the cells of origin for the SHH subgroup are the granule-neuron progenitors, whereas for Groups 3 and 4, early rhombic lip is considered the common source of origin [3–5].

Epidemiologically, the estimated annual incidence of the tumor in the US is approximately 500 cases per year and the median age of diagnosis is 6–8 years; it is very rarely diagnosed in adults [6].

Since 1990, when the estimated event-free survival (EFS) of MBs was 20–50% [7], and with the application of newer therapeutic techniques, the median overall survival of all subtypes is estimated to be 70% [8–10]. The tumor presents a significant biological heterogeneity, as it has been observed that about 30% of patients will be diagnosed with metastatic disease at presentation, and patients who survive may be diagnosed with subsequent malignancies during their life or develop treatment-related neurocognitive, endocrinological, or development disorders, highlighting the need for risk stratification of patients with MB. The aim of risk stratification is the appropriate selection and management of patients who can really benefit from treatment or who need treatment intensification. Clinical and histological factors were the initial determinants of prognosis and the main parameters used for patient categorization into standard and high risk [11,12]. However, the development of new molecular techniques has revolutionized the prognostication of MBs, creating new molecular subgroups with distinct clinical features, response to treatment options, and prognosis. Around 2010, several researchers reported that medulloblastomas comprise at least four distinct molecular subgroups: wingless signaling activated (WNT), Sonic-hedgehog signaling activated (SHH), Group 3, and Group 4, largely based on transcriptome profiles and a few known genetic alterations [13–15]. Thereafter, for the first time in 2016, molecular subgroups of MBs were incorporated into the WHO's MB stratification [16,17]. The WNT subgroup accounts for approximately 10% of all MBs, whereas the SHH subgroup is most common in infants and young adults, accounting for 25% of all MBs [15,18]. Group 3 and Group 4 constitute approximately 65% of medulloblastoma cases and are characterized by great heterogeneity in clinical phenotypes and survival rates [19,20]. The most recent edition of CNS tumor classification (CNS 5), from 2021, divided medulloblastomas into "molecularly" and "histologically" defined, denoting the diverse biology of the tumor [21].

However, although recent research has mainly focused on a thorough investigation of molecular mechanisms behind MB pathogenesis and their contribution to risk stratification of patients, clinicopathological characteristics are also important factors for both relapse and prognosis and have been involved in recently developed prognostic nomograms [22].

The main scope of our review is to summarize the evidence concerning clinical, pathological, and molecular factors affecting the prognosis of childhood medulloblastomas. We mainly focus on the interconnection between these factors and their role in risk stratification, aiming to prove that appropriate treatment selection in chosen patients is feasible.

2. Methodology

We searched the literature via PubMed, Scopus, and Cochrane for relevant studies, using specific keywords such as "medulloblastoma", "prognosis", and "prognostic factors" from inception to January 2023. Studies referring to clinicopathological and molecular factors associated with the prognosis of childhood medulloblastomas were included, whereas studies referring to adulthood or not referring to prognosis, as well as non-English papers, were excluded from the reviewing process. The primary outcome of our review was to investigate possible interactions between clinical, histologic, and molecular characteristics of MBs and the prognosis of the patients. In addition, the effect of the aforementioned factors on relapse occurrence and their association with post-relapse prognosis were set as secondary outcomes.

3. Results

3.1. Clinical and Histological Prognostic Factors

Before the establishment of molecular subgroups of MBs, patient risk stratification was mainly carried out based on their clinical characteristics, the histological features of the tumor, and the treatment approaches followed. Using the above factors as prognostic parameters, patients are categorized into two discrete subtypes: standard and high risk. Age < 3 years old, residual tumor > 1.5 cm^2, and large-cell/anaplastic histology are considered high-risk features, whereas patients not fulfilling the above criteria are considered standard risk [9,12,23].

3.2. Age

One of the clinical characteristics used for risk stratification is the age of the patient. In general, younger age at diagnosis seem to have a worse prognosis compared to older children and is considered a high-risk feature [24]. More precisely, infants and children <3 years showed the worst prognosis, and various studies have investigated survival rates of those patients [25]. Rutkowski et al. reported a hazard ratio (HR) of 4.02 (95% CI 1.28–12.96) for higher risk for relapse or death for children below 2 years of age compared to children 2–3 years old, whereas results from a Canadian study concluded that children older than 18 months had better survival rates compared to infants below that threshold [26,27].

A possible explanation could be the avoidance of craniospinal irradiation of the tumor in that age group due to the defects that radiotherapy cause in the developing brain. Despite that, a recently published meta-analysis and a retrospective study from Brazil did not reach a statistical significance for age as a poor prognostic factor [8,28,29]. On the other hand, MBs in adults demonstrate a lower mutational rate, are less aggressive, and are associated with better prognosis compared to younger patients [30].

3.3. Extent of Disease

Another significant factor that affects the prognosis of childhood MBs and is included in the risk-stratification system is the extent of disease. Chang's staging is the main clinical classification system for MB patients and evaluates the local extent (T stage) and the tumor's dissemination (M stage) [31,32]. Although the role of the local extent as a prognostic factor is debated, with some studies showing worse prognosis for tumors located in the midline or with involvement of the fourth ventricle and the brainstem [26,33–35] and others not demonstrating similar findings [36,37], the contribution of metastasis to prognosis is well established. It is estimated that 30% of patients present with metastatic disease at diagnosis, which is accompanied by significantly diminished survival rates, with an eight-year OS of 65% and 27% in non-metastatic and metastatic patients, respectively [26]. Special consideration is given to stage M1 (tumor cells disseminated to CFS), which exhibits decreased OS similar to other metastatic stages, implying the need for prompt diagnosis of M1 staging, incorporation into high-risk features, and the implementation of intensifying treatment plans [24,26,38,39].

3.4. Extent of Resection

Surgical resection comprises an important part of MB treatment plans, and the extent of resection poses a significant prognostic factor. The main goal of resection is the removal of the whole extent of the tumor, with gross total resection (GTR) demonstrating a favorable impact on both PFS and OS, as shown by observational studies and meta-analyses [8,26,34,40]. On the other hand, residual disease after surgery, and especially residual tumors > 1.5 cm^2, is considered a poor prognostic factor, leading to local tumor relapses and worst survival rates. However, the benefit of extensive surgical resections may be counterbalanced for post-surgical neurologically adverse events, ranging from endocrinologic abnormalities to neurologic complications such as cerebellar-mutism syndrome, which are present in a considerable percentage of patients after GTR [41]. The latter is of paramount importance mainly for centrally located tumors, in whom total resection might not be feasible and which are categorized as high-risk tumors with a need for treatment intensification. Despite that, Thompson et al., when examining the prognostic value of GTR compared to near-total resection (NTR), along with the integration of clinical and molecular factors, did not conclude significant survival differences, and similar results were also shown by other studies [42–44]. Consequently, GTR demonstrates a favorable impact on the prognosis of MB patients, but the EOR should be evaluated in combination with other parameters, such as tumor location and post-surgical complications.

3.5. Histological Variant

There are four main histological subtypes of MBs: desmoplastic/nodular (DMN), classic (CMB), MBs with extensive nodularity (MBEN), and large cell/anaplastic (LCA). Each of them is characterized by different histological patterns and is associated with distinct molecular and genetic alterations, exhibiting diverse prognosis [3,45,46]. Multiple studies have examined the role of histology as a prognostic factor of MBs. Firstly, DMN, which is characterized by desmoplasia with pericellular fibrinogen deposits, demonstrates better prognosis compared to the classic subtype ([8], desmoplastic vs. classic, HR 0.41, 95% CI 0.31–0.56, OS, and [26], DMN/MBEN vs. classic, HR 0.44, 95% CI 0.31–0.64). Similarly, MBEN histology, which is mainly found in the early years of life, exhibits and good to excellent prognosis [47]. The above survival advantage seems to be maintained even in the presence of adverse prognostic factors (i.e., metastatic setting). In a more detailed way, Leary et al. suggested a similar EFS in non-metastatic compared to metastatic DMN, whereas Gupta et al. showed a better OS in extracranial metastatic desmoplastic compared to non-desmoplastic subtypes [48,49]. On the other hand, LCA, which is characterized by the presence of anaplasia in histopathology, exhibits the worst prognosis compared to other subtypes [46]. Semantically, the degree of anaplasia seems to affect prognosis in a significant manner, where severe anaplasia leads to worse OS and EFS compared to mild. The poor prognosis of that subtype could be attributed to the association of LCA with high-risk features, as it usually affects patients at a younger age, is diagnosed with metastasis at presentation, and is associated with specific molecular and genetic alternations such as LOH, isochromosome 17q, and MYC-family genes [50–52]. Especially for the latter, Ellison et al. and Ryan et al. demonstrated the co-expression of c-MYC amplification with severe anaplasia and high-risk features, implying a worse prognosis [53,54].

Despite that, the latest WHO classification combines all the above histological subtypes into one category, called histologically defined MBs, which are associated with specific molecular pathways, suggesting the need for a multilayered evaluation of specific tumor characteristics.

3.6. Other Prognostic Factors

Except for the above-described clinicopathological and molecular factors, hematological and serum markers are also described in the literature, which can predict the survival of MB patients. Li et al. investigated the role of serum markers on prognosis and revealed that an elevated preoperative neutrophil-to-lymphocyte ratio (NLR) and platelet-to-lymphocyte ratio (PLR) were detected more frequently in Group 3 and Group 4 MBs and were associated independently with worse PFS and OS [55]. In addition, lower levels of lymphocytes during radiotherapy (RT) were associated with increased risk of recurrence [56]. In agreement with this, Zhu et al. evaluated the prognostic value of a systemic inflammatory index (SII) and nutritional status along with serum markers and advocated that high levels of inflammatory markers impaired OS in multivariable models [57].

Apart from serum markers, recent research has focused on the fast-growing field of radiomics, where the incorporation of image analysis into risk-prediction models, which are based on well-established factors, could evaluate the prognosis of each patient preoperatively and at diagnosis. The latter is of paramount importance, as it would assist with further understanding of the diverse nature of MBs and the designation of appropriate treatment strategies. Until recently, radiomic analysis had managed to indirectly predict the prognosis of patients, as MRI findings were associated with the molecular subgroup of the tumor [58,59] or the dissemination to the CSF [60]. However, the co-estimation of imaging findings, clinical characteristics, and molecular subgroup led to the development of nomograms, predicting both PFS [61] and OS [62].

4. Molecular Classification

During the last 20 years, knowledge about medulloblastoma biology has fiercely increased, primarily because of the advance of integrated genomics. The first approved classification of medulloblastomas concerning the molecular characteristics was performed by the WHO in 2016, resulting in four different molecular groups of MBs, each of which has a totally different molecular signature from both genetic and epigenetic aspects: WNT (wingless-related integration site) activated, SHH (sonic hedgehog)- activated, Group 3, and Group 4 [16,17,63]. The first two groups were identified and named based on the signaling pathways that were found to be activated in WNT MBs and SHH MBs, respectively: Wingless/Integration-1 (WNT) activated and sonic hedgehog (SHH) activated. It has been histologically proven that WNT MBs and SHH MBs arise from different cell types. It is well known that medulloblastomas are generated from cells that are related to some extent to cerebellar granule-neuron-precursor (CGNP) development and that some medulloblastoma cells retain primitive features equivalent to those of the precursors of the embryonic brain. Therefore, it seems that the acquisition of CGNP identity is a crucial determinant of progenitor cells' ability to form hedgehog-induced MBs [64]. Group 3 and Group 4 constitute approximately 65% of medulloblastoma cases and are characterized by great heterogeneity in clinical phenotypes and survival rates [20]. These different subtypes are associated with different demographic and clinical features, but this is not always the case. Lately, a unified lineage of origin for both Groups 3 and 4 within the human fetal RL^{SVZ} was defined. These recent data explain the underlying molecular signatures, biological and clinical overlap, and site of diagnosis that these two groups share [5].

The intention behind molecular classification is to better relate clinical phenotypes with the tumor biology and to identify new personalized, safer, therapeutic targets. The four main molecular groups describe in a vague manner the disease evolution and outcome. In the updated WHO classification of the CNS tumors, Group 3 and Group 4 are merged into one, called non-WNT/non-SHH MB. It is a very large category, to which the majority of pediatric MB patients belong [21]. The classification by Schwalbe et al. divides MBs into seven subtypes and impresses that the only group that remains intact is the WNT-MB class.

4.1. The WNT Group

The WNT group accounts for 10% of MBs and usually develops in the midline cerebellum but is also capable of spreading to the dorsal brainstem. The WNT group overall has the best prognosis out of all MB groups [65]. Mutations of the WNT-signaling pathway cause its fundamental activation [66]. Genomic analyses showed that the vast majority of patients (85–90%) with WNT MBs have a mutation in exon 3 of CTNNB1 [10]. As a result, β-catenin is stabilized, leading to constant activation of the WNT pathway [67]. Mutation in adenomatous polyposis coli (APC), a germline mutation, is also associated with WNT MBs [62].

There is a conflict about the subtypes within the WNT group; some studies have presented evidence for at least two distinct subgroups, whereas other researchers have reported only one [68–70]. One of the suggested subgroups is low risk, more than 90% survival, and typically non-metastatic [10]. The second suggested WNT subtype is mainly characterized by metastatic cases and anaplastic histology [68]. Because of the confusion concerning WNT-MB sub-classification, many subdivisions have been proposed. Some groups use both testing of gene-expression patterns with DNA-methylation arrays. A very recent and modern approach is the similarity-network-fusion (SFN) strategy, which constructs networks of combined data [70]. As a result, Cavalli et al. identified two different subtypes of WNT MBs: WNTα and WNTβ. Generally, WNT MBs are related to accumulated beta-catenin inside the nucleus, accumulation of mutations in CTNNB1, and, in most cases, monosomy in chromosome 6 [66]. The above-mentioned markers are used to identify WNT MBs, but 1 in 10 MBs can be missed [71].

4.2. The SHH-MB Group

SHH MBs are the most common group in infants, accounting for 25% of all medulloblastoma cases. Usually, it is found in cerebellar hemispheres but can also be found in the midline. It is characterized by mutations or copy-number alterations of SHH-pathway genes. According to Robinson et al., the infant-SHH group should be split into SHH-I and SHH-II, as it seems that the first one is enriched in SUFU aberrations and chromosome 2 gain [72–74]. Another study suggested the subclassification of the SHH group into α, β, γ, and δ subgroups [66,70]. According to the study, infant SHH-I and SHH-II correspond to SHH-β and SHH-γ, respectively. The prognosis of SHH-γ is better than that of SHH-β. SHHα can be of the LCA or ND subtype. It has been found to be enriched with MYCN, GLI2, and YAP1 amplifications, as well as TP53 mutations and copy-number alterations (9q, 10q, and 17p loss) [70,75,76].

4.3. Group 3 and Group 4

Group 3 has the highest rate of mortality, with only a 58% 5-year OS in children and an even lower, 45% 5-year OS in infants [19,65,77]. In fact, Group 3 has a variety of grim features, such as young age and metastasis even after diagnosis. Histologically, it is characterized by anaplastic large cells that can serve as a prognostic marker [78]. Concerning molecular events, an aberrant amplification of MYC takes place [79]. Group 3 seems to be highly heterogenous with patients developing MYC-amplified tumors, with a very short survival rate since only 20% survive up to 5 years. Group 3 MB tumors reappear as metastases far from the primary tumor, with a rate of metastases independent of the survival percentage. Tumors belonging to Group 4 usually demonstrate isochromosome 17q (i17q) [80]. The overlap in the mutational spectrum, the transcriptional profile, and the DNA-methylation pattern between Group 3 and Group 4 has led them to be considered the non-WNT/non-SHH group in the latest WHO classification [21]. Indeed, tumors belonging to this group have more of a molecular affinity with each other than with SHH or WNT MBs. Unlike WNT and SHH MBs, the reason for this molecular diversity and the large and confusing overlapping between Groups 3 and 4 remains obscure.

In summary, since the recognition of the four core MB groups in 2010, molecular subgrouping has experienced a revolutionary diversification. Nowadays, about 12 molecular subtypes are defined and new data come to light every day. Cavalli et al. analyzed more than 700 primary-MB tissue samples and showed that SHH MBs can be divided into four subclasses, with different copy-number aberrations, activated pathways, and—most importantly—different clinical outcomes. The SHHα subgroup has the worst prognosis of all four subgroups [70].

5. Medulloblastomas and Genetics

Medulloblastoma genetic analysis is a key component not only for risk stratification but also for prognosis [81]. Currently, the molecular classification of MB tumors is routinely performed not only because of the impact that variations have on treatment and clinical outcome but also because it is undeniable that the great progress in molecular analyses, such as high-throughput next-generation-sequencing (NGS) technologies, allows for better understanding of medulloblastomas' tumorigenesis and biology, which should ultimately enhance the application of tailored treatment therapies.

Each molecular subgroup of MBs can be identified by a unique signature of DNA alterations and copy-number variation, abnormal gene transcription, and various post-transcriptional modifications. These characteristics are associated with different clinical phenotypes and, when combined, could have an important prognostic value. TP53 R273H mutation, which lies within the DNA-binding domain of the tumor-suppressor protein Tp53, is responsible for the loss of DNA binding and decreased activation of Tp53 target gene expression. As a result, cells resist apoptosis and an aberrant transcriptional activation and increased cell migration take place. TP53 mutation in the R273H point is associated with poor follow-up in the SHHα subgroup and generally with worse prognosis [70]. In addition, it has been shown in mice models that TP53 R237H mutation is responsible for tumors with high metastatic potential [82,83]. TP53 germ-line mutations lead to mutations in hedgehog-signaling genes, resulting in medulloblastoma growth in patients with Li–Fraumeni syndrome. Cerebellum granule-cell precursors (GCPs) are the cells of origin of SHH medulloblastomas, indicating that GCPs are highly susceptible to tumorigenesis in the absence of P53.

Other genes, such as MYCN and GLI2, are frequently found in various cohorts to be over-expressed [84]. Indeed, both genes are risk factors for SHH MBs. TP53 could serve as a reliable prognostic marker in SHH MB cases, as it has been recently shown that patients with the above-mentioned mutations have a worse outcome compared with patients with wild-type TP53 [85]. From a histological perspective, mutations in the TP53, when present, reflect poor prognosis in all four groups [86]. A validated molecular marker used for Group 3 is NPR3 (natriuretic peptide receptor 3), a protein-coding gene, and for Group 4 it is

KCNA1 (potassium voltage-gated channel subfamily A member 1), another protein-coding gene [66]. Apart from the conventional genetic markers, it has been demonstrated that the incorporation of DNA-methylation biomarkers significantly ameliorates survival prediction for non-WNT medulloblastomas in patients 3 to 16 years old. The addition of MXI1- and IL8-methylation status with the currently used molecular and clinical features noticeably improved disease-risk stratification [87,88].

It may take years before genetic tests based on sequencing technologies can be incorporated as a part of standard care for our patients. Further studies are needed to validate their prognostic merit and lead to tailored therapies that are able to detect measurable, residual disease and prevent the fatal relapse of medulloblastomas.

6. Non-Coding RNAs

New reliable and affordable methods are needed to help prognosis and to suggest the most appropriate therapy to patients with MBs individually. MiRNAs could be the answer to that, as they have already been used in treating various diseases, including cancer. MicroRNAs (miRNAs or miRs) are small non-coding RNA molecules that have been identified as major regulators of cancer growth, functioning either as oncogenes or tumor suppressors. MiRNAs help tumor cells called oncomiRs to proliferate, but others inhibit cell proliferation and promote cell differentiation, known as tumor-suppressor miRs. MicroRNAs have been implicated in gene-expression regulation through different mechanisms. Usually, based on sequence-specific binding, they can inhibit the translation of messenger RNA (mRNA) or mark mRNA molecules for degradation [89]. Due to molecular-technique improvement, new and affordable methods are available, suggesting that miRNAs can be used as promising biomarkers of MBs [90,91]. MiRNAs can be readily detected in tumor biopsies, and they are also stable in body fluids due to being bound to lipoproteins, associated with the Argonaute 2 (Ago2) protein, packaged into microvesicles and other microparticles (such as apoptotic bodies, microvesicles, and exosome-like particles) as circulating miRNAs [92–94]. Therefore, they are protected from endogenous RNA activity, making them a reliable and stable marker [95].

Different miRNAs have different molecular signatures in the four distinct groups. It has also been found that downregulation of miR-204 expression is associated with poor survival in children diagnosed with Group 3 or Group 4 MBs [96]. Moreover, in Group 4 patients, there is generally an intermediate prognosis: Low expression of miR-204 marks out a distinct sub-group with remarkably poor survival. This is a rather important finding, as Group 4 is characterized by a lack of reliable prognostic markers [97].

The most important remark about miR-204 is probably that the replacement of downregulated expression levels could limit a tumor's metastatic potential and thus be a promising therapeutic approach. The improvement of RNA-sequencing platforms has led to the identification of several miRNAs that alter gene regulation and promote cancer and metastasis. Large cohort studies with the neuroblastoma pediatric population revealed the crucial role of miR-383, miR-206, miR-183, miR-128a/b, and miR-133b in WNT MBs, as they are downregulated significantly [98,99]. Identification of new molecular markers for diagnosis and prognosis is important. Long non-coding RNAs (lncRNAs) are now among the most promising diagnostic tool, as they play an important role in brain-tumor growth and metastasis [100]. Kesherwani et al. found that high expression of DLEU2 and DSCR8 in Group 3 and high expression of DLEU2 and low expression of XIST in Group 4 are associated with poor prognosis of MBs [101]. Gao et al. showed that LOXL1-AS1 (LOXL1 antisense RNA 1) promotes cell proliferation and migration in MBs [102–104]. In 2020, Joshi et al. conducted the first genome-wide analysis of lncRNAs' expression profile in MBs. The screening of 17 lncRNAs yielded positive results, with H19, lnc-RRM2-3, LINC01551, LINC00336, lnc-CDYL-1, FAM222A-AS1, and AL139393.2 associated with poor prognosis [105].

In 2022, Lee et al. showed in vitro that long non-coding RNA SPRIGHTLY promote the MB subgroup 4 [106]. SPRIGHTLY modulates the EGFR-signaling pathway through regulatory effects. These modifications affect cell growth through changes in the tumor microenvironment [106].

According to Zhang et al., HOTAIR (HOX transcript antisense RNA) is another LncRNA that promotes MB progression [104]. HOTAIR knockdown led to a reduction of tumor growth, cell proliferation, and increased cell apoptosis. HOTAIR act through bindings to miR-1 and miR-206, which lead to increased expression of YY1 (Yin Yang 1). It has been proven that non-coding RNAs regulate tumor metabolism involved in development and relapse. We estimate that future studies will enable a full investigation into ncRNA-associated prognostic potential and that it will be incorporated into the prognosis and stratification of medulloblastomas.

7. Recurrence

Recurrence of MB (relapsed MB, rMB) is considered a serious adverse event of the tumor, which is present in approximately 30% of patients and associated with poor prognosis. Recent studies have reported significantly diminished PFS and OS for rMBs (only 5% of patients will remain alive after 5 years), even in the presence of a wide range of therapeutic options, such as re-irradiation, surgery, chemotherapy, and targeted therapies [107]. The above observation prioritizes the need for the development of appropriate risk-stratification models based on clinical and molecular subgroups for relapsed patients, which could also assist with the selection of adequate treatment strategies.

Regarding prognostic factors of MB relapse, both clinical and histological characteristics of the tumor at diagnosis seem to affect the time and pattern of relapse and post-relapse survival rates. Concerning age, younger patients (<5 years old) have a higher rate of recurrence, and the role of histology is not clear. Although LCA was associated with reduced time to relapse and short time to death post-relapse [108], Sabel et al. argued that histology did not affect the aforementioned factors [109]. In addition, the detection of MYC amplification was characterized as a negative prognostic for both the development of recurrence and time to death after relapse [109]. Treatment modality at diagnosis was another significant factor in observational studies, where craniospinal irradiation of the primary tumor showed prolonged time to relapse and better survival rates afterwards [108–110]. Nevertheless, the site of recurrence seems not to be affected by treatment type and is mainly molecularly driven. On the other hand, presence of metastatic dissemination at diagnosis had no effect on survival after relapse [111].

Prospective studies also evaluated the existence of prognostic factors for MB recurrence in infants (iMB) and young children and investigated parameters associated with post-relapse survival (PRS). Gross total resection and the absence of residual disease or <1.5 cm^2 residual disease showed a better EFS compared to STR or residual > 1.5 cm^2 [112,113], whereas the time from diagnosis to relapse was not shown to affect survival [114]. From a histopathological perspective, DMEN/DN histology demonstrated a better PFS compared to CMB [112], and further molecular analysis revealed that a considerable number of patients within the SHH subgroup had DN/MBEN histology and were associated with better prognosis. However, Hicks et al. argued that in DN/MBEN SHH iMBs, there is a subset of patients with the SHH$_I$ molecular subtype that had a worse PFS (HR 3.8, 95% CI 1.00–11.8, $p = 0.038$), underlining the importance of an extended molecular subtyping for the better understanding of recurrence risk in iMBs [115]. In concordance with this, the SJYC07 trial reported similar results [72], whereas the HIT-2000 study [116] and ACNS1221 [117] did not reach statistical significance for the difference in PFS between the SHH$_I$ and SHH$_{II}$ subgroups. On the contrary, non-DN/MBEN histology or STR within the SHH subgroup were considered poor prognostic factors. On the other hand, Group 3 usually presented with a disseminated relapse pattern [115,118] and was characterized by MYC amplification and LCA histology, resulting in diminished PFS, whereas Group 4 demonstrated local relapse and a moderate prognosis. Regarding PRS and taking under consideration that CSI is often omitted in iMBs due to neurocognitive disorders, salvaging CSI led to improved survival after recurrence [114,118]. Other prognostic factors for PRS, as shown by multivariable models, were Group 3 and a disseminated pattern of relapse, which led to poor prognosis.

The observation of different treatment outcomes among MB patients, their diversity in histopathological and molecular characteristics, and the presence of different cells of origin, imply the detection of discrete molecular findings at relapse compared to the primary tumor. However, methylation data analysis performed at relapsed tumor specimens concluded that MBs maintain their primary characteristics also at recurrence ("tumor fidelity"), affecting all aspects of the disease, starting from time to relapse [119]. Differences in relapsed MBs are critical to the development of effective therapies. Research on primary and recurrent MB tumors has revealed that the variance in genomic changes between the two is the mutations on the driver that are present in around 41% of reoccurring tumors and various acquired somatic DNA alterations in around 53% of them [120,121]. The performance of methylation profiling indicates, once more, that in general, the molecular signature of the relapsed tumor resembles that of the original one, except, of course, for the prementioned alterations [122].

In the SHH MB group, it seems that age is being negatively correlated with differences between gene expression in the primary and in the relapsed tumor. Particularly, the youngest patients with SHH MB, develop relapsed tumors with copy-number variations and supreme transcriptome variability compared to the primary tumor. The majority of relapsed cases are characterized by the loss of 17p and, in a limited number of cases, by new TP53 mutation [123]. This finding suggests a model of bi-allelic gene inactivation, resulting in further accumulation of genomic changes. On the contrary, Groups 3 and 4 are presented with metastatic disease, which is associated with poor prognosis [124].

Richardson et al. studied more than 100 relapsed MBs, enabling the characterization of the molecular basis in medulloblastoma reoccurrence with the goal of the clinical exploitation of this knowledge. They found that molecular groups and the novel subtypes also remained consistent to the original stratification of the primary tumor. However, it was found that a small subset of Group 4 MBs switched subgroups when relapsing [125].

Hill et al. also proved that MBs show an altered molecular profile at relapse, which is predictive of disease prognosis but cannot be detected earlier. They pointed out the significance of P53-MYC interactions during tumor relapse and their prognostic value as predictors of clinically aggressive disease [126]. These findings enhance the need for biopsy in clinical practice during relapse and thus the development of improved and patient-tailored therapeutic strategies.

8. Applying the Knowledge Gained

The knowledge acquired from molecular data suggests that clinical risk is not enough for the reliable assessment of relapse risk. The intention behind molecular classification is to better relate clinical phenotypes with the tumor biology and to identify new personalized, safer, therapeutic targets. So far, randomized controlled trials focusing on older children, and SJYC07 including younger children (<3 years old), have evaluated both clinical prognostic factors and molecular subgroups to guide treatment decisions. More precisely, the ACNS0331 study concluded a non-inferior EFS in clinically defined average-risk patients with MB in whom a reduction of radiation-boost volume was preferred compared to posterior-fossa radiation therapy. In addition, that regimen decreased neurocognitive disorders attributed to RT, serving as an additional advantage in the treatment of patients lacking high-risk features. However, molecular subgrouping revealed a specific subgroup with inferior EFS when low-dose CSI was administered compared to the standard dose [127]. In concordance, the SJMB3 trial stratified patients into categories based on both clinical and molecular prognostic factors, pinpointing the importance of co-estimation of those parameters in the case of treatment de-intensification in favorable-risk groups (such as the WNT subgroup) or intensifying treatment in the presence of adverse prognostic factors such as metastatic disease or subtype III or MYC amplification in Group 3 patients [78]. Similarly for younger children enrolled in the SJYC07 trial, treatment selection according to clinically and histologically defined risk-adapted factors did not improve EFS, especially for the intermediate- and high-risk groups [78]. On the contrary, using molecular profiling led to a better survival outcome in the SHH$_{II}$ subgroup compared to SHH$_{I}$, in whom significant adverse genetic factors, such as SUFU aberration and isochromosome 2 gain, were detected. In addition, recent clinical trials have been designed (i.e., PNET 5 (NCT02066220) and SJMB12 (NCT01878617)) and enrolled pediatric patients based on both clinical and molecular data.

For the PNET 5 study, the only criterion for the assignment of patients was β-catenin status. Therefore, children positive for β-catenin endonucleic accumulation were assigned to treatment arm PNET5 MB-LR, whereas children with negative results were assigned to treatment arm PNET 5 MB-SR. It is worth mentioning that the initial diagnostic assessments (imaging, staging, histology, and tumor biology) needed for inclusion in the study were the same for both treatment arms. An amendment of the protocol permitted the entry of WNT-activated MB patients with high-risk characteristics to the PNET 5 MB WNT-HR study. Likewise, patients with high-risk SHH MB with TP53 mutation (somatic, germline, and mosaicism) were included in the PNET 5 MB SHH-TP53 study.

The second phase II clinical trial, called SJMB12, stratified MB treatment according to clinical risk (low, standard, intermediate, or high risk) and molecular subtype (WNT, SHH, or non-WNT/non-SHH). The main aim was to evaluate whether participants with low-risk WNT tumors could be treated with a lower dose of radiation and mild chemotherapy to achieve the same survival rates with fewer side effects. All children had surgery to remove as much of the primary tumor as was safely possible, radiation therapy, and chemotherapy. However, the amount of therapy (radiation and chemotherapy) was determined by the patient's treatment stratum. The treatment-stratum assignment had been planned based on the tumor's molecular subgroup and clinical risk.

Both studies are ongoing, and we have to wait for the results to fulfill the research community's ambitions for more efficient and safe treatment of MBs.

9. Conclusions

Until 2014, MB grading, like general grading in CNS tumors, was based exclusively on histological data. However, since then, a lot has changed in the diagnostics and therapeutics of cancer diseases. Undoubtedly, genomic and transcriptomic analyses shed light on the molecular and genetic pathways involved in the pathogenesis of MBs, evolving risk-stratification systems. Molecular markers can provide powerful prognostic knowledge, and this is why they have been added to the biomarker list of grading and prognosis estimation. Apart from the already-applied technologies, new molecular biomarkers have come into view. Recent studies have revealed the promising prognostic value of various analyses based on genomic approaches that use the cell-free DNA (cfDNA) of the cerebrospinal fluid (CSF) and the different structural variants and point mutations by multiplexed droplet digital PCR (ddPCR) [128]. Moreover, Cao et al. brought out the great potential of the MCM3 marker, a minichromosome-maintenance protein, through a multi-omics approach that combines single-cell RNA sequencing and proteomics analysis [129]. Undoubtedly, scientists are trying to combine state-of-the-art molecular analyses with modern mass-spectrometry imaging techniques that will allow for the identification of sub-group-specific tumor-cell populations whose unique functions can be exploited for future prognostic and therapeutic strategies.

Disparities among patients' clinical outcomes make the application of further subtypes of MB urgent and have been included in this study. Despite the prognostic value of the recent 2021 WHO molecular classification, it is obvious that there is a great heterogeneity within each of the four groups and their relevant subgroups. Therefore, there is a constant update of downstream classification from studies around the world, and this is only the beginning. As technology improves and permits wider and more complicated data interpretation, a more detailed subgroup analysis will appear. Furthermore, as the new molecular characterization in MBs remains independent and difficult to match with the histological data, we face problems of overlapping associations. That is the case for desmoplastic/nodular MB and MBEN, subtypes of the SHH group [130].

The new era in molecular-based medulloblastoma prognosis and stratification has arrived. It remains to be seen, while awaiting the first sets of data from the ongoing relevant clinical trials, how translational research can be integrated into clinical practice to balance survival with quality of survival.

Funding: This research received no external funding.

Conflicts of Interest: The authors declare no conflict of interest.

References

1. Smoll, N.R.; Drummond, K.J. The incidence of medulloblastomas and primitive neurectodermal tumours in adults and children. *J. Clin. Neurosci.* **2012**, *19*, 1541–1544. [CrossRef]
2. Salari, N.; Ghasemi, H.; Fatahian, R.; Mansouri, K.; Dokaneheifard, S.; Shiri, M.H.; Hemmati, M.; Mohammadi, M. The global prevalence of primary central nervous system tumors: A systematic review and meta-analysis. *Eur. J. Med. Res.* **2023**, *28*, 39. [CrossRef] [PubMed]
3. Massimino, M.; Biassoni, V.; Gandola, L.; Garrè, M.L.; Gatta, G.; Giangaspero, F.; Poggi, G.; Rutkowski, S. Childhood medulloblastoma. *Crit. Rev. Oncol. Hematol.* **2016**, *105*, 35–51. [CrossRef] [PubMed]
4. Millard, N.E.; De Braganca, K.C. Medulloblastoma. *J. Child Neurol.* **2016**, *31*, 1341–1353. [CrossRef] [PubMed]
5. Smith, K.S.; Bihannic, L.; Gudenas, B.L.; Haldipur, P.; Tao, R.; Gao, Q.; Li, Y.; Aldinger, K.A.; Iskusnykh, I.Y.; Chizhikov, V.V.; et al. Unified rhombic lip origins of group 3 and group 4 medulloblastoma. *Nature* **2022**, *609*, 1012–1020. [CrossRef]
6. Brandes, A.A.; Paris, M.K. Review of the prognostic factors in medulloblastoma of children and adults. *Crit. Rev. Oncol. Hematol.* **2004**, *50*, 121–128. [CrossRef]
7. Von Bueren, A.O.; Kortmann, R.D.; von Hoff, K.; Friedrich, C.; Mynarek, M.; Müller, K.; Goschzik, T.; Zur Mühlen, A.; Gerber, N.; Warmuth-Metz, M.; et al. Treatment of Children and Adolescents With Metastatic Medulloblastoma and Prognostic Relevance of Clinical and Biologic Parameters. *J. Clin. Oncol.* **2016**, *34*, 4151–4160. [CrossRef]
8. Liu, Y.; Xiao, B.; Li, S.; Liu, J. Risk Factors for Survival in Patients With Medulloblastoma: A Systematic Review and Meta-Analysis. *Front. Oncol.* **2022**, *12*, 827054. [CrossRef] [PubMed]
9. Hennika, T.; Gururangan, S. Childhood medulloblastoma: Current and future treatment strategies. *Expert. Opin. Orphan Drugs* **2015**, *3*, 1299–1317. [CrossRef]
10. Sursal, T.; Ronecker, J.S.; Dicpinigaitis, A.J.; Mohan, A.L.; Tobias, M.E.; Gandhi, C.D.; Jhanwar-Uniyal, M. Molecular Stratification of Medulloblastoma: Clinical Outcomes and Therapeutic Interventions. *Anticancer Res.* **2022**, *42*, 2225–2239. [CrossRef]
11. Tarbell, N.J.; Friedman, H.; Polkinghorn, W.R.; Yock, T.; Zhou, T.; Chen, Z.; Burger, P.; Barnes, P.; Kun, L. High-risk medulloblastoma: A pediatric oncology group randomized trial of chemotherapy before or after radiation therapy (POG 9031). *J. Clin. Oncol.* **2013**, *31*, 2936–2941. [CrossRef] [PubMed]
12. Gilbertson, R.; Wickramasinghe, C.; Hernan, R.; Balaji, V.; Hunt, D.; Jones-Wallace, D.; Crolla, J.; Perry, R.; Lunec, J.; Pearson, A.; et al. Clinical and molecular stratification of disease risk in medulloblastoma. *Br. J. Cancer* **2001**, *85*, 705–712. [CrossRef] [PubMed]
13. Kool, M.; Korshunov, A.; Remke, M.; Jones, D.T.; Schlanstein, M.; Northcott, P.A.; Cho, Y.J.; Koster, J.; Schouten-van Meeteren, A.; van Vuurden, D.; et al. Molecular subgroups of medulloblastoma: An international meta-analysis of transcriptome, genetic aberrations, and clinical data of WNT, SHH, Group 3, and Group 4 medulloblastomas. *Acta Neuropathol.* **2012**, *123*, 473–484. [CrossRef] [PubMed]
14. Kool, M.; Koster, J.; Bunt, J.; Hasselt, N.E.; Lakeman, A.; Van Sluis, P.; Troost, D.; Meeteren, N.S.-V.; Caron, H.N.; Cloos, J.; et al. Integrated Genomics Identifies Five Medulloblastoma Subtypes with Distinct Genetic Profiles, Pathway Signatures and Clinicopathological Features. *PLoS ONE* **2008**, *3*, e3088. [CrossRef] [PubMed]
15. Gibson, P.; Tong, Y.; Robinson, G.; Thompson, M.C.; Currle, D.S.; Eden, C.; Kranenburg, T.A.; Hogg, T.; Poppleton, H.; Martin, J.; et al. Subtypes of medulloblastoma have distinct developmental origins. *Nature* **2010**, *468*, 1095–1099. [CrossRef]
16. Sharma, T.; Schwalbe, E.C.; Williamson, D.; Sill, M.; Hovestadt, V.; Mynarek, M.; Rutkowski, S.; Robinson, G.W.; Gajjar, A.; Cavalli, F.; et al. Second-generation molecular subgrouping of medulloblastoma: An international meta-analysis of Group 3 and Group 4 subtypes. *Acta Neuropathol.* **2019**, *138*, 309–326. [CrossRef]
17. Louis, D.N.; Perry, A.; Reifenberger, G.; von Deimling, A.; Figarella-Branger, D.; Cavenee, W.K.; Ohgaki, H.; Wiestler, O.D.; Kleihues, P.; Ellison, D.W. The 2016 World Health Organization Classification of Tumors of the Central Nervous System: A summary. *Acta Neuropathol.* **2016**, *131*, 803–820. [CrossRef]
18. Perreault, S.; Ramaswamy, V.; Achrol, A.S.; Chao, K.; Liu, T.T.; Shih, D.; Remke, M.; Schubert, S.; Bouffet, E.; Fisher, P.G.; et al. MRI surrogates for molecular subgroups of medulloblastoma. *AJNR Am. J. Neuroradiol.* **2014**, *35*, 1263–1269. [CrossRef]
19. Williamson, D.; Schwalbe, E.C.; Hicks, D.; Aldinger, K.A.; Lindsey, J.C.; Crosier, S.; Richardson, S.; Goddard, J.; Hill, R.M.; Castle, J.; et al. Medulloblastoma group 3 and 4 tumors comprise a clinically and biologically significant expression continuum reflecting human cerebellar development. *Cell Rep.* **2022**, *40*, 111162. [CrossRef]

20. Northcott, P.A.; Shih, D.J.H.; Peacock, J.; Garzia, L.; Sorana Morrissy, A.; Zichner, T.; Stütz, A.M.; Korshunov, A.; Reimand, J.; Schumacher, S.E.; et al. Subgroup-specific structural variation across 1000 medulloblastoma genomes. *Nature* **2012**, *488*, 49–56. [CrossRef]
21. Louis, D.N.; Perry, A.; Wesseling, P.; Brat, D.J.; Cree, I.A.; Figarella-Branger, D.; Hawkins, C.; Ng, H.K.; Pfister, S.M.; Reifenberger, G.; et al. The 2021 WHO Classification of Tumors of the Central Nervous System: A summary. *Neuro Oncol.* **2021**, *23*, 1231–1251. [CrossRef] [PubMed]
22. Guo, C.; Yao, D.; Lin, X.; Huang, H.; Zhang, J.; Lin, F.; Mou, Y.; Yang, Q. External Validation of a Nomogram and Risk Grouping System for Predicting Individual Prognosis of Patients With Medulloblastoma. *Front. Pharm.* **2020**, *11*, 590348. [CrossRef] [PubMed]
23. Borowska, A.; Jóźwiak, J. Medulloblastoma: Molecular pathways and histopathological classification. *Arch. Med. Sci.* **2016**, *12*, 659–666. [CrossRef] [PubMed]
24. Hagel, C.; Sloman, V.; Mynarek, M.; Petrasch, K.; Obrecht, D.; Kühl, J.; Deinlein, F.; Schmid, R.; von Bueren, A.O.; Friedrich, C.; et al. Refining M1 stage in medulloblastoma: Criteria for cerebrospinal fluid cytology and implications for improved risk stratification from the HIT-2000 trial. *Eur. J. Cancer* **2022**, *164*, 30–38. [CrossRef] [PubMed]
25. Lafay-Cousin, L.; Smith, A.; Chi, S.N.; Wells, E.; Madden, J.; Margol, A.; Ramaswamy, V.; Finlay, J.; Taylor, M.D.; Dhall, G.; et al. Clinical, Pathological, and Molecular Characterization of Infant Medulloblastomas Treated with Sequential High-Dose Chemotherapy. *Pediatr. Blood Cancer* **2016**, *63*, 1527–1534. [CrossRef]
26. Rutkowski, S.; von Hoff, K.; Emser, A.; Zwiener, I.; Pietsch, T.; Figarella-Branger, D.; Giangaspero, F.; Ellison, D.W.; Garre, M.L.; Biassoni, V.; et al. Survival and prognostic factors of early childhood medulloblastoma: An international meta-analysis. *J. Clin. Oncol.* **2010**, *28*, 4961–4968. [CrossRef]
27. Johnston, D.L.; Keene, D.; Bartels, U.; Carret, A.S.; Crooks, B.; Eisenstat, D.D.; Fryer, C.; Lafay-Cousin, L.; Larouche, V.; Moghrabi, A.; et al. Medulloblastoma in children under the age of three years: A retrospective Canadian review. *J. Neurooncol.* **2009**, *94*, 51–56. [CrossRef]
28. Bleil, C.B.; Bizzi, J.W.J.; Bedin, A.; de Oliveira, F.H.; Antunes, Á.C.M. Survival and prognostic factors in childhood medulloblastoma: A Brazilian single center experience from 1995 to 2016. *Surg. Neurol. Int.* **2019**, *10*, 120. [CrossRef]
29. Walter, A.W.; Mulhern, R.K.; Gajjar, A.; Heideman, R.L.; Reardon, D.; Sanford, R.A.; Xiong, X.; Kun, L.E. Survival and neurodevelopmental outcome of young children with medulloblastoma at St Jude Children's Research Hospital. *J. Clin. Oncol.* **1999**, *17*, 3720–3728. [CrossRef]
30. Franceschi, E.; Giannini, C.; Furtner, J.; Pajtler, K.W.; Asioli, S.; Guzman, R.; Seidel, C.; Gatto, L.; Hau, P. Adult Medulloblastoma: Updates on Current Management and Future Perspectives. *Cancers* **2022**, *14*, 3708. [CrossRef]
31. Dufour, C.; Beaugrand, A.; Pizer, B.; Micheli, J.; Aubelle, M.S.; Fourcade, D.; Couanet, D.; Laplanche, A.; Kalifa, C.; Grill, J. Metastatic Medulloblastoma in Childhood: Chang's Classification Revisited. *Int. J. Surg. Oncol.* **2012**, *2012*, 245385. [CrossRef] [PubMed]
32. Chang, C.H.; Housepian, E.M.; Herbert, C., Jr. An operative staging system and a megavoltage radiotherapeutic technic for cerebellar medulloblastomas. *Radiology* **1969**, *93*, 1351–1359. [CrossRef] [PubMed]
33. Jiang, T.; Zhang, Y.; Wang, J.; Du, J.; Ma, Z.; Li, C.; Liu, R.; Zhang, Y. Impact of tumor location and fourth ventricle infiltration in medulloblastoma. *Acta Neurochir.* **2016**, *158*, 1187–1195. [CrossRef] [PubMed]
34. Zeltzer, P.M.; Boyett, J.M.; Finlay, J.L.; Albright, A.L.; Rorke, L.B.; Milstein, J.M.; Allen, J.C.; Stevens, K.R.; Stanley, P.; Li, H.; et al. Metastasis stage, adjuvant treatment, and residual tumor are prognostic factors for medulloblastoma in children: Conclusions from the Children's Cancer Group 921 randomized phase III study. *J. Clin. Oncol.* **1999**, *17*, 832–845. [CrossRef]
35. Qin, Q.; Huang, D.; Jiang, Y. Survival difference between brainstem and cerebellum medulloblastoma: The surveillance, epidemiology, and end results-based study. *Medicine* **2020**, *99*, e22366. [CrossRef]
36. Kumar, L.P.; Deepa, S.F.; Moinca, I.; Suresh, P.; Naidu, K.V. Medulloblastoma: A common pediatric tumor: Prognostic factors and predictors of outcome. *Asian J. Neurosurg.* **2015**, *10*, 50. [CrossRef]
37. Nalita, N.; Ratanalert, S.; Kanjanapradit, K.; Chotsampancharoen, T.; Tunthanathip, T. Survival and Prognostic Factors in Pediatric Patients with Medulloblastoma in Southern Thailand. *J. Pediatr. Neurosci.* **2018**, *13*, 150–157. [CrossRef]
38. Sanders, R.P.; Onar, A.; Boyett, J.M.; Broniscer, A.; Morris, E.B.; Qaddoumi, I.; Armstrong, G.T.; Boop, F.A.; Sanford, R.A.; Kun, L.E.; et al. M1 Medulloblastoma: High risk at any age. *J. Neurooncol.* **2008**, *90*, 351–355. [CrossRef]
39. Hoff, K.V.; Hinkes, B.; Gerber, N.U.; Deinlein, F.; Mittler, U.; Urban, C.; Benesch, M.; Warmuth-Metz, M.; Soerensen, N.; Zwiener, I.; et al. Long-term outcome and clinical prognostic factors in children with medulloblastoma treated in the prospective randomised multicentre trial HIT'91. *Eur. J. Cancer* **2009**, *45*, 1209–1217. [CrossRef]
40. Dietzsch, S.; Placzek, F.; Pietschmann, K.; von Bueren, A.O.; Matuschek, C.; Glück, A.; Guckenberger, M.; Budach, V.; Welzel, J.; Pöttgen, C.; et al. Evaluation of Prognostic Factors and Role of Participation in a Randomized Trial or a Prospective Registry in Pediatric and Adolescent Nonmetastatic Medulloblastoma—A Report From the HIT 2000 Trial. *Adv. Radiat. Oncol.* **2020**, *5*, 1158–1169. [CrossRef]
41. Ramaswamy, V.; Remke, M.; Bouffet, E.; Bailey, S.; Clifford, S.C.; Doz, F.; Kool, M.; Dufour, C.; Vassal, G.; Milde, T.; et al. Risk stratification of childhood medulloblastoma in the molecular era: The current consensus. *Acta Neuropathol.* **2016**, *131*, 821–831. [CrossRef] [PubMed]

42. Thompson, E.M.; Bramall, A.; Herndon, J.E., 2nd; Taylor, M.D.; Ramaswamy, V. The clinical importance of medulloblastoma extent of resection: A systematic review. *J. Neurooncol.* **2018**, *139*, 523–539. [CrossRef] [PubMed]
43. Thompson, E.M.; Hielscher, T.; Bouffet, E.; Remke, M.; Luu, B.; Gururangan, S.; McLendon, R.E.; Bigner, D.D.; Lipp, E.S.; Perreault, S.; et al. Prognostic value of medulloblastoma extent of resection after accounting for molecular subgroup: A retrospective integrated clinical and molecular analysis. *Lancet Oncol.* **2016**, *17*, 484–495. [CrossRef]
44. Sedano, P.; Segundo, C.G.; De Ingunza, L.; Cuesta-Álvaro, P.; Pérez-Somarriba, M.; Diaz-Gutiérrez, F.; Colino, C.G.; Lassaletta, A. Real-world data for pediatric medulloblastoma: Can we improve outcomes? *Eur. J. Pediatr.* **2021**, *180*, 127–136. [CrossRef]
45. Massimino, M.; Antonelli, M.; Gandola, L.; Miceli, R.; Pollo, B.; Biassoni, V.; Schiavello, E.; Buttarelli, F.R.; Spreafico, F.; Collini, P.; et al. Histological variants of medulloblastoma are the most powerful clinical prognostic indicators. *Pediatr. Blood Cancer* **2013**, *60*, 210–216. [CrossRef]
46. Orr, B.A. Pathology, diagnostics, and classification of medulloblastoma. *Brain Pathol.* **2020**, *30*, 664–678. [CrossRef] [PubMed]
47. Korshunov, A.; Sahm, F.; Stichel, D.; Schrimpf, D.; Ryzhova, M.; Zheludkova, O.; Golanov, A.; Lichter, P.; Jones, D.T.W.; von Deimling, A.; et al. Molecular characterization of medulloblastomas with extensive nodularity (MBEN). *Acta Neuropathol.* **2018**, *136*, 303–313. [CrossRef]
48. Leary, S.E.; Zhou, T.; Holmes, E.; Geyer, J.R.; Miller, D.C. Histology predicts a favorable outcome in young children with desmoplastic medulloblastoma: A report from the children's oncology group. *Cancer* **2011**, *117*, 3262–3267. [CrossRef]
49. Gupta, T.; Dasgupta, A.; Epari, S.; Shirsat, N.; Chinnaswamy, G.; Jalali, R. Extraneuraxial metastases in medulloblastoma: Is histology and molecular biology important? *J. Neurooncol.* **2017**, *135*, 419–421. [CrossRef]
50. Roussel, M.F.; Robinson, G.W. Role of MYC in Medulloblastoma. *Cold Spring Harb. Perspect. Med.* **2013**, *3*, a014308. [CrossRef]
51. von Hoff, K.; Hartmann, W.; von Bueren, A.O.; Gerber, N.U.; Grotzer, M.A.; Pietsch, T.; Rutkowski, S. Large cell/anaplastic medulloblastoma: Outcome according to myc status, histopathological, and clinical risk factors. *Pediatr. Blood Cancer* **2010**, *54*, 369–376. [CrossRef] [PubMed]
52. Eberhart, C.G.; Kratz, J.; Wang, Y.; Summers, K.; Stearns, D.; Cohen, K.; Dang, C.V.; Burger, P.C. Histopathological and molecular prognostic markers in medulloblastoma: C-myc, N-myc, TrkC, and anaplasia. *J. Neuropathol. Exp. Neurol.* **2004**, *63*, 441–449. [CrossRef] [PubMed]
53. Ellison, D.W.; Kocak, M.; Dalton, J.; Megahed, H.; Lusher, M.E.; Ryan, S.L.; Zhao, W.; Nicholson, S.L.; Taylor, R.E.; Bailey, S.; et al. Definition of disease-risk stratification groups in childhood medulloblastoma using combined clinical, pathologic, and molecular variables. *J. Clin. Oncol.* **2011**, *29*, 1400–1407. [CrossRef] [PubMed]
54. Ryan, S.L.; Schwalbe, E.C.; Cole, M.; Lu, Y.; Lusher, M.E.; Megahed, H.; O'Toole, K.; Nicholson, S.L.; Bognar, L.; Garami, M.; et al. MYC family amplification and clinical risk-factors interact to predict an extremely poor prognosis in childhood medulloblastoma. *Acta Neuropathol.* **2012**, *123*, 501–513. [CrossRef] [PubMed]
55. Li, K.; Duan, W.-C.; Zhao, H.-B.; Wang, L.; Wang, W.-W.; Zhan, Y.-B.; Sun, T.; Zhang, F.-J.; Yu, B.; Bai, Y.-H.; et al. Preoperative Neutrophil to Lymphocyte Ratio and Platelet to Lymphocyte Ratio are Associated with the Prognosis of Group 3 and Group 4 Medulloblastoma. *Sci. Rep.* **2019**, *9*, 13239. [CrossRef]
56. Grassberger, C.; Shinnick, D.; Yeap, B.Y.; Tracy, M.; Ellsworth, S.G.; Hess, C.B.; Weyman, E.A.; Gallotto, S.L.; Lawell, M.P.; Bajaj, B.; et al. Circulating Lymphocyte Counts Early During Radiation Therapy Are Associated With Recurrence in Pediatric Medulloblastoma. *Int. J. Radiat. Oncol. Biol. Phys.* **2021**, *110*, 1044–1052. [CrossRef]
57. Zhu, S.; Cheng, Z.; Hu, Y.; Chen, Z.; Zhang, J.; Ke, C.; Yang, Q.; Lin, F.; Chen, Y.; Wang, J. Prognostic Value of the Systemic Immune-Inflammation Index and Prognostic Nutritional Index in Patients With Medulloblastoma Undergoing Surgical Resection. *Front. Nutr.* **2021**, *8*, 754958. [CrossRef]
58. Dasgupta, A.; Gupta, T.; Pungavkar, S.; Shirsat, N.; Epari, S.; Chinnaswamy, G.; Mahajan, A.; Janu, A.; Moiyadi, A.; Kannan, S.; et al. Nomograms based on preoperative multiparametric magnetic resonance imaging for prediction of molecular subgrouping in medulloblastoma: Results from a radiogenomics study of 111 patients. *Neuro Oncol.* **2019**, *21*, 115–124. [CrossRef]
59. Iv, M.; Zhou, M.; Shpanskaya, K.; Perreault, S.; Wang, Z.; Tranvinh, E.; Lanzman, B.; Vajapeyam, S.; Vitanza, N.A.; Fisher, P.G.; et al. MR Imaging-Based Radiomic Signatures of Distinct Molecular Subgroups of Medulloblastoma. *AJNR Am. J. Neuroradiol.* **2019**, *40*, 154–161. [CrossRef]
60. Zheng, H.; Li, J.; Liu, H.; Wu, C.; Gui, T.; Liu, M.; Zhang, Y.; Duan, S.; Li, Y.; Wang, D. Clinical-MRI radiomics enables the prediction of preoperative cerebral spinal fluid dissemination in children with medulloblastoma. *World J. Surg. Oncol.* **2021**, *19*, 134. [CrossRef]
61. Liu, Z.M.; Zhang, H.; Ge, M.; Hao, X.L.; An, X.; Tian, Y.J. Radiomics signature for the prediction of progression-free survival and radiotherapeutic benefits in pediatric medulloblastoma. *Childs Nerv. Syst.* **2022**, *38*, 1085–1094. [CrossRef] [PubMed]
62. Yan, J.; Zhang, S.; Li, K.K.; Wang, W.; Li, K.; Duan, W.; Yuan, B.; Wang, L.; Liu, L.; Zhan, Y.; et al. Incremental prognostic value and underlying biological pathways of radiomics patterns in medulloblastoma. *EBioMedicine* **2020**, *61*, 103093. [CrossRef] [PubMed]
63. Pietsch, T.; Schmidt, R.; Remke, M.; Korshunov, A.; Hovestadt, V.; Jones, D.T.; Felsberg, J.; Kaulich, K.; Goschzik, T.; Kool, M.; et al. Prognostic significance of clinical, histopathological, and molecular characteristics of medulloblastomas in the prospective HIT2000 multicenter clinical trial cohort. *Acta Neuropathol.* **2014**, *128*, 137–149. [CrossRef] [PubMed]
64. Schüller, U.; Heine, V.M.; Mao, J.; Kho, A.T.; Dillon, A.K.; Han, Y.G.; Huillard, E.; Sun, T.; Ligon, A.H.; Qian, Y.; et al. Acquisition of granule neuron precursor identity is a critical determinant of progenitor cell competence to form Shh-induced medulloblastoma. *Cancer Cell* **2008**, *14*, 123–134. [CrossRef] [PubMed]

65. Northcott, P.A.; Jones, D.T.; Kool, M.; Robinson, G.W.; Gilbertson, R.J.; Cho, Y.J.; Pomeroy, S.L.; Korshunov, A.; Lichter, P.; Taylor, M.D.; et al. Medulloblastomics: The end of the beginning. *Nat. Rev. Cancer* **2012**, *12*, 818–834. [CrossRef]
66. Taylor, M.D.; Northcott, P.A.; Korshunov, A.; Remke, M.; Cho, Y.J.; Clifford, S.C.; Eberhart, C.G.; Parsons, D.W.; Rutkowski, S.; Gajjar, A.; et al. Molecular subgroups of medulloblastoma: The current consensus. *Acta Neuropathol.* **2012**, *123*, 465–472. [CrossRef]
67. Parsons, D.W.; Li, M.; Zhang, X.; Jones, S.; Leary, R.J.; Lin, J.C.; Boca, S.M.; Carter, H.; Samayoa, J.; Bettegowda, C.; et al. The genetic landscape of the childhood cancer medulloblastoma. *Science* **2011**, *331*, 435–439. [CrossRef]
68. Menyhárt, O.; Győrffy, B. Molecular stratifications, biomarker candidates and new therapeutic options in current medulloblastoma treatment approaches. *Cancer Metastasis Rev.* **2020**, *39*, 211–233. [CrossRef]
69. Schwalbe, E.C.; Lindsey, J.C.; Nakjang, S.; Crosier, S.; Smith, A.J.; Hicks, D.; Rafiee, G.; Hill, R.M.; Iliasova, A.; Stone, T.; et al. Novel molecular subgroups for clinical classification and outcome prediction in childhood medulloblastoma: A cohort study. *Lancet Oncol.* **2017**, *18*, 958–971. [CrossRef]
70. Cavalli, F.M.G.; Remke, M.; Rampasek, L.; Peacock, J.; Shih, D.J.H.; Luu, B.; Garzia, L.; Torchia, J.; Nor, C.; Morrissy, A.S.; et al. Intertumoral Heterogeneity within Medulloblastoma Subgroups. *Cancer Cell* **2017**, *31*, 737–754. [CrossRef]
71. Northcott, P.A.; Buchhalter, I.; Morrissy, A.S.; Hovestadt, V.; Weischenfeldt, J.; Ehrenberger, T.; Gröbner, S.; Segura-Wang, M.; Zichner, T.; Rudneva, V.A.; et al. The whole-genome landscape of medulloblastoma subtypes. *Nature* **2017**, *547*, 311–317. [CrossRef] [PubMed]
72. Robinson, G.W.; Rudneva, V.A.; Buchhalter, I.; Billups, C.A.; Waszak, S.M.; Smith, K.S.; Bowers, D.C.; Bendel, A.; Fisher, P.G.; Partap, S.; et al. Risk-adapted therapy for young children with medulloblastoma (SJYC07): Therapeutic and molecular outcomes from a multicentre, phase 2 trial. *Lancet Oncol.* **2018**, *19*, 768–784. [CrossRef] [PubMed]
73. Robinson, G.W.; Orr, B.A.; Wu, G.; Gururangan, S.; Lin, T.; Qaddoumi, I.; Packer, R.J.; Goldman, S.; Prados, M.D.; Desjardins, A.; et al. Vismodegib Exerts Targeted Efficacy Against Recurrent Sonic Hedgehog-Subgroup Medulloblastoma: Results From Phase II Pediatric Brain Tumor Consortium Studies PBTC-025B and PBTC-032. *J. Clin. Oncol.* **2015**, *33*, 2646–2654. [CrossRef] [PubMed]
74. Robinson, G.; Parker, M.; Kranenburg, T.A.; Lu, C.; Chen, X.; Ding, L.; Phoenix, T.N.; Hedlund, E.; Wei, L.; Zhu, X.; et al. Novel mutations target distinct subgroups of medulloblastoma. *Nature* **2012**, *488*, 43–48. [CrossRef]
75. Gröbner, S.N.; Worst, B.C.; Weischenfeldt, J.; Buchhalter, I.; Kleinheinz, K.; Rudneva, V.A.; Johann, P.D.; Balasubramanian, G.P.; Segura-Wang, M.; Brabetz, S.; et al. The landscape of genomic alterations across childhood cancers. *Nature* **2018**, *555*, 321–327. [CrossRef]
76. Menyhárt, O.; Győrffy, B. Principles of tumorigenesis and emerging molecular drivers of SHH-activated medulloblastomas. *Ann. Clin. Transl. Neurol.* **2019**, *6*, 990–1005. [CrossRef]
77. DeSouza, R.M.; Jones, B.R.; Lowis, S.P.; Kurian, K.M. Pediatric medulloblastoma—Update on molecular classification driving targeted therapies. *Front. Oncol.* **2014**, *4*, 176. [CrossRef]
78. Gajjar, A.; Robinson, G.W.; Smith, K.S.; Lin, T.; Merchant, T.E.; Chintagumpala, M.; Mahajan, A.; Su, J.; Bouffet, E.; Bartels, U.; et al. Outcomes by Clinical and Molecular Features in Children With Medulloblastoma Treated With Risk-Adapted Therapy: Results of an International Phase III Trial (SJMB03). *J. Clin. Oncol.* **2021**, *39*, 822–835. [CrossRef]
79. Shrestha, S.; Morcavallo, A.; Gorrini, C.; Chesler, L. Biological Role of MYCN in Medulloblastoma: Novel Therapeutic Opportunities and Challenges Ahead. *Front. Oncol.* **2021**, *11*, 694320. [CrossRef]
80. Rausch, T.; Jones, D.T.; Zapatka, M.; Stütz, A.M.; Zichner, T.; Weischenfeldt, J.; Jäger, N.; Remke, M.; Shih, D.; Northcott, P.A.; et al. Genome sequencing of pediatric medulloblastoma links catastrophic DNA rearrangements with TP53 mutations. *Cell* **2012**, *148*, 59–71. [CrossRef]
81. Bosse, K.R.; Maris, J.M. Advances in the translational genomics of neuroblastoma: From improving risk stratification and revealing novel biology to identifying actionable genomic alterations. *Cancer* **2016**, *122*, 20–33. [CrossRef] [PubMed]
82. Heinlein, C.; Krepulat, F.; Löhler, J.; Speidel, D.; Deppert, W.; Tolstonog, G.V. Mutant p53(R270H) gain of function phenotype in a mouse model for oncogene-induced mammary carcinogenesis. *Int. J. Cancer* **2008**, *122*, 1701–1709. [CrossRef] [PubMed]
83. Olive, K.P.; Tuveson, D.A.; Ruhe, Z.C.; Yin, B.; Willis, N.A.; Bronson, R.T.; Crowley, D.; Jacks, T. Mutant p53 gain of function in two mouse models of Li-Fraumeni syndrome. *Cell* **2004**, *119*, 847–860. [CrossRef]
84. Korshunov, A.; Remke, M.; Kool, M.; Hielscher, T.; Northcott, P.A.; Williamson, D.; Pfaff, E.; Witt, H.; Jones, D.T.; Ryzhova, M.; et al. Biological and clinical heterogeneity of MYCN-amplified medulloblastoma. *Acta Neuropathol.* **2012**, *123*, 515–527. [CrossRef] [PubMed]
85. Zhukova, N.; Ramaswamy, V.; Remke, M.; Pfaff, E.; Shih, D.J.; Martin, D.C.; Castelo-Branco, P.; Baskin, B.; Ray, P.N.; Bouffet, E.; et al. Subgroup-specific prognostic implications of TP53 mutation in medulloblastoma. *J. Clin. Oncol.* **2013**, *31*, 2927–2935. [CrossRef]
86. Martin, A.M.; Raabe, E.; Eberhart, C.; Cohen, K.J. Management of pediatric and adult patients with medulloblastoma. *Curr. Treat. Options Oncol.* **2014**, *15*, 581–594. [CrossRef]
87. Schwalbe, E.C.; Williamson, D.; Lindsey, J.C.; Hamilton, D.; Ryan, S.L.; Megahed, H.; Garami, M.; Hauser, P.; Dembowska-Baginska, B.; Perek, D.; et al. DNA methylation profiling of medulloblastoma allows robust subclassification and improved outcome prediction using formalin-fixed biopsies. *Acta Neuropathol.* **2013**, *125*, 359–371. [CrossRef]

88. Pizer, B.L.; Clifford, S.C. The potential impact of tumour biology on improved clinical practice for medulloblastoma: Progress towards biologically driven clinical trials. *Br. J. Neurosurg.* **2009**, *23*, 364–375. [CrossRef]
89. Hamam, S.M.; Abdelzaher, E.; Fadel, S.H.; Nassra, R.A.; Sharafeldin, H.A. Prognostic value of microRNA-125a expression status in molecular groups of pediatric medulloblastoma. *Childs Nerv. Syst.* **2023**. [CrossRef]
90. Jiang, D.; Zhao, N. A clinical prognostic prediction of lymph node-negative breast cancer by gene expression profiles. *J. Cancer Res. Clin. Oncol.* **2006**, *132*, 579–587. [CrossRef]
91. Shen, J.; Stass, S.A.; Jiang, F. MicroRNAs as potential biomarkers in human solid tumors. *Cancer Lett.* **2013**, *329*, 125–136. [CrossRef] [PubMed]
92. Ashby, J.; Flack, K.; Jimenez, L.A.; Duan, Y.; Khatib, A.K.; Somlo, G.; Wang, S.E.; Cui, X.; Zhong, W. Distribution profiling of circulating microRNAs in serum. *Anal. Chem.* **2014**, *86*, 9343–9349. [CrossRef] [PubMed]
93. Arroyo, J.D.; Chevillet, J.R.; Kroh, E.M.; Ruf, I.K.; Pritchard, C.C.; Gibson, D.F.; Mitchell, P.S.; Bennett, C.F.; Pogosova-Agadjanyan, E.L.; Stirewalt, D.L.; et al. Argonaute2 complexes carry a population of circulating microRNAs independent of vesicles in human plasma. *Proc. Natl. Acad. Sci. USA* **2011**, *108*, 5003–5008. [CrossRef]
94. Qu, H.; Xu, W.; Huang, Y.; Yang, S. Circulating miRNAs: Promising biomarkers of human cancer. *Asian Pac. J. Cancer Prev.* **2011**, *12*, 1117–1125.
95. Laneve, P.; Po, A.; Favia, A.; Legnini, I.; Alfano, V.; Rea, J.; Di Carlo, V.; Bevilacqua, V.; Miele, E.; Mastronuzzi, A.; et al. The long noncoding RNA linc-NeD125 controls the expression of medulloblastoma driver genes by microRNA sponge activity. *Oncotarget* **2017**, *8*, 31003–31015. [CrossRef] [PubMed]
96. Li, W.; Jin, X.; Zhang, Q.; Zhang, G.; Deng, X.; Ma, L. Decreased expression of miR-204 is associated with poor prognosis in patients with breast cancer. *Int. J. Clin. Exp. Pathol.* **2014**, *7*, 3287–3292. [PubMed]
97. Bharambe, H.S.; Paul, R.; Panwalkar, P.; Jalali, R.; Sridhar, E.; Gupta, T.; Moiyadi, A.; Shetty, P.; Kazi, S.; Deogharkar, A.; et al. Downregulation of miR-204 expression defines a highly aggressive subset of Group 3/Group 4 medulloblastomas. *Acta Neuropathol. Commun.* **2019**, *7*, 52. [CrossRef] [PubMed]
98. Venkataraman, S.; Alimova, I.; Fan, R.; Harris, P.; Foreman, N.; Vibhakar, R. MicroRNA 128a increases intracellular ROS level by targeting Bmi-1 and inhibits medulloblastoma cancer cell growth by promoting senescence. *PLoS ONE* **2010**, *5*, e10748. [CrossRef]
99. Weeraratne, S.D.; Amani, V.; Teider, N.; Pierre-Francois, J.; Winter, D.; Kye, M.J.; Sengupta, S.; Archer, T.; Remke, M.; Bai, A.H.; et al. Pleiotropic effects of miR-183~96~182 converge to regulate cell survival, proliferation and migration in medulloblastoma. *Acta Neuropathol.* **2012**, *123*, 539–552. [CrossRef]
100. Latowska, J.; Grabowska, A.; Zarębska, Ż.; Kuczyński, K.; Kuczyńska, B.; Rolle, K. Non-coding RNAs in Brain Tumors, the Contribution of lncRNAs, circRNAs, and snoRNAs to Cancer Development-Their Diagnostic and Therapeutic Potential. *Int. J. Mol. Sci.* **2020**, *21*, 7001. [CrossRef]
101. Kesherwani, V.; Shukla, M.; Coulter, D.W.; Sharp, J.G.; Joshi, S.S.; Chaturvedi, N.K. Long non-coding RNA profiling of pediatric Medulloblastoma. *BMC Med. Genomics* **2020**, *13*, 87. [CrossRef]
102. Gao, R.; Zhang, R.; Zhang, C.; Liang, Y.; Tang, W. LncRNA LOXL1-AS1 Promotes the Proliferation and Metastasis of Medulloblastoma by Activating the PI3K/AKT Pathway. *Anal. Cell Pathol.* **2018**, *2018*, 9275685. [CrossRef]
103. Gao, R.; Zhang, R.; Zhang, C.; Zhao, L.; Zhang, Y. Long noncoding RNA CCAT1 promotes cell proliferation and metastasis in human medulloblastoma via MAPK pathway. *Tumori* **2018**, *104*, 43–50. [CrossRef] [PubMed]
104. Zhang, J.; Li, N.; Fu, J.; Zhou, W. Long noncoding RNA HOTAIR promotes medulloblastoma growth, migration and invasion by sponging miR-1/miR-206 and targeting YY1. *Biomed. Pharm.* **2020**, *124*, 109887. [CrossRef] [PubMed]
105. Joshi, P.; Jallo, G.; Perera, R.J. In silico analysis of long non-coding RNAs in medulloblastoma and its subgroups. *Neurobiol. Dis.* **2020**, *141*, 104873. [CrossRef] [PubMed]
106. Lee, B.; Katsushima, K.; Pokhrel, R.; Yuan, M.; Stapleton, S.; Jallo, G.; Wechsler-Reya, R.J.; Eberhart, C.G.; Ray, A.; Perera, R.J. The long non-coding RNA SPRIGHTLY and its binding partner PTBP1 regulate exon 5 skipping of SMYD3 transcripts in group 4 medulloblastomas. *Neurooncol. Adv.* **2022**, *4*, vdac120. [CrossRef]
107. Hill, R.M.; Plasschaert, S.L.A.; Timmermann, B.; Dufour, C.; Aquilina, K.; Avula, S.; Donovan, L.; Lequin, M.; Pietsch, T.; Thomale, U.; et al. Relapsed Medulloblastoma in Pre-Irradiated Patients: Current Practice for Diagnostics and Treatment. *Cancers* **2021**, *14*, 126. [CrossRef]
108. Hill, R.M.; Richardson, S.; Schwalbe, E.C.; Hicks, D.; Lindsey, J.C.; Crosier, S.; Rafiee, G.; Grabovska, Y.; Wharton, S.B.; Jacques, T.S.; et al. Time, pattern, and outcome of medulloblastoma relapse and their association with tumour biology at diagnosis and therapy: A multicentre cohort study. *Lancet Child Adolesc. Health* **2020**, *4*, 865–874. [CrossRef]
109. Sabel, M.; Fleischhack, G.; Tippelt, S.; Gustafsson, G.; Doz, F.; Kortmann, R.; Massimino, M.; Navajas, A.; von Hoff, K.; Rutkowski, S.; et al. Relapse patterns and outcome after relapse in standard risk medulloblastoma: A report from the HIT-SIOP-PNET4 study. *J. Neurooncol.* **2016**, *129*, 515–524. [CrossRef]
110. Huybrechts, S.; Le Teuff, G.; Tauziède-Espariat, A.; Rossoni, C.; Chivet, A.; Indersie, É.; Varlet, P.; Puget, S.; Abbas, R.; Ayrault, O.; et al. Prognostic Clinical and Biologic Features for Overall Survival after Relapse in Childhood Medulloblastoma. *Cancers* **2020**, *13*, 53. [CrossRef]
111. Koschmann, C.; Bloom, K.; Upadhyaya, S.; Geyer, J.R.; Leary, S.E. Survival After Relapse of Medulloblastoma. *J. Pediatr. Hematol. Oncol.* **2016**, *38*, 269–273. [CrossRef] [PubMed]

112. Von Bueren, A.O.; von Hoff, K.; Pietsch, T.; Gerber, N.U.; Warmuth-Metz, M.; Deinlein, F.; Zwiener, I.; Faldum, A.; Fleischhack, G.; Benesch, M.; et al. Treatment of young children with localized medulloblastoma by chemotherapy alone: Results of the prospective, multicenter trial HIT 2000 confirming the prognostic impact of histology. *Neuro Oncol.* **2011**, *13*, 669–679. [CrossRef] [PubMed]
113. Dhall, G.; Grodman, H.; Ji, L.; Sands, S.; Gardner, S.; Dunkel, I.J.; McCowage, G.B.; Diez, B.; Allen, J.C.; Gopalan, A.; et al. Outcome of children less than three years old at diagnosis with non-metastatic medulloblastoma treated with chemotherapy on the "Head Start" I and II protocols. *Pediatr. Blood Cancer* **2008**, *50*, 1169–1175. [CrossRef]
114. Müller, K.; Mynarek, M.; Zwiener, I.; Siegler, N.; Zimmermann, M.; Christiansen, H.; Budach, W.; Henke, G.; Warmuth-Metz, M.; Pietsch, T.; et al. Postponed is not canceled: Role of craniospinal radiation therapy in the management of recurrent infant medulloblastoma—An experience from the HIT-REZ 1997 & 2005 studies. *Int. J. Radiat. Oncol. Biol. Phys.* **2014**, *88*, 1019–1024. [CrossRef] [PubMed]
115. Hicks, D.; Rafiee, G.; Schwalbe, E.C.; Howell, C.I.; Lindsey, J.C.; Hill, R.M.; Smith, A.J.; Adidharma, P.; Steel, C.; Richardson, S.; et al. The molecular landscape and associated clinical experience in infant medulloblastoma: Prognostic significance of second-generation subtypes. *Neuropathol. Appl. Neurobiol.* **2021**, *47*, 236–250. [CrossRef] [PubMed]
116. Mynarek, M.; von Hoff, K.; Pietsch, T.; Ottensmeier, H.; Warmuth-Metz, M.; Bison, B.; Pfister, S.; Korshunov, A.; Sharma, T.; Jaeger, N.; et al. Nonmetastatic Medulloblastoma of Early Childhood: Results From the Prospective Clinical Trial HIT-2000 and An Extended Validation Cohort. *J. Clin. Oncol.* **2020**, *38*, 2028–2040. [CrossRef] [PubMed]
117. Lafay-Cousin, L.; Bouffet, E.; Strother, D.; Rudneva, V.; Hawkins, C.; Eberhart, C.; Horbinski, C.; Heier, L.; Souweidane, M.; Williams-Hughes, C.; et al. Phase II Study of Nonmetastatic Desmoplastic Medulloblastoma in Children Younger Than 4 Years of Age: A Report of the Children's Oncology Group (ACNS1221). *J. Clin. Oncol.* **2020**, *38*, 223–231. [CrossRef]
118. Erker, C.; Mynarek, M.; Bailey, S.; Mazewski, C.M.; Baroni, L.; Massimino, M.; Hukin, J.; Aguilera, D.; Cappellano, A.M.; Ramaswamy, V.; et al. Outcomes of Infants and Young Children With Relapsed Medulloblastoma After Initial Craniospinal Irradiation-Sparing Approaches: An International Cohort Study. *J. Clin. Oncol.* **2023**, *41*, 1921–1932. [CrossRef]
119. Zhao, X.; Liu, Z.; Yu, L.; Zhang, Y.; Baxter, P.; Voicu, H.; Gurusiddappa, S.; Luan, J.; Su, J.M.; Leung, H.C.; et al. Global gene expression profiling confirms the molecular fidelity of primary tumor-based orthotopic xenograft mouse models of medulloblastoma. *Neuro Oncol.* **2012**, *14*, 574–583. [CrossRef]
120. Morrissy, A.S.; Garzia, L.; Shih, D.J.; Zuyderduyn, S.; Huang, X.; Skowron, P.; Remke, M.; Cavalli, F.M.; Ramaswamy, V.; Lindsay, P.E.; et al. Divergent clonal selection dominates medulloblastoma at recurrence. *Nature* **2016**, *529*, 351–357. [CrossRef]
121. Wang, X.; Dubuc, A.M.; Ramaswamy, V.; Mack, S.; Gendoo, D.M.; Remke, M.; Wu, X.; Garzia, L.; Luu, B.; Cavalli, F.; et al. Medulloblastoma subgroups remain stable across primary and metastatic compartments. *Acta Neuropathol.* **2015**, *129*, 449–457. [CrossRef] [PubMed]
122. Kumar, R.; Smith, K.S.; Deng, M.; Terhune, C.; Robinson, G.W.; Orr, B.A.; Liu, A.P.Y.; Lin, T.; Billups, C.A.; Chintagumpala, M.; et al. Clinical Outcomes and Patient-Matched Molecular Composition of Relapsed Medulloblastoma. *J. Clin. Oncol.* **2021**, *39*, 807–821. [CrossRef]
123. Zakrzewska, M.; Rieske, P.; Debiec-Rychter, M.; Zakrzewski, K.; Polis, L.; Fiks, T.; Liberski, P.P. Molecular abnormalities in pediatric embryonal brain tumors–analysis of loss of heterozygosity on chromosomes 1, 5, 9, 10, 11, 16, 17 and 22. *Clin. Neuropathol.* **2004**, *23*, 209–217.
124. Okonechnikov, K.; Federico, A.; Schrimpf, D.; Sievers, P.; Sahm, F.; Koster, J.; Jones, D.T.W.; von Deimling, A.; Pfister, S.M.; Kool, M.; et al. Comparison of transcriptome profiles between medulloblastoma primary and recurrent tumors uncovers novel variance effects in relapses. *Acta Neuropathol. Commun.* **2023**, *11*, 7. [CrossRef] [PubMed]
125. Richardson, S.; Hill, R.M.; Kui, C.; Lindsey, J.C.; Grabovksa, Y.; Keeling, C.; Pease, L.; Bashton, M.; Crosier, S.; Vinci, M.; et al. Emergence and maintenance of actionable genetic drivers at medulloblastoma relapse. *Neuro Oncol.* **2022**, *24*, 153–165. [CrossRef] [PubMed]
126. Hill, R.M.; Kuijper, S.; Lindsey, J.C.; Petrie, K.; Schwalbe, E.C.; Barker, K.; Boult, J.K.; Williamson, D.; Ahmad, Z.; Hallsworth, A.; et al. Combined MYC and P53 defects emerge at medulloblastoma relapse and define rapidly progressive, therapeutically targetable disease. *Cancer Cell* **2015**, *27*, 72–84. [CrossRef]
127. Michalski, J.M.; Janss, A.J.; Vezina, L.G.; Smith, K.S.; Billups, C.A.; Burger, P.C.; Embry, L.M.; Cullen, P.L.; Hardy, K.K.; Pomeroy, S.L.; et al. Children's Oncology Group Phase III Trial of Reduced-Dose and Reduced-Volume Radiotherapy With Chemotherapy for Newly Diagnosed Average-Risk Medulloblastoma. *J. Clin. Oncol.* **2021**, *39*, 2685–2697. [CrossRef]
128. Arthur, C.; Jylhä, C.; de Ståhl, T.D.; Shamikh, A.; Sandgren, J.; Rosenquist, R.; Nordenskjöld, M.; Harila, A.; Barbany, G.; Sandvik, U.; et al. Simultaneous Ultra-Sensitive Detection of Structural and Single Nucleotide Variants Using Multiplex Droplet Digital PCR in Liquid Biopsies from Children with Medulloblastoma. *Cancers* **2023**, *15*, 1972. [CrossRef]

129. Cao, L.; Zhao, Y.; Liang, Z.; Yang, J.; Wang, J.; Tian, S.; Wang, Q.; Wang, B.; Zhao, H.; Jiang, F.; et al. Systematic analysis of MCM3 in pediatric medulloblastoma via multi-omics analysis. *Front. Mol. Biosci.* **2022**, *9*, 815260. [CrossRef]
130. Eibl, R.H.; Schneemann, M. Medulloblastoma: From TP53 Mutations to Molecular Classification and Liquid Biopsy. *Biology* **2023**, *12*, 267. [CrossRef]

Disclaimer/Publisher's Note: The statements, opinions and data contained in all publications are solely those of the individual author(s) and contributor(s) and not of MDPI and/or the editor(s). MDPI and/or the editor(s) disclaim responsibility for any injury to people or property resulting from any ideas, methods, instructions or products referred to in the content.

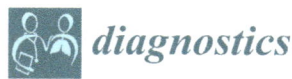

Article

The Prognostic Effect of CDKN2A/2B Gene Deletions in Pediatric Acute Lymphoblastic Leukemia (ALL): Independent Prognostic Significance in BFM-Based Protocols

Mirella Ampatzidou [1,*], Stefanos I. Papadhimitriou [2], Anna Paisiou [3], Georgios Paterakis [4], Marianna Tzanoudaki [5], Vassilios Papadakis [1], Lina Florentin [6] and Sophia Polychronopoulou [1]

[1] Department of Pediatric Hematology-Oncology (TAO), "Aghia Sophia" Children's Hospital, 11527 Athens, Greece
[2] Laboratory of Hematology, Unit of Molecular Cytogenetics, "G. Gennimatas" General Hospital, 11527 Athens, Greece
[3] Bone Marrow Transplantation Unit, "Aghia Sophia" Children's Hospital, 11527 Athens, Greece
[4] Laboratory of Flow Cytometry, Department of Immunology, "G. Gennimatas" General Hospital, 11527 Athens, Greece
[5] Department of Immunology, "Aghia Sophia" Children's Hospital, 11527 Athens, Greece
[6] Alfa Laboratory Diagnostic Center, YGEIA Hospital, 11524 Athens, Greece
* Correspondence: mirellaaba@yahoo.gr

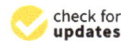

Citation: Ampatzidou, M.; Papadhimitriou, S.I.; Paisiou, A.; Paterakis, G.; Tzanoudaki, M.; Papadakis, V.; Florentin, L.; Polychronopoulou, S. The Prognostic Effect of CDKN2A/2B Gene Deletions in Pediatric Acute Lymphoblastic Leukemia (ALL): Independent Prognostic Significance in BFM-Based Protocols. *Diagnostics* 2023, 13, 1589. https://doi.org/10.3390/diagnostics13091589

Academic Editor: Chung-Che (Jeff) Chang

Received: 31 March 2023
Revised: 21 April 2023
Accepted: 27 April 2023
Published: 28 April 2023

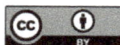

Copyright: © 2023 by the authors. Licensee MDPI, Basel, Switzerland. This article is an open access article distributed under the terms and conditions of the Creative Commons Attribution (CC BY) license (https://creativecommons.org/licenses/by/4.0/).

Abstract: One of the most frequent genes affected in pediatric ALL is the CDKN2A/2B gene, acting as a secondary cooperating event and playing an important role in cell-cycle regulation and chemosensitivity. Despite its inclusion in combined CNA (copy-number alterations) classifiers, like the IKZF1plus entity and the UKALL CNA profile, the prognostic impact of the individual gene deletions outside the context of a combined CNA evaluation remains controversial. Addressing the CDKN2A/2B deletions' additive prognostic effect in current risk-stratification algorithms, we present a retrospective study of a Greek pediatric ALL cohort comprising 247 patients studied over a 24-year period (2000–2023). Herein, we provide insight regarding the correlation with disease features, MRD clearance, and independent prognostic significance for this ALL cohort treated with contemporary BFM-based treatment protocols. Within an extended follow-up time of 135 months, the presence of the CDKN2A/2B deletions (biallelic or monoallelic) was associated with inferior EFS rates (65.1% compared to 91.8% for the gene non-deleted subgroup, $p < 0.001$), with the relapse rate accounting for 22.2% and 5.9%, respectively ($p < 0.001$). The presence of the biallelic deletion was associated with the worst outcomes (EFS 57.2% vs. 89.6% in the case of any other status, monoallelic or non-deleted, $p < 0.001$). Survival differences were demonstrated for B-ALL cases (EFS 65.3% vs. 93.6% for the non-deleted B-ALL subgroup, $p < 0.001$), but the prognostic effect was not statistically significant within the T-ALL cohort (EFS 64.3 vs. 69.2, $p = 0.947$). The presence of the CDKN2A/2B deletions clearly correlated with inferior outcomes within all protocol-defined risk groups (standard risk (SR): EFS 66.7% vs. 100%, $p < 0.001$, intermediate risk (IR): EFS 77.1% vs. 97.9%, $p < 0.001$, high risk (HR): EFS 42.1% vs. 70.5% $p < 0.001$ for deleted vs non-deleted cases in each patient risk group); additionally, in this study, the presence of the deletion differentiated prognosis within both MRD-positive and -negative subgroups on days 15 and 33 of induction. In multivariate analysis, the presence of the CDKN2A/2B deletions was the most important prognostic factor for relapse and overall survival, yielding a hazard ratio of 5.2 (95% confidence interval: 2.59–10.41, $p < 0.001$) and 5.96 (95% confidence interval: 2.97–11.95, $p < 0.001$), respectively, designating the alteration's independent prognostic significance in the context of modern risk stratification. The results of our study demonstrate that the presence of the CDKN2A/2B deletions can further stratify all existing risk groups, identifying patient subgroups with different outcomes. The above biallelic deletions could be incorporated into future risk-stratification algorithms, refining MRD-based stratification. In the era of targeted therapies, future prospective controlled clinical trials will further explore the possible use of cyclin-dependent kinase inhibitors (CDKIs) in CDKN2A/2B-affected ALL pediatric subgroups.

Keywords: acute lymphoblastic leukemia (ALL); child; genetics; CDKN2A/2B deletions; fluorescent in situ hybridization (FISH); multiple-ligation probe amplification (MLPA); copy-number alterations (CNAs); risk stratification; minimal residual disease (MRD)

1. Introduction

Major survival improvements in pediatric acute lymphoblastic leukemia (ALL) have been accomplished through the refinement of the risk-adapted approach [1–3] and MRD-guided treatment [1,3,4], as well as due to the enhanced delineation of the underlying disease biology [5–12]. Apart from the well-established adverse genetic aberrations, like the BCR::ABL1 fusion and KMT2A gene rearrangements, modern therapeutic protocols are currently incorporating the combined evaluation of the copy-number status of selected genes, which may also serve as adverse modifiers [11,13,14]. Hence, although CNA classifiers like the IKZF1plus entity [13] and the UKALL CNA profile [14] are constantly gaining relevance as potential risk-stratification markers [15,16], the prognostic impact of individual single-gene deletions remains controversial in most cases.

One of the genes that has a disputable effect on prognosis in pediatric ALL is the cyclin-dependent kinase inhibitor 2A/2B (CDKN2A/2B), located on the 9p21 chromosomal region and comprising two tumor-suppressor genes lying adjacent to each other, which encode for three proteins: (a) $p16^{INK4A}$ (inhibitor of CDK4), (b) $p14^{ARF}$ (alternative reading frame) by CDKN2A, and (c) $p15^{INK4B}$ by CDKN2B [17]. As a secondary cooperating event, inactivation of the CDKN2A/2B genes can play an important role in leukemogenesis, regulating the cell cycle, chemosensitivity, and apoptosis [17–19].

Although CDKN2A/B deletions are detected in approximately 20–25% of pediatric B-cell precursor (BCP) ALL cases and 38.5–50% of T-ALL patients [19–21], with the percentage rising to more than 80% in cases of B-other and BCR/ABL1-like ALL [22,23], results on the prognostic impact of the biallelic or monoallelic deletion remain inconclusive [24–34]. In addition, the use of cyclin-dependent kinase inhibitors (CDKIs) in CDKN2A/2B-affected ALL pediatric subgroups requires prospective evaluation in the framework of targeted therapies and controlled clinical trials. Herein, we present a retrospective study of a Greek pediatric ALL cohort studied over a 24-year period (2000–2023), with a median follow-up time of 135 months, providing insight regarding the deletion's correlation with disease features and disease clearance and its independent prognostic significance in the context of contemporary BFM-based treatment protocols. Additionally, our study demonstrates that, in the absence of NGS technologies, the combination of iFISH and MLPA could be a simple, feasible, and validated approach for identifying the majority of CDKN2A/2B deletions.

2. Materials and Methods

2.1. Patients

During the years 2000–2023, 247 ALL patients (151 males/96 females, median age 5.0 years (range 0.2–17.5)) were consecutively diagnosed and homogeneously treated according to BFM-based protocols in a single center, the Department of Pediatric Hematology-Oncology (T.A.O.) of "Aghia Sophia" Children's Hospital in Athens, Greece. The diagnosis of B-cell- or T-cell-precursor origin was established according to conventional FAB and immunophenotypic criteria. A total of 220 patients (89.1%) were diagnosed with B-cell-precursor ALL and 27 patients (10.9%) with T-cell-precursor ALL.

2.2. Diagnosis; Morphologic, Molecular, and Cytogenetic Testing

All patients were evaluated by morphology of bone-marrow (BM) smears, histochemistry, immunophenotyping, conventional cytogenetics (G-banding), FISH, and RT-PCR for the presence of common ALL translocations.

2.3. Flow Cytometry (FC)

BM samples were investigated for leukemia-associated immunophenotypes and were assessed by flow-cytometry (FC) using 3–5-color antibody combinations, adapted to the published AIEOP-BFM Consensus Guidelines 2016 for Flow Cytometric Immunophenotyping of Pediatric ALL for patients treated after 2016 [35]. Follow-up samples for minimal-residual-disease (MRD) study were collected from BM at days 15, 33, and 78; weeks 22–24 before initiation; and at the end of maintenance therapy. All high-risk (HR) patients were also evaluated before each HR block. MRD was detected by flow cytometry, initially using 5 colors and, since 2019, 9 and 10 colors for B-ALL and T-ALL phenotypes, respectively. Sample analysis was performed with FC-500 and NAVIOS (Beckman-Coulter, Miami, FL, USA) flow cytometers using CXP-Analysis or Kaluza (versions 1.3 and 2.1) software. For MRD detection, a minimum of 500,000 events was collected with count extrapolation of up to 3,600,000 events if needed. Sensitivity of 0.1 to 0.01% was achieved in most cases, with an acquisition of a minimum of 20 events in the MRD gate.

2.4. G-Banding, FISH, and RT-PCR

Bone-marrow cells were cultured for 24, 48, and 72 h prior to G-banding. A 300-banding resolution technique (300 bands per haploid set—300 bphs) was applied. FISH evaluation using commercial probe sets was performed in non-cultured cells for the detection of ETV6::RUNX1, TCF3::PBX1, and BCR::ABL1 fusion genes; KMT2A gene rearrangements; and CDKN2A/2B, ETV6, and RUNX1 duplications, deletions, or amplifications. Bone-marrow cells were analyzed with interphase FISH according to the probe manufacturer' instructions (Abbott Molecular Inc., Abbott Park, IL, USA). The probe set employed consists of a centromeric probe for chromosome 9, plus a locus-specific identifier, measuring 222 kilobases (kb) and spanning the entire length of CDKN2A (INK4A and ARF) and CDKN2B (INK4B), as well as the entire length of the methylthioadenosine phosphorylase (MTAP) gene in the centromeric direction in the 9p21.3 chromosome region. Based on results from normal bone-marrow smears, the cutoff level for any kind of deletion or monosomy was set to 10%, and at least 300 cells were analyzed in each test. Cases with two different deleted populations (one biallelic and one monoallelic) were classified as having a biallelic deletion.

Ficoll-Hypaque-purified BM samples (Sigma-Aldrich, Saint-Louis, MO, USA, and Merck, Darmstadt, Germany) were studied by RT-PCR for the presence of the common translocations ETV6::RUNX1, TCF3::PBX1, BCR::ABL1, and KMT2A::AFF1.

2.5. MLPA (Multiple-Ligation Probe Amplification)

MLPA (multiple-ligation probe amplification) was applied using the SALSA-MLPA P335 kit (MRC Holland, Amsterdam, the Netherlands). Among the 247 ALL patients consecutively treated in our department (54 SR, 130 IR, 63 HR), BM samples from 95 non-selected patients were MLPA analyzed (retrospective: 45 patients, prospective and consecutively diagnosed since 2015: 50 patients), evaluating the copy-number status detection of 8 genes: IKZF1, CDKN2A/2B, PAR1, BTG1, EBF1, PAX5, ETV6, and RB1. The Salsa-MLPA-P335Kit was used according to the manufacturer's instructions [36,37].

2.6. Conventional Risk Stratification, Therapy Groups, and Treatment Protocol

All patients were treated according to AIEOP-BFM-ALL-based protocols (BFM 1995/2000 and ALLIC-BFM 2009) [38–40]. Initial risk stratification was conducted according to protocol criteria [39,40]. All patients were stratified as good or poor prednisone responders (GPR or PPR) according to peripheral-blood (PB) smears on day 8 of remission-induction therapy (absolute-blast count < or $\geq 1000/\mu L$).

Non-T ALL patients with WBC < 20,000/μL at diagnosis and age ≥ 1 to <6 years who lacked high-risk criteria and had an FC-MRD load on day 15 of <0.1% when treated on the ALLIC-BFM 2009 protocol were characterized as standard-risk (SR) patients according to protocol stratification. The high-risk (HR) group included patients with any of the following: detection of KMT2A/AFF1, detection of BCR/ABL1, poor prednisone response on day +8, inability to achieve complete remission (CR) on day +33, hypodiploidy, and FC-MRD ≥ 10% on day 15 for patients treated on the ALLIC-BFM 2009 protocol. All other patients were allocated to the intermediate-risk (IR) group by protocol stratification.

The remission induction, consolidation, and reinduction therapy was applied according to the BFM backbone, as previously described [41,42], using a two-arm BFM backbone applied before 2009 and following the three-arm ALLIC BFM 2009 stratification afterwards [41–43].

2.7. Statistical Analysis

Event-free survival (EFS) and overall-survival (OS) estimates were calculated using the Kaplan–Meier method and standard errors of the estimates were calculated using Greenwood's formula. Time to relapse was calculated as the time from diagnosis to first relapse, whereas time to event was estimated as the time from diagnosis to the first adverse event (relapse, refractory disease, secondary malignancy, or death). Patients were censored at the time of last follow-up. OS was defined as the time from diagnosis to death from any cause, and patients were censored at the time of last follow-up. The log-rank test was used for comparison of survival curves between different groups. Multivariate analysis was conducted, and prognostic factors for EFS and OS were identified using the Cox proportional-hazard regression model. The significance of covariate or factor effects was tested using the Wald tests. Associations between categorical variables were tested using the x^2 test. All tests were conducted with a significance level of 5% (p-values of ≤0.05 were considered statistically significant). Analysis was performed using IBM SPSS v29.0 software.

3. Results

3.1. FISH and MLPA Concordance in CDKN2A/2B Evaluation

In our cohort of 247 ALL patients, 63/247 patients (25.5%) harbored CDKN2A/2B deletions. The majority of CDKN2A/2B deletions were identified by FISH (55/63), with the rest of the cases detected by MLPA or karyotype. G-banding cytogenetics captured the deletion in only eight cases.

Among the 95 samples analyzed by MLPA in the whole cohort, 29 referred to the CDKN2A/2B-deleted subgroup, as identified by any method. Out of the 29 CDKN2A/2B-deleted samples evaluated, the deletion was identified in 23 cases by FISH and in 20 cases by MLPA. Concordance between FISH and MLPA was evidenced in 15 cases, eight cases were identified by FISH only, and five cases were detected by MLPA only, with negative FISH results.

3.2. The Incidence of CDKN2A/2B Deletions and Comparative Description of Clinical and Genetic Disease Features between the CDKN2A/2B Deleted and Non-Deleted Subgroup

Sixty-three out of 247 patients (25.5%) harbored CDKN2A/2B deletions, either biallelic ($n = 35$) or monoallelic ($n = 28$). Among 220 B-ALL patients, the presence of CDKNA/2B deletions was identified in 49/220 (22.3%), and within the 27 T-ALL subsets, CDKN2A/2B deletions were present in 14/27 patients (51.8%). The detection of CDKN2A/2B deletions was associated with older age at diagnosis (median age: 5.9 years vs. 4.3 years, $p = 0.04$), higher WBC count (median WBC: 22.15×10^9/L vs. 9.33×10^9/L, $p < 0.001$), and non-significant difference regarding CNS infiltration (12/63, 19.0% vs. 14.1% 26/184, $p = 0.37$) compared to the subgroup with non-deleted CDKN2A/2B. Regarding protocol risk stratification, patients harboring CDKN2A/2B deletions presented with a trend towards IR- and HR-group stratification, compared to patients without evidence of the aberration, with the SR group accounting for 14.3% within the deleted subgroup vs. 24.5% when analyzing the CDKN2A/2B-non-deleted subgroup. The presence of the deletion was associated with a higher co-occurrence of the BCR::ABL1 fusion transcript (4.8% vs. 1.1%) and the PAX5 gene deletion (13.8% vs. 6.1%). Comparative description of the deleted and non-deleted CDKN2A/2B subgroup and coexistence with other genetic aberrations is described in Table 1.

Table 1. Comparison of baseline demographic, clinical, immunophenotypic, genetic, and treatment characteristics of ALL patients with or without the presence of CDKN2A/2B deletions.

Characteristics	Total (N = 247) n (%)	Patients with CDKN2A/2B Deletions (N = 63) n (%)	Patients without CDKN2A/2B Deletions (N = 184) n (%)	p-Value
Gender				
• Male	151 (61.1)	40 (63.5)	110 (59.8)	
• Female	96 (38.9)	23 (36.5)	74 (40.2)	0.92
Age				
• Median, years	5.0	5.9	4.3	0.04
Immunophenotype				
• B-ALL	220 (89.1)	49 (77.8)	171 (92.9)	
• T-ALL	27 (10.9)	14 (22.2)	13 (7.1)	<0.001
White-Blood-Cell Count				
• Median ($\times 10^9$/L)	12.21	22.15	9.33	<0.001
CNS Infiltration				
• Yes (CN2, CN3)	38 (15.4)	12 (19.0)	26 (14.1)	0.37
Genetics				
• ETV6::RUNX1	50 (20.2)	10 (15.9)	40 (21.7)	0.32
• KMT2A rearrangements	12 (4.8)	1 (1.6)	11 (6.0)	0.03
• BCR::ABL1	5 (2.0)	3 (4.8)	2 (1.1)	0.04
• TCF3::PBX1	10 (4.0)	3 (4.8)	7 (3.8)	0.97
• iAMP21	3 (0.8)	1 (1.6)	2 (1.1)	0.78
• Hyperdiploidy	61 (24.7)	10 (15.9)	51 (27.7)	0.06
• Hypodiploidy	2 (0.8)	1 (1.6)	1 (1.1)	0.90
• IKZF1deletion	13 (13.7) *	2 (6.9) **	11 (16.7) ***	0.02
• IKZF1plus	1 (1.0) *	0 (0.0)	1 (1.5) ***	0.31
• PAX5 deletion	8 (8.4) *	4 (13.8) **	4 (6.1) ***	0.04
Treatment Protocol				
• BFM 95/2000 modified	119 (48.2)	31 (49.2)	88 (47.8)	0.95
• ALLIC BFM 2009	128 (51.8)	32 (50.8)	96 (52.2)	0.65
Protocol Risk Group				
• Standard risk	54 (21.9)	9 (14.3)	45 (24.5)	0.03
• Intermediate risk	130 (52.6)	35 (55.6)	95 (51.6)	0.08
• High risk	63 (25.5)	19 (30.1)	44 (23.9)	0.09
Therapy Risk Group				
• Standard risk	7 (2.8)	0 (0)	7 (3.8)	0.04
• Intermediate risk	167 (67.6)	43 (68.3)	124 (67.4)	0.09
• High risk	73 (29.6)	20 (31.7)	53 (28.8)	0.06
FC-MRD status				
• FC-MRDd15 positive ($MRD_{d15} > 10^{-4}$)	185 (74.9)	47 (74.6)	138 (75.0)	0.84
• FC-MRDd33 positive ($MRD_{d33} > 10^{-4}$)	59 (23.9)	14 (22.2)	45 (24.4)	0.94
Complete Remission (EOI-CR #)				
• Yes	230 (93.1)	61 (96.8)	167 (90.8)	0.08
• No	17 (6.9)	2 (3.2)	17 (9.2)	0.06

* Results out of 95 BM samples evaluated by MLPA; ** results out of 29 BM samples evaluated by MLPA; *** results out of 66 BM samples evaluated by MLPA; FC-MRD: flow cytometry–minimal residual disease; EOI-CR: end of induction–complete remission; # complete remission, defined as flow-cytometric evaluation of <1% lymphoblasts by the end of induction.

3.3. Impact of CDKN2A/2B Deletions in Treatment Response and MRD Clearance

A higher rate of poor prednisone response on day 8 of induction therapy was observed within the CDKN2A/2B-deleted subgroup (19.0% vs. 12.5% for non-deleted patients, $p = 0.3$), but the results were not statistically significant. No statistically significant differences were noted between the two genetic groups (CDKN2A/2B deleted vs. CDKN2A/2B non-deleted) regarding the prevalence of MRD positivity on days 15 and 33 (74.6% vs. 75.0% on day 15, $p = 0.84$ and 22.2% vs. 24.4% on day 33, $p = 0.94$). There was a trend for a higher percentage of end-induction complete remission (CR) in the CDKN2A/2B-deleted subgroup but with no statistically significant difference ($p = 0.08$).

The effect of the CDKN2A/2B deletions on early treatment response and MRD clearance is shown in Table 1.

3.4. Prognostic Impact of CDKN2A/2B Deletions on Survival Rates and Outcome

With a median follow-up time of 135 months, overall survival (OS) and event-free survival (EFS) for the whole cohort were 89.9% and 85.0%, respectively. EFS rates for B-ALL and T-ALL patients were 87.3% and 66.7%, respectively ($p = 0.002$).

The presence of the CDKN2A/2B deletion (biallelic or monoallelic) was associated with inferior EFS of 65.1% compared to 91.8% for the gene-non-deleted subgroup ($p < 0.001$), with a relapse rate of 22.2% and 5.9% for the deleted and non-deleted cases, respectively ($p < 0.001$).

Patients that harbored a biallelic deletion had EFS rates of 57.2% vs. 89.6% in the case of any other status (monoallelic or non-deleted) ($p < 0.001$). In the case of patients in whom the deletion was monoallelic, EFS was 73.1% compared to 86.4% for the rest of the cohort ($p = 0.124$). Focusing solely on the CDKN2A/2B-deleted subgroup and further analyzing the gene-allelic status within the deleted sub-cohort, biallelic deletion was associated with adverse outcomes compared to the monoallelic aberration (EFS of 57.1% vs. 75.0%, $p = 0.002$).

Among the B-ALL cohort, the presence of the CDKN2A/2B deletion was associated with inferior outcomes (EFS 65.3% vs. 93.6% for the non-deleted B-ALL subgroup, $p < 0.001$) and a relapse rate of 24.5% vs. 5.8%, respectively ($p < 0.001$).

Analyzing the T-ALL cohort separately, CDKN2A/2B-deleted patients had non-statistically significant survival differences compared to their T-ALL non-deleted counterparts (EFS 64.3 vs. 69.2, $p = 0.947$).

Survival rates of specific cohorts by the presence of CDKN2A/2B deletion are presented in Figure 1.

3.5. Prognostic Impact of CDKN2A/2B Deletions by Risk Stratification and Integration of MRD Status

The presence of the CDKN2A/2B deletion also further stratified patients within all conventional risk groups, as defined by the BFM-protocol stratification. Within the SR group, the presence of the deletion was associated with inferior outcomes of only 66.7% vs. 100% for the rest of the SR patients ($p < 0.001$). Similarly, within the IR and HR groups, EFS for the CDKN2A/2B-deleted subgroup was 77.1% and 42.1%, respectively, compared to 97.9% and 70.5%, respectively, for IR and HR patients who did not harbor the deletion ($p < 0.001$). Survival rates by CDKN2A/2B deletion within separate therapy risk groups are shown in Figure 2.

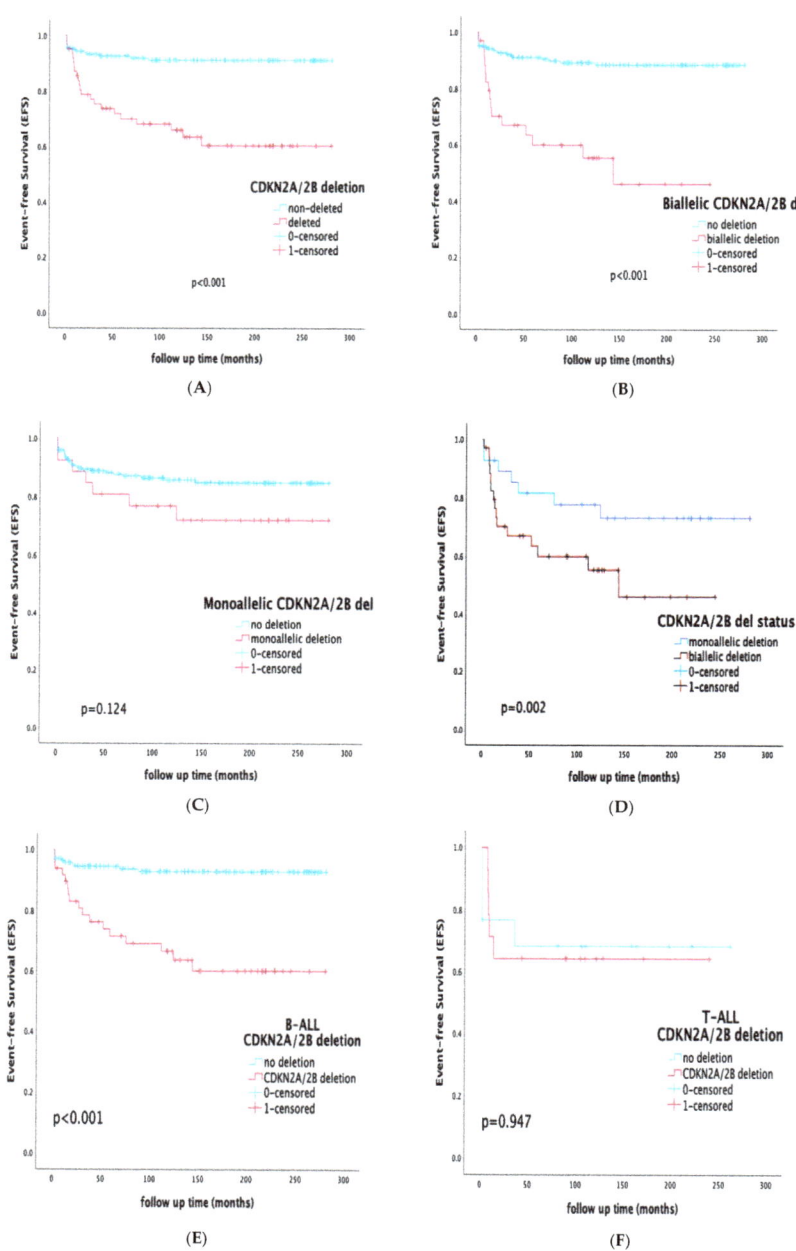

Figure 1. Event-free survival (EFS) rates in specific cohorts: (**A**) whole cohort, EFS of the CDKN2A/2B-deleted vs. -non-deleted subgroup; (**B**) whole cohort, EFS of the CDKN2A/2B-biallelic-deleted vs. -non-deleted subgroup; (**C**) whole cohort, EFS of the CDKN2A/2B-monoallelic-deleted vs. -non-deleted subgroup; (**D**) CDKN2A/2B-deleted subgroup, EFS by the status of CDKN2A/2B deletion, biallelic vs. monoallelic; (**E**) B-ALL cohort, EFS of the CDKN2A/2B-deleted vs. -non-deleted subgroup; (**F**) T-ALL cohort, EFS of the CDKN2A/2B-deleted vs. -non-deleted subgroup.

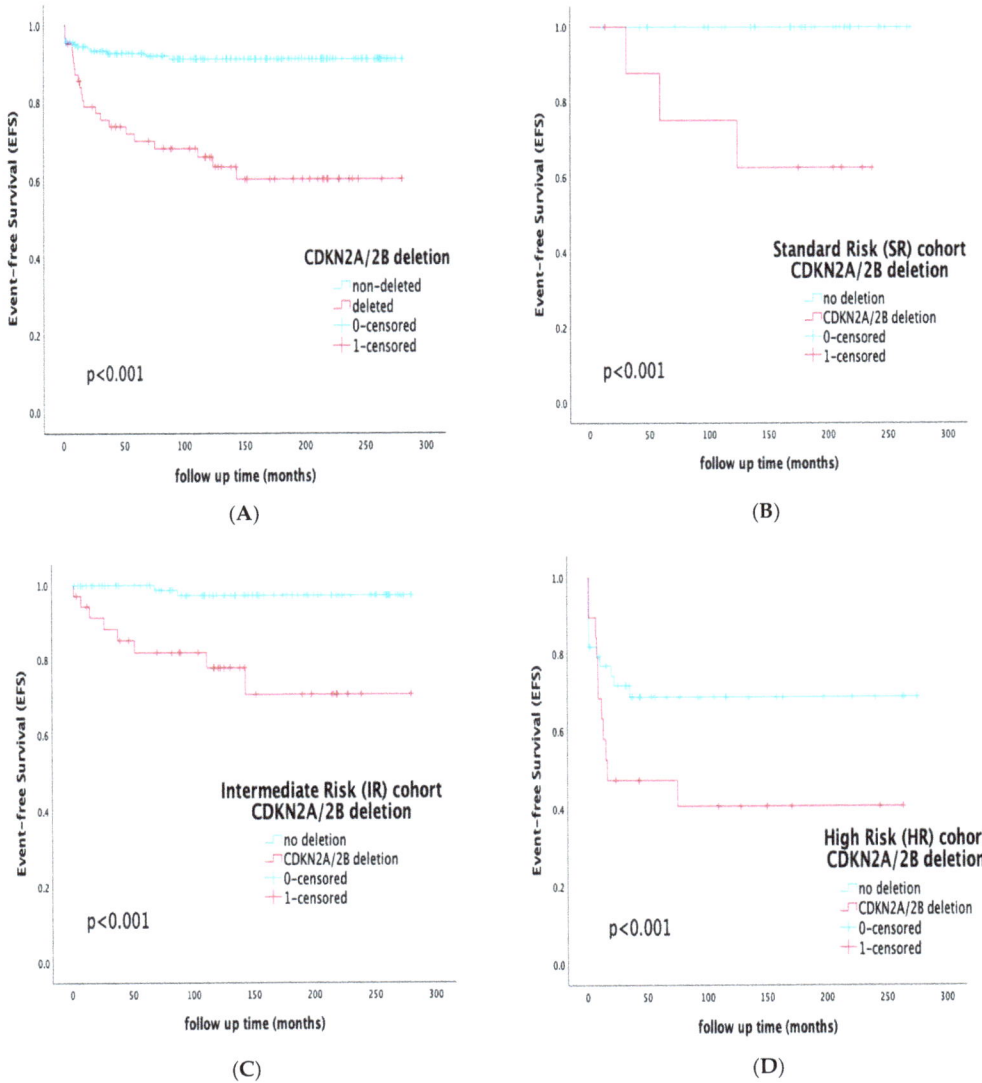

Figure 2. Event-free survival (EFS) rates by CDKN2A/2B deletion within separate therapy risk groups: (**A**) whole cohort, EFS of the CDKN2A/2B-deleted vs. -non-deleted subgroup, (**B**) standard-risk-group (SR) cohort, EFS of the CDKN2A/2B-deleted vs. -non-deleted subgroup, (**C**) intermediate-risk-group (IR) cohort, EFS of the CDKN2A/2B-deleted vs. -non-deleted subgroup, (**D**) high-risk-group (HR) cohort, EFS of the CDKN2A/2B-deleted vs. -non-deleted subgroup.

To evaluate the prognostic effect of the CDKN2A/2B deletion within distinct MRD subgroups, we analyzed the presence of the deletion within MRD-positive and -negative subgroups on days 15 and 33 of induction therapy. The detection of CDKN2A/2B deletion further stratified patients both within the MRDd15-positive subgroup on day 15 (EFS 59.6% vs. 90.6%, $p < 0.001$) and within the MRDd15-negative subgroup (EFS 78.6% vs. 95.6%, $p = 0.035$). Additionally, analyzing the cohort by MRD status at the end of induction (day

33), the presence of CDKN2A/2B deletion further stratified both the MRDd33-positive and MRDd33-negative subgroups, respectively. Within the MRDd33-positive subgroup, CDKN2A/2B-deleted cases had inferior outcomes (EFS 42.9% vs. 72.3% for the non-deleted MRDd33-positive cases, $p = 0.02$), and similar statistically significant differences were found within the MRDd33-negative sub-cohort (EFS 71.5% vs. 97.8%, $p < 0.001$). Survival rates by CDKN2A/2B deletion within separate MRD subgroups are displayed in Figure 3.

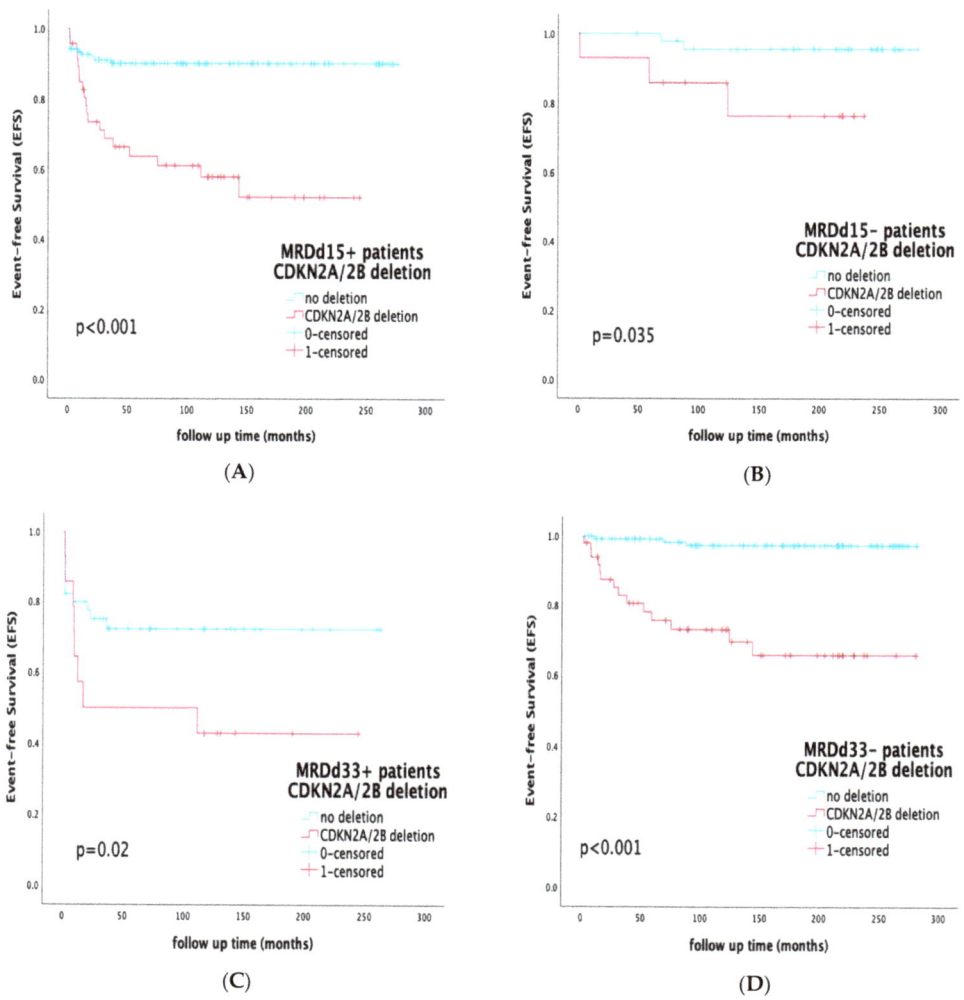

Figure 3. Event-free survival (EFS) rates by CDKN2A/2B deletion within separate MRD subgroups: (A) MRDd15+ patients on day 15 of induction, EFS of the CDKN2A/2B-deleted vs. -non-deleted subgroup; (B) MRDd15− patients on day 15 of induction, EFS of the CDKN2A/2B-deleted vs. -non-deleted subgroup; (C) MRDd33+ patients on day 33 of induction, EFS of the CDKN2A/2B-deleted vs. -non-deleted subgroup; (D) MRDd33− patients on day 33 of induction, EFS of the CDKN2A/2B-deleted vs. -non-deleted subgroup.

3.6. Mutivariate Analysis and Correlation with Protocol Conventional Risk Factors

In an attempt to define the interaction between the presence of the CDKN2A/2B deletion, MRD, and other conventional risk factors, multivariate analysis was conducted and Cox regression analysis for EFS and OS was performed with the following covariables: presence of CDKN2A/2B deletions, FC-MRD status on day 15, FC-MRD status on day 33, BCR/ABL1 status, KMT2A status, and protocol-risk-group stratification.

The presence of the CDKN2A/2B deletions was the most important prognostic factor for relapse, yielding a hazard ratio of 5.2 (95% confidence interval: 2.59–10.41, $p < 0.001$). Treatment-risk-group allocation and positive FC-MRDd33 status at the end of induction were also prognostic for relapse, with a hazard ratio of 3.85 (95% confidence interval: 1.58–9.35, $p = 0.003$) and 2.5 (95% confidence interval: 1.13–5.53, $p = 0.024$), respectively.

Regarding OS, the presence of the CDKN2A/2B deletion was the most important prognostic factor for survival, yielding a hazard ratio of 5.96 (95% confidence interval: 2.97–11.95, $p < 0.001$), with risk-group allocation also retaining prognostic significance for survival, with a hazard ratio of 5.66 (95% confidence interval: 2.18–14.64, $p < 0.001$).

Details regarding multivariate Cox-regression analysis are shown in Table 2.

Table 2. (**A**) EFS multivariate Cox-regression analysis; (**B**) OS multivariate Cox-regression analysis, with inclusion of the covariables listed in the table.

(A)						
	SE	Wald	Sig. p-Value	Hazard Ratio (HR)	95.0% CI for HR	
					Lower	Upper
CDKN2A/2B deletion	0.354	21.641	<0.001	5.199	2.596	10.412
BCR/ABL1+	0.656	0.003	0.958	0.966	0.267	3.493
KMT2A+	0.637	0.140	0.708	1.269	0.364	4.421
T vs. B ALL	0.416	0.000	1.000	1.000	0.443	2.258
MRDd15 positivity	0.564	0.046	0.830	0.886	0.293	2.678
MRDd33 positivity	0.405	5.118	0.024	2.501	1.130	5.535
Therapy risk group	0.453	8.867	0.003	3.851	1.585	9.353
(B)						
	SE	Wald	Sig. p-Value	Hazard Ratio (HR)	95.0% CI for HR	
					Lower	Upper
CDKN2A/2B deletion	0.355	25.260	<0.001	5.958	2.970	11.949
BCR/ABL1+	0.688	0.161	0.688	0.759	0.197	2.920
KMT2A+	0.645	0.064	0.800	1.177	0.332	4.170
T vs. B ALL	0.430	0.054	0.817	0.905	0.389	2.104
MRDd15 positivity	0.570	0.001	0.979	1.015	0.332	3.102
MRDd33 positivity	0.407	3.355	0.067	2.106	0.949	4.674
Therapy risk group	0.485	12.755	<0.001	5.657	2.186	14.640

4. Discussion

During the past decade, the evolution of genome-wide technologies and the identification of gene copy-number alterations (CNAs) implicated in leukemogenesis have led to a constant decoding of the underlying biology of pediatric ALL [5,6,8,12]. One of the most frequent genes affected is the CDKN2A/2B gene, acting as a secondary cooperating event and playing an important role in cell-cycle regulation and chemosensitivity [8,11,18].

In the current study, we addressed CDKN2A/2B deletions' disputable prognostic significance [17,24–34] and provided evidence on its additive prognostic effect in current risk-stratification algorithms. We showed that the presence of the deletion is an independent prognostic factor and can further stratify all existing risk groups, integrating with MRD and identifying patient subgroups with different outcomes.

The CDKN2A/2B deletions are the most frequent CNAs in pediatric ALL, with most published studies reporting incidence rates of 20–25% in B-cell-precursor (BCP) ALL and 38.5–50% in T-ALL cases [17–19,21]. In our study, the CDKN2A/2B deletion accounted for 25.5% of the whole cohort (22.3% among B-ALL cases), with the prevalence of the deletion rising to 51.8% when evaluated within the T-ALL subgroup. As expected, the percentage detected directly correlates with the genomic-methodology technique applied, since the deletion can be detected by conventional cytogenetics, iFISH, MLPA, array-based comparative genomic hybridization (aCGH), and single-nucleotide polymorphism arrays (SNP-arrays) [19,20,44–46]. Some homozygous deletions in the 9p21 region might be the result of a heterozygous deletion followed by a copy-neutral loss of heterozygosity (CN-LOH), often referred to as uniparental disomy (UPD) [18,20,30]. This is an underappreciated chromosomal defect by conventional cytogenetics tools [18]. In our study, apart from cytogenetics, combined iFISH and MLPA evaluation was used, with iFISH identifying the CNAs in 87.3% of the positive cases; concordance between the two methods was 51.7%. The discordance in the identified results could be attributed to differences in cut-off sensitivity, presence of the deletion in minor subclones, or very small deletions that could be missed due to the size of probes used. The major limitations concern the MLPA method, which may not be sensitive enough for the detection of low-level (<20%) or mixed-cell populations, for which FISH is a more reliable technique [18,36,37,46]. Nevertheless, despite the fact that novel technologies such as aCGH and SNP-arrays could possibly overcome technique limitations [20,44], our study suggests that the combination of iFISH and MLPA could be a simple, feasible, and validated approach for identifying the majority of deletions.

In concordance with previously published reports [17–19], the presence of CDKN2A/2B deletions was associated with older age (median: 5.9 vs. 4.3 years, $p = 0.04$), higher WBC count upon diagnosis (median WBC: 22.15×10^9/L vs. 9.33×10^9/L, $p < 0.001$), and a trend towards IR- and HR-group stratification. The presence of the deletion was also associated with a higher co-occurrence of the BCR/ABL1 fusion transcript (4.8% vs. 1.1%, $p = 0.04$) and PAX5 gene deletion (13.8% vs. 6.1%, $p = 0.04$). The extent to which the presence of the abovementioned disease features translates to inferior outcomes of the CDKN2A/2B-deleted subgroup was one of the main scopes of our study.

CDKN2A/2B deletion has recently been incorporated into combined can-risk algorithms and classifiers, like the IKZF1plus entity [13] and the UKALL CNA profile [14]. The evaluation of CDKN2A/2B-deletion status, allocating patients to the CNA-poor-risk (CNA-PR) genomic subgroup, was part of a combined CNA algorithm introduced by Moorman et al. in the UKALL trials [14]. In the previously published study of our group [15], we demonstrated that the implementation of this can-profile risk index, including CDKN2A/2B gene status, could be feasible in BFM-based protocols, effectively stratifying patients within all conventional risk subgroups and identifying subsets of different prognosis. Despite its inclusion in combined algorithms, depending on the presence or absence of concurrent deletions, the prognostic impact of individual gene deletions outside the context of combined CNA evaluation remains controversial [17–21]. Many researchers have supported that CDKN2A/B deletions in childhood ALL were associated with an increased probability of relapse and impaired outcome [17–19,21,24–31], whereas Mirebeau et al. [32], Kim et al. [33], and van Zutven et al. [34] concluded that the presence of the deletion was not a poor prognostic factor in childhood B-ALL. In our study, within an extended follow-up time of 135 months, the presence of the CDKN2A/2B deletion (biallelic or monoallelic) was associated with inferior EFS rates (65.1% compared to 91.8% for the gene-non-deleted subgroup, $p < 0.001$), with the relapse rate accounting for 22.2% and 5.9% of the deleted and non-deleted cases, respectively ($p < 0.001$). Although the presence of the deletion was associated with a higher CR rate by the end of induction, this was not statistically significant, and the impact on EFS comes from the higher incidence of relapses, possibly due to acquired chemoresistance and clonal evolution. When addressing the specific prognostic value based on allelic status, many studies have supported that any loss of CDKN2A/2B tumor-suppressor genes may serve as an adverse prognostic marker [17,19,21,26,29], with others disputing the independent prognostic significance in the case of heterozygosity and coexisting aberrations [25,30,32–34]. Our results demonstrate that the presence of the biallelic deletion was associated with worst outcomes, (EFS 57.2% vs. 89.6% in the case of any other status, monoallelic or non-deleted, $p < 0.001$), and direct comparison between biallelic and monoallelic status revealed statistically significant differences in outcome and relapse prediction (EFS 57.1% vs. 75.0%, respectively $p = 0.002$).

Another interesting finding of our study was the fact that the presence of CDKN2A/2B deletions served as an important prognostic marker in B-ALL (EFS 65.3% vs. 93.6% for the non-deleted B-ALL subgroup, $p < 0.001$), but the prognostic effect was not statistically significant within the T-ALL cohort (EFS 64.3 vs. 69.2, $p = 0.947$). Although many studies have supported the independent prognostic significance of CDKN2A/2B deletions in adult T-ALL [47,48], the spectrum of genomic heterogeneity in pediatric T-ALL has still not been fully explored [49–51]. It is possible that the adverse prognosis in T-ALL is mainly driven by a variety of initiating and cooperating events, coinciding with heterogenous underlying mechanisms. These mechanisms may include CDKN2A/2B gene-promoter hypermethylation leading to downregulation, the absence of a biallelic deletion (ABD), variable co-deletion of contiguous genes like the methylthioadenosine phosphorylase (MTAP) cluster that are not always identified, and impaired myocyte enhancer factor 2C (MEF2C) expression, all associated with various impacts on chemosensitivity and drug resistance [52–54].

The major challenge in our study was to demonstrate CDKN2A/2B deletions' prognostic significance within all already-established risk groups. It is noteworthy that the majority of ALL recurrences were still observed in the large group of IR patients. In the AIEOP-BFM ALL 2000 protocol, 69% of relapses occurred in IR patients [55], highlighting the need for additional prognostic markers in this heterogenous, not-well-defined spectrum of IR subsets. In our studied cohort, the presence of the deletion was not associated with statistically significant differences in terms of MRD clearance and CR achievement (Table 1), but it clearly correlated with inferior outcomes within all protocol-defined risk groups (EFS SR: 66.7% vs. 100%, $p < 0.001$, IR: 77.1% vs. 97.9%, $p < 0.001$, HR: 42.1% vs. 70.5% $p < 0.001$). The results of our study demonstrate that the evaluation of CDKN2A/2B deletions can identify a subgroup of adverse-prognosis patients within the SR and IR treatment groups who may benefit from early treatment intensification. In the context of MRD-guided treatment protocols and integrating with MRD, the presence of the deletion in our patient cohort also effectively stratified MRD-positive and -negative subgroups on days 15 and 33 of induction therapy (Figure 3), suggesting that even among MRD-negative patients, by the end of induction the presence of the deletion served as an adverse modifier, moderating prognosis and outcome.

In multivariate analysis, the presence of CDKN2A/2B deletions was the most important prognostic factor for relapse and overall survival, yielding a hazard ratio of 5.2 (95% confidence interval: 2.59–10.41, $p < 0.001$) and 5.96 (95% confidence interval: 2.97–11.95, $p < 0.001$), respectively, designating the deletion's independent prognostic significance in the context of modern risk stratification.

5. Conclusions

In the current study, the presence of CDKN2A/2B deletion, especially in the case of biallelic status, was associated with inferior outcomes in B-ALL, with subcohorts of different prognosis identified within all conventional risk groups. In multivariate analysis, the presence of CDKN2A/2B deletion retained independent prognostic significance, representing a novel proposed factor for predicting relapse and survival. The identification of the deletion is low cost, simple, and feasible via a combination of iFISH and MLPA, leading to early identification of distinct patient subgroups with different prognosis. The results indicate that biallelic CDKN2A/2B deletion can be a genomic feature incorporated into future risk-stratification algorithms in an effort to further genetically refine MRD-based stratification and improve treatment-group allocation and ultimate patient outcome. In the frame of targeted therapies, future prospective controlled clinical trials should explore the use of cyclin-dependent kinase inhibitors (CDKIs) [56–58] in CDKN2A/2B-affected ALL pediatric subgroups.

Author Contributions: Conceptualization, M.A., S.I.P. and S.P.; methodology, M.A., A.P. and S.P.; software, M.A.; validation, M.A. and S.P.; formal analysis, M.A.; investigation, S.I.P., L.F., G.P. and M.T.; resources, M.A. and S.P.; data curation, M.A.; writing—original draft preparation, M.A.; writing—review and editing, V.P., S.I.P. and S.P.; visualization, M.A. and S.P.; supervision, S.P.; project administration, S.P.; funding acquisition, S.P. All authors have read and agreed to the published version of the manuscript.

Funding: This research received no external funding.

Institutional Review Board Statement: Ethical review and approval were waived for this study for the following reasons: The patient' parents or legal guardians have already consented to the process of biological and genetic studies from blood and bone-marrow diagnostic samples for research purposes. Genetic studies included G-banding, FISH, PCR, and MLPA. Additionally, the parents consented to the anonymous use and publication of produced data and genetic results.

Informed Consent Statement: Informed consent was obtained from all subjects involved in the study. Written informed consent has been obtained from the patients or parents to publish this paper or any other anonymous data and results.

Data Availability Statement: The authors ensure that the data shared are in accordance with consent provided by participants on the use of confidential data. The data presented in this study are available on request from the corresponding author. Hard copies of all data and results are also available in the patients' files and collaborating involved laboratories. The data are not publicly available due to privacy and ethical restrictions.

Conflicts of Interest: The authors have no conflict of interest to declare.

References

1. Pui, C.-H.; Yang, J.J.; Hunger, S.P.; Pieters, R.; Schrappe, M.; Biondi, A.; Vora, A.; Baruchel, A.; Silverman, L.B.; Schmiegelow, K.; et al. Childhood acute lymphoblastic leukemia: Progress through collaboration. *J. Clin. Oncol.* **2015**, *33*, 2938–2948. [CrossRef] [PubMed]
2. Hunger, S.P.; Mullighan, C.G. Redefining ALL classification: Toward detecting high-risk ALL and implementing precision medicine. *Blood* **2015**, *125*, 3977–3987. [CrossRef] [PubMed]
3. Inaba, H.; Mullighan, C.G. Pediatric Acute Lymphoblastic Leukemia. *Haematologica* **2020**, *105*, 2524–2539. [CrossRef] [PubMed]
4. Ampatzidou, M.; Paterakis, G.; Vasdekis, V.; Papadhimitriou, S.I.; Papadakis, V.; Vassilopoulos, G.; Polychronopoulou, S. Prognostic significance of flow cytometry MRD log reduction during induction treatment of childhood ALL. *Leuk. Lymphoma* **2018**, *60*, 258–261. [CrossRef]
5. Brady, S.W.; Roberts, K.G.; Gu, Z.; Shi, L.; Pounds, S.; Pei, D.; Cheng, C.; Dai, Y.; Devidas, M.; Qu, C.; et al. The genomic landscape of pediatric acute lymphoblastic leukemia. *Nat. Genet.* **2022**, *54*, 1376–1389. [CrossRef]
6. Iacobucci, I.; Mullighan, C.G. Genetic basis of acute lymphoblastic leukemia. *J. Clin. Oncol.* **2017**, *35*, 975–983. [CrossRef]
7. Moorman, A.V. New and emerging prognostic and predictive genetic biomarkers in B-cell precursor acute lymphoblastic leukemia. *Haematologica* **2016**, *101*, 407–416. [CrossRef]
8. Kuiper, R.P.; Schoenmakers, E.F.P.M.; Van Reijmersdal, S.V.; Hehir-Kwa, J.Y.; Van Kessel, A.G.; Van Leeuwen, F.N.; Hoogerbrugge, P.M. High-resolution genomic profiling of childhood ALL reveals novel recurrent genetic lesions affecting pathways involved in lymphocyte differentiation and cell cycle progression. *Leukemia* **2007**, *21*, 1258–1266. [CrossRef]
9. Kiss, R.; Gángó, A.; Benard-Slagter, A.; Egyed, B.; Haltrich, I.; Hegyi, L.; de Groot, K.; Kiraly, P.A.; Krizsan, S.; Kajtar, B.; et al. Comprehensive profiling of disease-relevant copy number aberrations for advanced clinical diagnostics of pediatric acute lymphoblastic leukemia. *Mod. Pathol.* **2020**, *33*, 812–824. [CrossRef]
10. Ampatzidou, M.; Kelaidi, C.; Dworzak, M.N.; Polychronopoulou, S. Adolescents and young adults with acute lymphoblastic and acute myeloid leukemia. *MEMO-Mag. Eur. Med. Oncol.* **2018**, *11*, 47–53.
11. Steeghs, E.M.P.; Boer, J.M.; Hoogkamer, A.Q.; Boeree, A.; de Haas, V.; de Groot-Kruseman, H.A.; Horstmann, M.A.; Escherich, G.; Pieters, R.; Boer, M.L.D. Copy number alterations in B-cell development genes, drug resistance, and clinical outcome in pediatric B-cell precursor acute lymphoblastic leukemia. *Sci. Rep.* **2019**, *9*, 4634. [CrossRef]

12. O'Connor, D.; Enshaei, A.; Bartram, J.; Hancock, J.; Harrison, C.J.; Hough, R.; Samarasinghe, S.; Schwab, C.; Vora, A.; Wade, R.; et al. Genotype specific minimal residual disease interpretation improves stratification in pediatric acute lymphoblastic leukemia. *J. Clin. Oncol.* **2018**, *36*, 34–43. [CrossRef] [PubMed]
13. Stanulla, M.; Dagdan, E.; Zaliova, M.; Möricke, A.; Palmi, C.; Cazzaniga, G.; Eckert, C.; Te Kronnie, G.; Bourquin, J.P.; Bornhauser, B.; et al. IKZF1(plus) defines a new minimal residual disease-dependent very-poor prognostic profile in pediatric B-cell precursor acute lymphoblastic leukemia. *J. Clin. Oncol.* **2018**, *36*, 1240–1249. [CrossRef]
14. Moorman, A.V.; Enshaei, A.; Schwab, C.; Wade, R.; Chilton, L.; Elliott, A.; Richardson, S.; Hancock, J.; Kinsey, S.E.; Mitchell, C.D.; et al. A novel integrated cytogenetic and genomic classification refines risk stratification in pediatric acute lymphoblastic leukemia. *Blood* **2014**, *124*, 1434–1444. [CrossRef] [PubMed]
15. Ampatzidou, M.; Florentin, L.; Papadakis, V.; Paterakis, G.; Tzanoudaki, M.; Bouzarelou, D.; Papadhimitriou, S.I.; Polychronopoulou, S. Copy number alteration profile provides additional prognostic value for acute lymphoblastic leukemia patients treated on BFM protocols. *Cancers* **2021**, *13*, 3289. [CrossRef]
16. Gupta, S.K.; Bakhshi, S.; Kumar, L.; Kamal, V.K.; Kumar, R. Gene copy number alteration profile and its clinical correlation in B-cell acute lymphoblastic leukemia. *Leuk. Lymphoma* **2017**, *58*, 333–342. [CrossRef] [PubMed]
17. Zhang, W.; Kuang, P.; Liu, T. Prognostic significance of CDKN2A/B deletions in acute lymphoblastic leukaemia: A meta-analysis. *Ann. Med.* **2019**, *51*, 28–40. [CrossRef] [PubMed]
18. Carrasco Salas, P.; Fernandez, L.; Vela, M.; Bueno, D.; Gonzalez, B.; Valentin, J.; Lapunzina, P.; Perez-Martinez, A. The role of CDKN2A/B deletions in pediatric acute lymphoblastic leukemia. *Pediatr. Hematol. Oncol.* **2016**, *33*, 415–422. [CrossRef]
19. Feng, J.; Guo, Y.; Yang, W.; Zou, Y.; Zhang, L.; Chen, Y.; Zhang, Y.; Zhu, X.; Chen, X. Childhood Acute B-Lineage Lymphoblastic Leukemia With CDKN2A/B Deletion Is a Distinct Entity With Adverse Genetic Features and Poor Clinical Outcomes. *Front. Oncol.* **2022**, *12*, 878098. [CrossRef] [PubMed]
20. Sulong, S.; Moorman, A.V.; Irving, J.A.E.; Strefford, J.C.; Konn, Z.J.; Case, M.C.; Minto, L.; Barber, K.E.; Parker, H.; Wright, S.L.; et al. A comprehensive analysis of the CDKN2A gene in childhood acute lymphoblastic leukemia reveals genomic deletion, copy number neutral loss of heterozygosity, and association with specific cytogenetic subgroups. *Blood* **2009**, *113*, 100–107. [CrossRef]
21. Agarwal, M.; Bakhshi, S.; Dwivedi, S.N.; Kabra, M.; Shukla, R.; Seth. R. Cyclin dependent kinase inhibitor 2A/B gene deletions are markers of poor prognosis in Indian children with acute lymphoblastic leukemia. *Pediatr. Blood Cancer* **2018**, *65*, e27001. [CrossRef] [PubMed]
22. Tasian, S.K.; Loh, M.L.; Hunger, S.P. Philadelphia chromosome-like acute lymphoblastic leukemia. *Blood* **2017**, *130*, 2064–2072. [CrossRef] [PubMed]
23. Gupta, S.K.; Bakhshi, S.; Chopra, A.; Kamal, V.K. Molecular genetic profile in BCR-ABL1 negative pediatric B-cell acute lymphoblastic leukemia can further refine outcome prediction in addition to that by end-induction minimal residual disease detection. *Leuk. Lymphoma* **2017**, *59*, 1899–1904. [CrossRef] [PubMed]
24. Graf Einsiedel, H.; Taube, T.; Hartmann, R.; Eckert, C.; Seifert, G.; Wellmann, S.; Henze, G.; Seeger, K. Prognostic value of p16(INK4a) gene deletions in pediatric acute lymphoblastic leukemia. *Blood* **2001**, *97*, 4002–4004. [CrossRef] [PubMed]
25. Kees, U.R.; Burton, P.R.; Lu, C.; Baker, D.L. Homozygous deletion of the p16/MTS1 gene in pediatric acute lymphoblastic leukemia is associated with unfavorable clinical outcome. *Blood* **1997**, *89*, 4161–4166. [CrossRef] [PubMed]
26. Carter, T.L.; Watt, P.M.; Kumar, R.; Burton, P.R.; Reaman, G.H.; Sather, H.N.; Baker, D.L.; Kees, U.R. Hemizygous p16(INK4A) deletion in pediatric acute lymphoblastic leukemia predicts independent risk of relapse. *Blood* **2001**, *97*, 572–574. [CrossRef]
27. Dalle, J.H.; Fournier, M.; Nelken, B.; Mazingue, F.; Lai, J.-L.; Bauters, F.; Fenaux, P.; Quesnel, B. p16(Ink4a) immunocytochemical analysis is an independent prognostic factor in childhood acute lymphoblastic leukemia. *Blood* **2002**, *99*, 2620–2623. [CrossRef] [PubMed]
28. Calero Moreno, T.M.; Gustafsson, G.; Garwicz, S.; Grander, D.; Jonmundsson, G.K.; Frost, B.-M.; Makipernaa, A.; Rasool, O.; Savolainen, E.-R.; Schmiegelow, K.; et al. Deletion of the Ink4-locus (the p16ink4a, p14ARF and p15ink4b genes) predicts relapse in children with ALL treated according to the Nordic protocols NOPHO-86 and NOPHO-92. *Leukemia* **2002**, *16*, 2037–2045. [CrossRef] [PubMed]
29. Kathiravan, M.; Singh, M.; Bhatia, P.; Trehan, A.; Varma, N.; Sachdeva, M.S.; Bansal, D.; Jain, R.; Naseem, S. Deletion of CDKN2A/B is Associated with Inferior Relapse Free Survival in Pediatric B Cell Acute Lymphoblastic Leukemia. *Leuk. Lymphoma* **2019**, *60*, 433–441. [CrossRef]
30. Braun, M.; Pastorczak, A.; Fendler, W.; Madzio, J.; Tomasik, B.; Taha, J.; Bielska, M.; Sedek, L.; Szczepanski, T.; Matysiak, M.; et al. Biallelic Loss of CDKN2A is Associated with Poor Response to Treatment in Pediatric Acute Lymphoblastic Leukemia. *Leuk. Lymphoma* **2017**, *58*, 1162–1171. [CrossRef]
31. Papadhimitriou, S.I.; Polychronopoulou, S.; Tsakiridou, A.A.; Androutsos, G.; Paterakis, G.S.; Athanassiadou, F. p16 inactivation associated with aggressive clinical course and fatal outcome in TEL/AML1-positive acute lymphoblastic leukemia. *J. Pediatr. Hematol. Oncol.* **2005**, *27*, 675–677. [CrossRef] [PubMed]
32. Mirebeau, D.; Acquaviva, C.; Suciu, S.; Bertin, R.; Dastugue, N.; Robert, A.; Boutard, P.; Méchinaud, F.; Plouvier, E.; Otten, J.; et al. The prognostic significance of CDKN2A, CDKN2B and MTAP inactivation in B-lineage acute lymphoblastic leukemia of childhood. Results of the EORTC studies 58881 and 58951. *Haematologica* **2006**, *91*, 881–885.

33. Kim, M.; Yim, S.-H.; Cho, N.-S.; Kang, S.-H.; Ko, D.-H.; Oh, B.; Kim, T.Y.; Min, H.J.; She, C.J.; Kang, H.J.; et al. Homozygous Deletion of CDKN2A (P16, P14) and CDKN2B (P15) Genes is a Poor Prognostic Factor in Adult But Not in Childhood B-Lineage Acute Lymphoblastic Leukemia: A Comparative Deletion and Hypermethylation Study. *Cancer Genet. Cytogenet.* **2009**, *195*, 59–65. [CrossRef]
34. van Zutven, L.J.; van Drunen, E.; de Bont, J.M.; Wattel, M.M.; Boer, M.L.D.; Pieters, R.; Hagemeijer, A.; Slater, R.M.; Beverloo. H.B. CDKN2 deletions have no prognostic value in childhood precursor-B acute lymphoblastic leukaemia. *Leukemia* **2005**, *19*, 1281–1284. [CrossRef]
35. Dworzak, M.N.; Buldini, B.; Gaipa, G.; Ratei, R.; Hrusak, O.; Luria, D.; Rosenthal, E.; Bourquin, J.-P.; Sartor, M.; Schumich, A.; et al. AIEOP-BFM Consensus Guidelines 2016 for Flow Cytometric Immunophenotyping of Pediatric Acute Lymphoblastic Leukemia. *Cytom. Part B Clin. Cytom.* **2018**, *94*, 82–93. [CrossRef]
36. Schwab, C.J.; Jones, L.R.; Morrison, H.; Ryan, S.L.; Yigittop, H.; Schouten, J.P.; Harrison, C.J. Evaluation of multiplex ligation dependent probe amplification as a method for the detection of copy number abnormalities in B-cell precursor acute lymphoblastic leukemia. *Genes Chromosom. Cancer* **2009**, *49*, 1104–1113. [CrossRef]
37. Konialis, C.; Savola, S.; Karapanou, S.; Markaki, A.; Karabela, M.; Polychronopoulou, S.; Ampatzidou, M.; Voulgarelis, M.; Viniou, N.-A.; Variami, E.; et al. Routine application of a novel MLPA-based first-line screening test uncovers clinically relevant copy number aberrations in haematological malignancies undetectable by conventional cytogenetics. *Hematology* **2014**, *19*, 217–224. [CrossRef]
38. Riehm, H.; Schrappe, M.; Reiter, A. Trial ALL-BFM 95. Treatment protocol ALL-BFM 95 for children and adolescents with acute lymphoblastic leukemia: A cooperative multicenter trial of the German Society for Pediatric Hematology and Oncology. *Blood* **2008**, *111*, 4477–4489.
39. Möricke, A.; Zimmermann, M.; Reiter, A.; Henze, G.; Schrauder, A.; Gadner, H.; Ludwig, W.D.; Ritter, J.; Harbott, J.; Mann, G.; et al. Long-term results of five consecutive trials in childhood acute lymphoblastic leukemia performed by the ALL-BFM study group from 1981 to 2000. *Leukemia* **2010**, *24*, 265–284. [CrossRef]
40. ALL IC 2009 Trial of the I-BFM Study Group. 2009. Available online: https://bfminternational.wordpress.com/clinical-trials/ongoing-trials/ (accessed on 1 March 2023).
41. Papadakis, V.; Panagiotou, J.P.; Polychronopoulou-Androulakaki, S.; Mikraki, V.; Paecharidou, A.; Tsitsikas, C.; Vrachnou, E.; Paterakis, G.; Mavrou, A.; Sambani, C.; et al. Results of childhood acute lymphoblastic leukemia treatment in Greek patients using a BFM-based protocol. *HAEMA* **2003**, *6*, 208–216.
42. Ampatzidou, M.; Panagiotou, J.P.; Paterakis, G.; Papadakis, V.; Papadhimitriou, S.I.; Parcharidou, A.; Papargyri, S.; Rigatou, E.; Avgerinou, G.; Tsitsikas, K.; et al. Childhood acute lymphoblastic leukemia: 12 years of experience, using a Berlin-Frankfurt-Münster approach, in a Greek center. *Leuk. Lymphoma* **2014**, *56*, 251–255. [CrossRef] [PubMed]
43. Ampatzidou, M.; Papadhimitriou, S.I.; Paterakis, G.; Pavlidis, D.; Tsitsikas, K.; Kostopoulos, I.V.; Papadakis, V.; Vassilopoulos, G.; Polychronopoulou, S. ETV6/RUNX1-positive childhood acute lymphoblastic leukemia (ALL): The spectrum of clonal heterogeneity and its impact on prognosis. *Cancer Genet.* **2018**, *224–225*, 1–11. [CrossRef] [PubMed]
44. Usvasalo, A.; Savola, S.; Räty, R.; Vettenranta, K.; Harila-Saari, A.; Koistinen, P.; Savolainen, E.-R.; Elonen, E.; Saarinen-Pihkala, U.M.; Knuutila, S. CDKN2A Deletions in Acute Lymphoblastic Leukemia of Adolescents and Young Adults—An Array CGH Study. *Leukemia Res.* **2008**, *32*, 1228–1235. [CrossRef] [PubMed]
45. Karrman, K.; Castor, A.; Behrendtz, M.; Forestier, E.; Olsson, L.; Ehinger, M.; Biloglav, A.; Fioretos, T.; Paulsson, K.; Johansson, B. Deep sequencing and SNP array analyses of pediatric T-cell acute lymphoblastic leukemia reveal NOTCH1 mutations in minor subclones and a high incidence of uniparental isodisomies affecting CDKN2A. *J. Hematol. Oncol.* **2015**, *8*, 42. [CrossRef]
46. Gardiner, R.B.; Morash, B.A.; Riddell, C.; Wang, H.; Fernandez, C.V.; Yhap, M.; Berman, J.N. Using MS-MLPA as an efficient screening tool for detecting 9p21 abnormalities in pediatric acute lymphoblastic leukemia. *Pediatr. Blood Cancer* **2012**, *58*, 852–859. [CrossRef]
47. Wang, H.; Zhou, Y.; Huang, X.; Zhang, Y.; Qian, J.; Li, J.; Li, X.; Li, C.; Lou, Y.; Mai, W.; et al. CDKN2A deletions are associated with poor outcomes in 101 adults with T-cell acute lymphoblastic leukemia. *Am. J. Hematol.* **2021**, *96*, 312–319. [CrossRef]
48. Jang, W.; Park, J.; Kwon, A.; Choi, H.; Kim, J.; Lee, G.D.; Han, E.; Jekarl, D.W.; Chae, H.; Han, K.; et al. CDKN2B downregulation and other genetic characteristics in T-acute lymphoblastic leukemia. *Exp. Mol. Med.* **2019**, *51*, 1–15. [CrossRef]
49. Yu, H.; Du, Y.; Xu, J.; Zhang, M. Prognostic relevance of genetic variations in T-cell acute lymphoblastic leukemia/lymphoma. *Transl. Cancer Res.* **2019**, *8*, 2485–2495. [CrossRef]
50. Kumari, S.; Ali, M.S.; Singh, J.; Arora, M.; Verma, D.; Pandey, A.K.; Benjamin, M.; Bakhshi, S.; Palanichamy, J.K.; Sharma, A.; et al. Prognostic utility of key copy number alterations in T cell acute lymphoblastic leukemia. *Hematol. Oncol.* **2022**, *40*, 577–587. [CrossRef]
51. Liu, Y.; Easton, J.; Shao, Y.; Maciaszek, J.; Wang, Z.; Wilkinson, M.R.; McCastlain, K.; Edmonson, M.; Pounds, S.B.; Shi, L.; et al. The genomic landscape of pediatric and young adult T-lineage acute lymphoblastic leukemia. *Nat. Genet.* **2017**, *49*, 1211–1218. [CrossRef]
52. Tsellou, E.; Troungos, C.; Moschovi, M.; Athanasiadou-Piperopoulou, F.; Polychronopoulou, S.; Kosmidis, H.; Kalmanti, M.; Hatzakis, A.; Dessypris, N.; Kalofoutis, A.; et al. Hypermethylation of CpG islands in the promoter region of the p15INK4B gene in childhood acute leukaemia. *Eur. J. Cancer* **2005**, *41*, 584–589. [CrossRef] [PubMed]

53. Kumari, S.; Singh, J.; Arora, M.; Ali, M.S.; Pandey, A.K.; Benjamin, M.; Palanichamy, J.K.; Bakhshi, S.; Qamar, I.; Chopra, A. Copy Number Alterations in CDKN2A/2B and MTAP Genes Are Associated with Low MEF2C Expression in T-cell Acute Lymphoblastic Leukemia. *Cureus* **2022**, *14*, e32151. [CrossRef] [PubMed]
54. Colomer-Lahiguera, S.; Pisecker, M.; König, M.; Nebral, K.; Pickl, W.F.; Kauer, M.O.; Haas, O.A.; Ullmann, R.; Attarbaschi, A.; Dworzak, M.N.; et al. MEF2C-dysregulated pediatric T-cell acute lymphoblastic leukemia is associated with CDKN1B deletions and a poor response to glucocorticoid therapy. *Leuk. Lymphoma* **2017**, *58*, 2895–2904. [CrossRef] [PubMed]
55. Conter, V.; Bartram, C.R.; Valsecchi, M.G.; Schrauder, A.; Panzer-Grümayer, R.; Möricke, A.; Aricò, M.; Zimmermann, M.; Mann, G.; De Rossi, G.; et al. Molecular response to treatment redefines all prognostic factors in children and adolescents with B-cell precursor acute lymphoblastic leukemia: Results in 3184 patients of the AIEOP-BFM ALL 2000 study. *Blood* **2010**, *115*, 3206–3214. [CrossRef] [PubMed]
56. Sherr, C.J.; Beach, D.; Shapiro, G.I. Targeting CDK4 and CDK6: From discovery to therapy. *Cancer Discov.* **2016**, *6*, 353–367. [CrossRef]
57. Richter, A.; Schoenwaelder, N.; Sender, S.; Junghanss, C.; Maletzki, C. Cyclin-Dependent Kinase Inhibitors in Hematological Malignancies—Current Understanding, (Pre)Clinical Application and Promising Approaches. *Cancers* **2021**, *13*, 2497. [CrossRef]
58. Bride, K.L.; Hu, H.; Tikhonova, A.; Fuller, T.J.; Vincent, T.L.; Shraim, R.; Li, M.M.; Carroll, W.L.; Raetz, E.A.; Aifantis, I.; et al. Rational Drug Combinations With CDK4/6 Inhibitors in Acute Lymphoblastic Leukemia. *Haematologica* **2021**, *107*, 1746–1757. [CrossRef]

Disclaimer/Publisher's Note: The statements, opinions and data contained in all publications are solely those of the individual author(s) and contributor(s) and not of MDPI and/or the editor(s). MDPI and/or the editor(s) disclaim responsibility for any injury to people or property resulting from any ideas, methods, instructions or products referred to in the content.

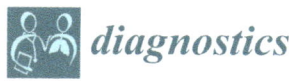

Review

Nutritional Status at Diagnosis as Predictor of Survival from Childhood Cancer: A Review of the Literature

Maria A. Karalexi [1,2,*], Georgios Markozannes [1,3], Christos F. Tagkas [1], Andreas Katsimpris [2], Xanthippi Tseretopoulou [1,4], Konstantinos K. Tsilidis [1,3], Logan G. Spector [5], Joachim Schüz [6], Tania Siahanidou [7], Eleni Th. Petridou [2,8] and Evangelia E. Ntzani [1,9]

1. Department of Hygiene and Epidemiology, School of Medicine, University of Ioannina, 45110 Ioannina, Greece
2. Hellenic Society for Social Pediatrics and Health Promotion, 11527 Athens, Greece
3. Department of Epidemiology and Biostatistics, School of Public Health, Imperial College London, London SW7 2BX, UK
4. Department of Pediatric Endocrinology, Addenbrooke's Hospital, Cambridge CB2 0QQ, UK
5. Department of Pediatrics, Division of Epidemiology & Clinical Research, University of Minnesota, Minneapolis, MN 55455, USA
6. Section of Environment and Radiation, International Agency for Research on Cancer (IARC), 69372 Lyon, France
7. First Department of Pediatrics, National and Kapodistrian University of Athens, 11527 Athens, Greece
8. Department of Hygiene, Epidemiology, and Medical Statistics, School of Medicine, National and Kapodistrian University of Athens, 11527 Athens, Greece
9. Center for Evidence Synthesis in Health, Brown University School of Public Health, Providence, RI 02903, USA
* Correspondence: marykaralexi@windowslive.com; Tel.: +30-69850-31991; Fax: +30-26510-07853

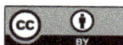

Abstract: Few studies so far have examined the impact of nutritional status on the survival of children with cancer, with the majority of them focusing on hematological malignancies. We summarized published evidence reporting the association of nutritional status at diagnosis with overall survival (OS), event-free survival (EFS), relapse, and treatment-related toxicity (TRT) in children with cancer. Published studies on children with leukemia, lymphoma, and other solid tumors have shown that both under-nourished and over-nourished children at cancer diagnosis had worse OS and EFS. Particularly, the risk of death and relapse increased by 30–50% among children with leukemia with increased body mass index at diagnosis. Likewise, the risk of TRT was higher among malnourished children with osteosarcoma and Ewing sarcoma. Nutritional status seems to play a crucial role in clinical outcomes of children with cancer, thus providing a significant modifiable prognostic tool in childhood cancer management. Future studies with adequate power and longitudinal design are needed to further evaluate the association of nutritional status with childhood cancer outcomes using a more standardized definition to measure nutritional status in this population. The use of new technologies is expected to shed further light on this understudied area and give room to person-targeted intervention strategies.

Keywords: undernutrition; obesity; nutritional status; childhood cancer; overall survival; event-free survival; relapse; treatment-related toxicity; review

1. Introduction

Cancer is the leading cause of death in children and adolescents worldwide [1]. Every year, just over 150,000 children are diagnosed with cancer [2]. Since a large proportion of childhood cancers in low- and middle-income countries are never diagnosed, the more realistic annual number is estimated to be at least twice as high, i.e., above 360,000 children [3]. Given these caveats, the age-standardized incidence (ASR) of the disease, estimated at 140.6 per million person-years in children aged 0–14 years, is increasing, with leukemia being the most common cancer site (ASR: 46.4), followed by central nervous system (CNS) tumors (ASR: 28.2) and lymphomas (ASR: 15.2) [4]. Over the past decades, advances in childhood cancer care, including novel imaging techniques for diagnostics and risk stratification, as well as multimodal novel therapies and supportive healthcare, have led to impressive increases in five-year survival, which exceeds 80% for all cancer types and 90% for acute lymphoblastic leukemia (ALL) in many European and North American countries nowadays [5]. However, severe or life-threatening long-term consequences may occur in up to 80% of childhood cancer survivors [5,6]. Indeed, a recent report showed that mortality among cancer patients is higher than that in the general population, mainly attributed to increased cardiotoxicity and risk of second neoplasms [7]. Poor nutritional status, defined as undernutrition (body mass index (BMI) < 5th percentile) or overnutrition (BMI $\geq$ 85th percentile) by the World Health Organization (WHO), seems to be a poor prognostic indicator linked to treatment-related toxicities in adults with solid tumors [8]. Recent research suggests that nutritional factors may also adversely affect outcomes in children and adolescents treated for cancer [9]. However, few studies have examined the impact of nutritional status on the survival of children with cancer, with the majority of them focusing on hematological malignancies [10,11].

Undernutrition is commonly reported in children treated for cancer, with a prevalence rate estimated as high as 50% in some populations [12]. Multimodal dose-intense antineoplastic therapies, surgery, and radiotherapy may cause serious complications that synergistically enhance poor nutritional status [13]. Treating undernutrition in children with cancer will assist them in tolerating traditional and novel therapies and thus plays a crucial role in improving outcomes and quality of life [13–15].

Overnutrition has long been associated with treatment-related complications. Such examples include the increased risk for thrombo-hemorrhagic fatal events in children with acute promyelocytic leukemia, the increased risk for infections (i.e., urinary tract infections and infections of central lines) in patients with ALL, as well as increased nephrotoxicity and post-operative complications in patients with osteosarcoma [15–18].

We aimed to review published literature and summarize evidence reporting the association of nutritional status at diagnosis with overall survival (OS), event-free survival (EFS), relapse, and treatment-related toxicity (TRT) in children treated for different types of cancer.

2. Methods

An independent and blinded literature search of the Medline database (via PubMed) was conducted from inception up to October 18 2021 using an algorithm based on relative key terms, such as "nutritional", "undernutrition", "obesity", "BMI", "prognostic", "survival", "relapse", "toxicity", "complications", "childhood malignancies", and "childhood cancer". The reference lists of identified studies were searched for additional eligible articles potentially missed through the initial literature search in a procedure called "snowball" procedure. Eligible were studies that examined the association of nutritional status at diagnosis with clinical outcomes, such as OS, EFS, relapse, histological response, and TRT in children (0–14 years) with cancer. We considered both systematic reviews and meta-analyses, as well as primary publications eligible for inclusion. Other types of publications, such as letters to the editor, commentaries, and editorials, were excluded. Case reports, case series, in vitro, or animal studies were also excluded. Nutritional status was defined by each study based on body mass index (BMI), weight change, or other body composition indices that defined under- or over-nutrition. We included studies reporting on any type of pediatric cancer.

The identified articles were independently screened by two reviewers to identify those that met the pre-determined inclusion criteria. Disagreements in the selection of studies or snowball procedure were resolved by team consensus. In articles with overlapping populations, the most recent or most complete publication was considered eligible. We extracted data based on a pre-defined form, including the name of the first author, publication year, study type, childhood population characteristics (including the studied cancer sites), the definition of the nutritional status based on the study, outcomes of interest (OS, EFS, relapse, TRT) along with the accompanying effect estimates (relative risk, hazard ratio, etc.) and their corresponding 95% confidence intervals (CI) and/or p-values.

Due to the large heterogeneity in exposure and outcome definitions across the identified studies, no quantitative synthesis of the results was feasible. Thus, a narrative presentation of the eligible studies by cancer type was performed (Table 1).

Table 1. Summary of studies reporting the association between nutritional status at diagnosis and outcomes of children with cancer *.

Cancer Site	N Studies	Outcomes
Leukemia	Meta-analyses (N = 5); 5 more recent original studies	- ALL: increased BMI associated with higher mortality, risk of relapse, and poorer EFS - AML: increased BMI associated with poorer OS and EFS - Post HSCT: malnutrition linked to poorer OS, progression-free survival, and higher risk of GvHD; lower BMI associated with poorer OS and EFS
Hodgkin lymphoma	2	- Malnutrition associated with worse OS (75–79%)
Ewing sarcoma	3	- Undernutrition associated with increased cardiotoxicity risk - No association between low BMI and TRT - Abnormal BMI (high or low) associated with poor histological response and OS
Osteosarcoma	2	- High BMI associated with increased risk of complications (arterial thrombosis, nephrotoxicity) - Low BMI associated with increased risk of wound infection and slough - High BMI linked to worse OS and EFS
Rhabdomyosarcoma	2	- Over 10% weight loss associated with increased number of hospitalization days - Patient weight ($\geq$50 kg) associated with worse EFS
Neuroblastoma and Wilms tumors	2	- Non-significant associations

* Abbreviations: ALL, acute lymphoblastic leukemia; AML, acute myeloid leukemia; BMI, body mass index; EFS, event-free survival; GvHD, graft versus host disease; HSCT, hematopoietic stem cell transplantation; OS, overall survival; TRT, treatment-related toxicity.

3. Results

The search strategy identified 4927 records, and after title, abstract, and full-text screening we included 22 publications in the present review (Figure 1). We identified 4 systematic reviews and meta-analyses and 18 primary studies. The most commonly studied cancer site was acute leukemia, reported in six publications (27%), followed by all cancer sites as a combined variable, which was reported in four primary studies (18%). The most commonly studied outcome was OS (n = 17 studies; 77%), followed by EFS (n = 10 studies; 45%), while treatment-related complications were studied as outcome in seven publications (32%).

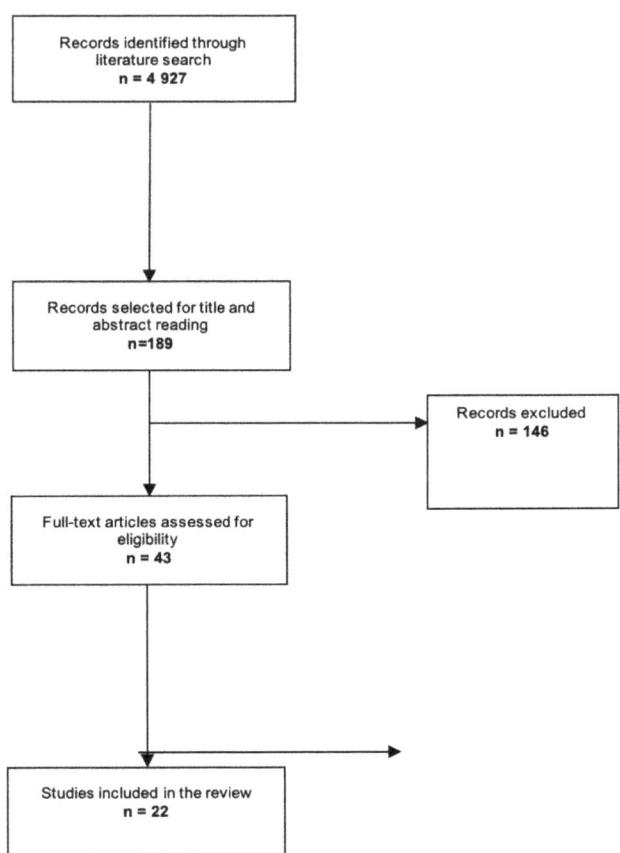

Figure 1. Flow chart of the selection process.

3.1. Hematological Malignancies

A previous meta-analysis of 11 articles found poorer EFS in children with ALL who had higher BMI (≥85th percentile; relative risk [RR]: 1.35; 95% CI: 1.20, 1.51; n = 6 studies; I^2: 34%, $p = 0.18$) compared to those with lower BMI at diagnosis (Table 1). In addition, children with higher BMI at diagnosis had significantly higher mortality (RR: 1.31; 95% CI: 1.09, 1.58; n = 4 studies; I^2: 49%, $p = 0.12$) [19]. Between-study heterogeneity was non-significant in all meta-analyses, whereas no evidence of publication bias was shown. Children with acute myeloid leukemia (AML) and higher BMI at diagnosis were also associated with poorer EFS (RR: 1.36; 95% CI: 1.16, 1.60; I^2: 0%, $p = 0.99$) and OS (RR: 1.56; 95% CI: 1.32, 1.86; I^2: 0%, $p = 0.66$) compared to children with lower BMI [19]. Similarly, two other meta-analyses showed significant associations between obesity and childhood leukemia survival outcomes. In particular, a meta-analysis including 11 studies found a statistically significant association between obesity, as defined by high BMI at diagnosis, and poorer OS (hazard ratio [HR]: 1.30, 95% CI: 1.16, 1.46; n = 7 studies; I^2: 71%; $p = 0.002$); however, statistically significant between-study heterogeneity was noted in this meta-analysis. High BMI at diagnosis was also associated with poorer EFS (HR: 1.46, 95% CI: 1.29, 1.64; n = 7 studies; I^2: 39%, $p = 0.13$) among children with acute leukemia [20]. A more recent meta-analysis (2018) showed an increased mortality rate (HR: 1.79, 95% CI: 1.03, 3.10; n = 3 studies; I^2: 0%, $p = 0.37$), as well as increased risk for relapse (HR: 1.28, 95% CI: 1.04, 1.57; n = 2 studies; I^2: 0%, $p = 0.59$) for children older than 10 years with ALL. However, these meta-analyses included a limited number of studies (n = 2–3) [21]. A statistically significant association between obesity and increased mortality for AML was also shown (HR: 1.64, 95% CI: 1.32, 2.04; n = 3 studies; I^2: 0%, $p = 0.73$), whereas no effect sizes were reported for AML relapse [21]. A recent study from Brazil assessed the impact of nutritional status on outcomes of children (n = 148) undergoing allogeneic hematopoietic stem cell transplantation (HSCT). Severe malnutrition was linked to a statistically significantly increased risk of acute graft versus host disease (HR: 1.68, 95% CI: 1.02, 2.74), as well as increased mortality (HR: 3.63, 95% CI: 1.76, 7.46), poorer progression-free survival (HR: 2.12, 95% CI: 1.25, 3.60), and poorer OS (HR: 3.27, 95% CI: 1.90, 5.64) [22]. A meta-analysis including 24 studies (18 on adolescents and 6 on children) examined the association between BMI and clinical outcomes after HSCT in patients with hematological malignancies. Compared to normal, lower BMI before or during transplantation was significantly linked to poorer OS ($RR_{pre\text{-}HSCT\ stage}$: 1.17, 95% CI: 1.08, 1.27; n = 11 studies; I^2: 0%, $p = 0.67$/$RR_{HSCT\ stage}$: 1.34, 95% CI: 1.01, 1.78; n = 5 studies; I^2: 60%, $p = 0.04$), as well as to poorer EFS ($RR_{pre\text{-}HSCT\ stage}$: 1.29, 95% CI: 0.96, 1.72; n = 5 studies; I^2: 18%, $p = 0.30$/$RR_{HSCT\ stage}$: RR: 1.53, 95% CI: 1.09, 2.06; n = 2 studies; I^2: 31%, $p = 0.23$). Again, the small number of included studies in some meta-analyses should be acknowledged. By contrast, there was no impact of high BMI on clinical outcomes among these patients at any transplantation stage [23].

A recent study in Pakistan showed that OS in children with Hodgkin lymphoma significantly decreased in cases of moderate (79%) and severe malnutrition (75%) compared to no malnutrition (96%; $p = 0.006$) [24]. By contrast, a 2021 study including 191 children with leukemia and lymphoma showed no impact of malnutrition on clinical outcomes [25].

The small sample sizes and the retrospective design of the identified studies should be acknowledged when interpreting these results. However, overall evidence from published studies suggests that poor nutritional status, especially over nutrition at diagnosis, may be a significant predictor of poor outcomes among children with leukemia, particularly ALL. Further research is needed to investigate the association with other leukemia subtypes, especially the rarer AML subtype, as well as the potential association with lymphomas, where evidence remains inconclusive.

3.2. Ewing Sarcoma

A USA cohort study including data from the University of California, San Francisco (UCSF) and Stanford University Medical Centers (n = 142 patients with Ewing sarcoma) showed non-statistically significant correlations between BMI at diagnosis and TRT ($p = 0.43$), specifically grade 3 and grade 4 non-hematologic toxicities during follow-up [26] (Table 1). With regards to clinical outcomes, in a study from Israel, abnormal BMI, defined as high or low BMI combined into one category, was statistically significantly associated with poor histologic response, namely tumor necrosis < 90% (odds ratio [OR]: 4.33, 95% CI: 1.12, 19.14), as well as worse OS (HR: 2.76, 95% CI: 1.19, 9.99) [27], whereas no correlations were found with EFS in this population (n = 50 patients). Lastly, regarding TRT, a study from Canada (n = 71 patients) reported significant correlations between low BMI at diagnosis and cardiotoxicity among children receiving anthracycline chemotherapy for Ewing sarcoma ($p = 0.03$), though this association was non-significant in multivariate logistic regression models ($p = 0.35$) after adjusting for potential covariates [28]. Given the limited sample sizes and the retrospective design of the identified studies, further research is needed to allow firm conclusions to be drawn regarding the association of nutritional status with Ewing sarcoma outcomes.

3.3. Osteosarcoma

Two longitudinal cohort studies derived from the Children's Oncology Group (COG) examined the impact of nutritional status on TRT and clinical outcomes in patients with osteosarcoma [29,30] (Table 1). Regarding TRT, the first study (n = 498) showed that high

BMI was significantly associated with an increased risk of arterial thrombosis in the postoperative period (OR: 9.40, $p = 0.03$) [29]. The second study showed that children with high BMI had increased odds of developing grade III–IV nephrotoxicity (OR = 2.70, 95% CI: 1.20, 6.40). Regarding clinical outcomes, children in the high BMI group had a significantly poorer 5-year OS of 70% compared to children with normal BMI (OS: 80%; HR: 1.60, 95% CI: 1.14, 2.24). There was also a trend towards worse EFS at 3 years from diagnosis in children with high BMI compared to those with normal BMI (66% versus 75%; HR: 1.30, 95% CI: 0.90, 1.80), whereas there was no impact of low BMI on OS and EFS among these patients [30].

3.4. Rhabdomyosarcoma

Two studies based on prospective data obtained from the COG assessed the association between nutritional status and rhabdomyosarcoma outcomes [31,32] (Table 1). In the first study, nutritional status was not a prognostic indicator for infections or survival. However, patients with more than 10% weight loss at 24 weeks of follow-up had a significantly increased number of hospitalization days (OR: 1.24, 95% CI: 1.00, 1.54) [32] and a trend towards a higher risk of grade 3 and grade 4 toxicity (OR: 1.16, 95% CI: 0.99, 1.35) at 42 weeks of follow-up. Children with low BMI (<10th percentile) did not have significantly worse OS compared to those with normal BMI at baseline (HR: 1.70, 95% CI: 0.98, 2.96; $p = 0.0596$). The second USA study on 570 children with intermediate-risk rhabdomyosarcoma examined the impact of tumor volume and patient weight on EFS based on a partitioning algorithm and accounting for age and greatest tumor dimension. The results of the algorithm showed that tumor volume (≥ 20 cm^3), histology, and patient weight (≥ 50 kg) were statistically significantly associated with twofold worse EFS (HR: 2.12, 95% CI: 1.12, 4.02) [31].

3.5. Other Cancer Sites

Two studies reported non-statistically significant associations between nutritional status and OS in children with neuroblastoma and Wilms tumor [33,34] (Table 1). A study from Turkey evaluated the impact of nutritional status on the survival of children with all types of cancer. Though malnutrition was a significant complication in this population, with a prevalence of 30% at diagnosis increased to 38% three months later, there was no impact of malnutrition on survival outcomes [35]. Likewise, a study on 139 children with Ewing sarcoma and osteosarcoma reported high proportions of malnutrition 2 years after treatment initiation (43% of osteosarcoma and 25% of Ewing sarcoma) [36]; again, malnutrition had non-significant effects on survival outcomes. A more recent study assessed the prognostic effect of sarcopenia, defined by the BMI-z score, the prognostic nutritional index (PNI), and the total psoas muscle area (tPMA), on the survival of children with bone and soft tissue sarcomas [37]. This study showed that the decrease in PNI ($p = 0.03$) and tPMA of more than 25% ($p = 0.04$) were associated with worse one-year OS; yet, more research is needed to evaluate the prognostic significance of tPMA in children with sarcomas. A study on pediatric cancer patients in Hungary showed that undernutrition at diagnosis, defined by the BMI Z-score and the ideal body weight percent (IBW%), was associated with worse 5-year OS only in patients with solid tumors [38]. Lastly, a study from the Netherlands, including 269 children with all types of cancer, found a significant impact of malnutrition on OS (HR: 3.63, 95% CI: 1.52–8.70), whereas increased weight loss (>5%) was also linked to increased risk of febrile neutropenia and subsequent bacteremia during the first year following diagnosis (OR: 3.05, 95% CI: 1.27, 7.30) [39]. Similar findings have been reported by a recent study in Italy which showed that weight loss of more than 5% at 3 months following diagnosis was associated with poorer OS (HR: 2.75, 95% CI: 1.12, 6.79) and a higher risk of infections requiring hospitalization (HR: 7.72, 95% CI: 2.27, 26.2) [40].

4. Discussion

The present review identified 22 published studies reporting associations between nutritional status and survival outcomes in children diagnosed with cancer. Despite the large heterogeneity in studied exposures and outcomes, the present findings suggest that malnutrition is a significant predictor of outcomes in childhood cancer. In particular, published studies on children with acute leukemia, lymphoma, and other solid tumors have shown that both under-nourished and over-nourished children at cancer diagnosis had worse OS and EFS. Of note is that the risk of death and relapse increased by 30–50% among children with leukemia with increased BMI at diagnosis. Likewise, the risk of TRT was higher among malnourished children with osteosarcoma and Ewing sarcoma.

Over the last decades, epidemiological and clinical research has aimed to identify prognostic indicators of childhood cancer with the ultimate goal of optimal risk stratification and targeted therapeutic interventions. Several sociodemographic and clinical factors have been reported to affect the prognosis of childhood cancer, such as age, socioeconomic status, disease subtype, cytogenetic and molecular markers, laboratory markers, predisposing syndromes, tumor size, presence of metastases, etc. [41,42]. However, very few environmental factors have been investigated as potential predictors of outcomes in children with cancer [43,44]. Among these factors, nutritional status is a modifiable marker that has long been postulated to affect survival in both adult and pediatric malignancies [45]. Potential underlying mechanisms that may underlie the association between nutritional status and health outcomes include its impact on body composition makeup, modification of tumor microenvironment, and potential alteration of chemotherapy pharmacokinetics [46]. In particular, changes in lean tissue and fat mass can alter the distribution of chemotherapeutic agents, modify their metabolism, and subsequently affect their clearance, especially the clearance of hydrophilic and/or lipophilic drugs from systemic circulation.

4.1. Undernutrition and Cancer Outcomes

Undernutrition has been associated with treatment-related adverse effects and survival among adult patients with cancer [46]. Several underlying biological mechanisms have been proposed to explain this association. Weight loss and decreased muscle and fat mass can be induced by cancer progression, and they both result in a negative balance between synthetic and degradative protein pathways. Moreover, weight and muscle loss are responsible for the activation of inflammatory response and apoptosis of myocytes, as well as for the decreased muscle regeneration capacity [47]. In addition, muscle loss may decrease the excretion of anabolic hormones, such as testosterone and insulin-like growth factor (IGF)-1 [48]. Such phenomena may alter drug pharmacokinetics and thus contribute to the increased risk of dose-response toxicity, which is often observed in cancer patients with low muscle and lean tissue mass [48]. Though evidence in children with cancer is limited, previous studies have shown significant skeletal muscle mass wasting with a concurrent fat mass increase in children with ALL following treatment initiation [49]. Muscle wasting has been related to reductions in chemotherapeutic doses, delays of treatment, and/or premature treatment cessation [50]. Similar findings have been reported by studies on children with several types of solid cancer, concluding that body composition markers seem to be crucial prognostic indicators among pediatric oncology patients [49,51].

4.2. Overnutrition and Cancer Outcomes

With regard to overnutrition at diagnosis and survival from childhood cancer, several potential mechanisms have been proposed. There is clinical evidence suggesting that obese patients may have altered pharmacokinetics in the metabolism of chemotherapeutic agents, although prospective trials have not confirmed such variations [52,53]. Overnutrition may also affect both the tumor microenvironment and the microenvironment of the host [54]. In particular, the adipose tissue microenvironment physiology in obese patients is characterized by increased inflammation, as well as disruptions in vascularity and fibrosis which may contribute to tumor progression [54]. Moreover, obesity is associated with hyperinsulinemia and peripheral insulin resistance, which result in reduced growth hormone (GH) secretion and subsequent activation of the IGF-I system as a response to the decreased GH [55]. The association of the IGF-II axis with obesity remains less clear. Low IGF-II levels have been reported in obese children, especially in those with insulin resistance and increased inflammatory markers, such as IL-6 and TNF-a [56]. The overexpression of the IGF-I and -II axis in obese individuals seems to also play a crucial pathogenetic role in the first (initiating) "molecular hit" that contributes not only to leukemia development but also to the disease clinical course [57,58]. Indeed, numerous epidemiologic studies have supported this hypothesis, showing that both children of high birthweight and patients with diabetes have high expression of the IGF-I and II systems and are at increased risk of developing leukemia [18,59]. In addition, these metabolic and chronic inflammatory changes in obese cancer patients may result in the activation of multiple molecular cancer pathways, which subsequently increase the risk of disease resistance and progression [60].

4.3. Nutritional Interventions

Apart from the direct effect of cancer itself on nutritional status, several factors can also affect both appetite and food intake among cancer patients. Such factors include some common complications of cancer treatment, such as nausea, vomiting, mucositis (oral, esophageal, and bowel), diarrhea, and/or constipation [61]. Thus, targeted interventions to improve the nutritional status of children with cancer remain challenging. Dietary support and physical exercise recommendations both aim to maintain and improve the normal physical growth of patients before and during treatment [62]. A recent study evaluated the nutritional status following the implementation of a nutritional algorithm in children with cancer from low- and middle-income countries [63]. This study showed an increase in the mid-upper-arm circumference in children enrolled in the algorithm protocol compared to those receiving the standard nutritional care provided by their institution ($p = 0.02$); however, a non-significant difference in weight change was noted between the two comparison groups ($p = 0.15$) [63]. Two other trials assessed the prognostic effect of ω-3 fatty acids and black seed oil on methotrexate-induced toxicity in children with ALL showing a decrease in the risk of hepatotoxicity during the maintenance treatment phase [64,65]. Other interventions that have been explored include the use of glutamine in order to sustain the integrity of the mucosal cell and gut barrier, which is often damaged in chemotherapy-related mucositis [66]. Though evidence is scarce in pediatric patients, one study has shown a significant decrease in the use of parenteral feeding in children with cancer after the exogeneous administration of glutamine without any adverse effects; yet the incidence of mucositis was not reduced in the intervention group [66]. Novel alternative avenues to be explored include the potential beneficial effect of antioxidants or a ketogenic diet on clinical outcomes of children with cancer; however, further research is warranted in this understudied area [67].

Overall, treatment of under- and over-nutrition in cancer patients is not easy on clinical grounds. Interventions should be proactive, aiming to prevent the nutritional depletion before it becomes clinically apparent [68]. Parents and guardians of patients are important components in supporting the nutritional status of children with cancer throughout therapy [69]. Educational and dietician's support is also crucial in optimizing the health care support of little patients with cancer [70]. Currently, several approaches are being implemented targeting the family-based nutrition and cooking education of parents and guardians of children with cancer [71–73]. Among such interventions, web-based dietary and cooking intervention approaches have gained great attention among parents and young patients [74–76]. Preliminary results have shown that early interventions resulted in better nutrition practices, i.e., lower sodium consumption [73]. However, obstacles to the participation of families have been noted by several studies, mainly due to treatment-related complications affecting the child's health, requirement of parents' presence at the hospital, as well as time, financial and other logistics restraints [71,72]. Future research is thus needed to address these barriers and encourage nutrition and cooking education in a family-based manner.

4.4. Methodological Considerations

The limited power of published studies is an important methodological issue when evaluating the potential association between malnutrition and survival of pediatric cancer. Even in the case of meta-analysis, the limited number of included studies (less than 10 studies) in the majority of meta-analyses performed should be acknowledged. Moreover, most studies focused on the most frequent cancer site, acute leukemia, whereas evidence on the remaining cancer sites is scarce, thus not allowing firm conclusions to be drawn. In addition, the large heterogeneity in exposure and outcome definition should be acknowledged. The majority of identified studies considered nutritional status by measuring BMI. Other nutritional indices were weight change, BMI z-score, prognostic nutritional index (PNI), and total psoas muscle area (tPMA). Of note is that recent research argues for the use of BMI-related measures to evaluate the lean mass in cancer patients. By contrast, recent studies have proposed other mainly imaging-based measures, such as cross-sectional computed tomography, which seem to assess sarcopenia and obesity in this population more accurately [50,77,78]. However, only a few studies have evaluated the impact of such measures on the clinical outcomes of adult patients with cancer [77,79,80]. Moreover, the prognostic significance of imaging-based measures in children with cancer needs to be further explored, also addressing the potential harms, i.e., those related to exposure to radiation [80]. Additionally, while in developing countries, "underweight" is certainly occurring in the normal population at a certain high percentage, "overweight" is basically the norm in highly developed countries. For example, the USA population shows an overweight prevalence of >40% [81]. So, maybe the occurrence of underweight and overweight children with cancer reflects the situation in the respective countries and is hence a "larger problem". Regarding the outcome assessment, the identified studies assessed the impact of nutritional status on various clinical endpoints, such as OS, EFS, TRT, or specific treatment-related toxicities (cardiotoxicity, nephrotoxicity, etc.). Such heterogeneity did not allow the quantitative synthesis of the results in the context of a meta-analysis. Lastly, the retrospective design of several studies is another limitation, which increases the risk of misclassification bias; indeed, misclassification might be differential in retrospective studies, leading to recall bias, namely reports of higher exposures in children with the disease.

5. Conclusions

Despite the large heterogeneity of published literature and several other limitations reported herein, nutritional status seems to play a crucial role in the survival and clinical outcomes of children with cancer, thus providing a significant modifiable prognostic tool in childhood cancer management. Interventions targeting the optimal nutrition and normal development of children with cancer are thus necessary. Future studies with adequate power and longitudinal design are still needed to further evaluate the association of nutritional status with childhood cancer outcomes using a more standardized definition to measure nutritional status in this population. The use of new technologies to longitudinally and accurately assess the nutritional status on a large scale from diagnosis onwards is expected to shed further light on this understudied area and to give room to individualized person-targeted intervention strategies.

Author Contributions: M.A.K. and E.E.N. conceived and designed the study. M.A.K., G.M. and E.E.N. acquired and collected the data. M.A.K. analyzed the data. M.A.K. drafted the initial version of the manuscript. G.M., C.F.T., A.K., X.T., K.K.T., L.G.S., J.S., T.S., E.T.P. and E.E.N. drafted and critically revised the manuscript for important intellectual content and gave final approval of the version to be published. E.E.N. is the guarantor. All authors have read and agreed to the published version of the manuscript.

Funding: The present study is co-financed by Greece and the European Union (European Social Fund-ESF) through the Operational Programme «Human Resources Development, Education and Lifelong Learning» in the context of the project "Reinforcement of Postdoctoral Researchers—2nd Cycle" (MIS-5033021), implemented by the State Scholarships Foundation (IKY). None of the funders had any influence on the study design; in the collection, analysis, and interpretation of data; in the writing of the report; and in the decision to submit the article for publication. All authors had access to the data in the study and had final responsibility for the decision to submit for publication. Where authors are identified as personnel of the International Agency for Research on Cancer/World Health Organization, the authors alone are responsible for the views expressed in this article and they do not necessarily represent the decisions, policy or views of the International Agency for Research on Cancer/World Health Organization.

Institutional Review Board Statement: Not required.

Informed Consent Statement: The lead author (M.A.K.) affirms that the manuscript is an honest, accurate, and transparent account of the study being reported; that no important aspects of the study have been omitted; and that any discrepancies from the study as planned have been explained.

Data Availability Statement: No additional data are available.

Conflicts of Interest: The authors declare no conflict of interest.

References

1. Steliarova-Foucher, E.; Colombet, M.; Ries, L.A.G.; Moreno, F.; Dolya, A.; Bray, F.; Hesseling, P.; Shin, H.Y.; Stiller, C.A.; IICC-3 Contributors; et al. International incidence of childhood cancer, 2001–2010: A population-based registry study. *Lancet Oncol.* **2017**, *18*, 719–731. [CrossRef]
2. American Cancer Society's (ACS) publications. Cancer Facts & Figures 2020 and Cancer Facts & Figures 2016, and the ACS Website (January 2020). 2020. Available online: https://www.cancer.org/research/cancer-facts-statistics/all-cancer-facts-figures/cancer-facts-figures-2020.html (accessed on 1 January 2020).
3. Johnston, W.; Erdmann, F.; Newton, R.; Steliarova-Foucher, E.; Schüz, J.; Roman, E. Childhood cancer: Estimating regional and global incidence. *Cancer Epidemiol.* **2020**, *71*, 101662. [CrossRef] [PubMed]
4. Force, L.M.; Abdollahpour, I.; Advani, S.M.; Agius, D.; Ahmadian, E.; Alahdab, F.; Alam, T.; Alebel, A.; Alipour, V.; Allen, C.A.; et al. The global burden of childhood and adolescent cancer in 2017: An analysis of the Global Burden of Disease Study 2017. *Lancet Oncol.* **2019**, *20*, 1211–1225. [CrossRef]
5. Erdmann, F.; Frederiksen, L.E.; Bonaventure, A.; Mader, L.; Hasle, H.; Robison, L.L.; Winther, J.F. Childhood cancer: Survival, treatment modalities, late effects and improvements over time. *Cancer Epidemiol.* **2020**, *71*, 101733. [CrossRef] [PubMed]
6. Gibson, T.M.; Mostoufi-Moab, S.; Stratton, K.L.; Leisenring, W.M.; Barnea, D.; Chow, E.J.; Donaldson, S.S.; Howell, R.M.; Hudson, M.M.; Mahajan, A.; et al. Temporal patterns in the risk of chronic health conditions in survivors of childhood cancer diagnosed 1970–99: A report from the Childhood Cancer Survivor Study cohort. *Lancet Oncol.* **2018**, *19*, 1590–1601. [CrossRef]
7. World Health Organization. Double Burden of Malnutrition. Available online: https://www.who.int/nutrition/double-burden-malnutrition/en/ (accessed on 15 September 2018).
8. Rogers, P.C.; Melnick, S.J.; Ladas, E.J.; Halton, J.; Baillargeon, J.; Sacks, N. Children's Oncology Group (COG) Nutrition Committee. *Pediatr. Blood Cancer* **2008**, *50*, 447–450. [CrossRef]
9. Co-Reyes, E.; Li, R.; Huh, W.; Chandra, J. Malnutrition and obesity in pediatric oncology patients: Causes, consequences, and interventions. *Pediatr. Blood Cancer* **2012**, *59*, 1160–1167. [CrossRef]
10. Brinksma, A.; Huizinga, G.; Sulkers, E.; Kamps, W.; Roodbol, P.; Tissing, W. Malnutrition in childhood cancer patients: A review on its prevalence and possible causes. *Crit. Rev. Oncol. Hematol.* **2012**, *83*, 249–275. [CrossRef]
11. Iniesta, R.R.; Paciarotti, I.; Davidson, I.; McKenzie, J.M.; Brougham, M.F.; Wilson, D.C. Nutritional status of children and adolescents with cancer in Scotland: A prospective cohort study. *Clin. Nutr. ESPEN* **2019**, *32*, 96–106. [CrossRef]
12. Ladas, E.J.; Sacks, N.; Meacham, L.; Henry, D.; Enriquez, L.; Lowry, G.; Hawkes, R.; Dadd, G.; Rogers, P. A Multidisciplinary Review of Nutrition Considerations in the Pediatric Oncology Population: A Perspective from Children's Oncology Group. *Nutr. Clin. Pract.* **2005**, *20*, 377–393. [CrossRef]
13. Hamilton, E.C.; Curtin, T.; Slack, R.S.; Ge, C.; Slade, A.D.; Hayes-Jordan, A.; Lally, K.P.; Austin, M.T. Surgical Feeding Tubes in Pediatric and Adolescent Cancer Patients: A Single-institution Retrospective Review. *J. Pediatr. Hematol. Oncol.* **2017**, *39*, e342–e348. [CrossRef] [PubMed]
14. Brinksma, A.; Sanderman, R.; Roodbol, P.F.; Sulkers, E.; Burgerhof, J.G.M.; De Bont, E.S.J.M.; Tissing, W.J.E. Malnutrition is associated with worse health-related quality of life in children with cancer. *Support. Care Cancer* **2015**, *23*, 3043–3052. [CrossRef] [PubMed]
15. Fu, A.B.; Hodgman, E.I.; Burkhalter, L.S.; Renkes, R.; Slone, T.; Alder, A.C. Long-term central venous access in a pediatric leukemia population. *J. Surg. Res.* **2016**, *205*, 419–425. [CrossRef]

16. Li, M.-J.; Chang, H.-H.; Yang, Y.-L.; Lu, M.-Y.; Shao, P.-L.; Fu, C.-M.; Chou, A.-K.; Liu, Y.-L.; Lin, K.-H.; Huang, L.-M.; et al. Infectious complications in children with acute lymphoblastic leukemia treated with the Taiwan Pediatric Oncology Group protocol: A 16-year tertiary single-institution experience. *Pediatr. Blood Cancer* **2017**, *64*, e26535. [CrossRef]
17. Abla, O.; Ribeiro, R.C.; Testi, A.M.; Montesinos, P.; Creutzig, U.; Sung, L.; Di Giuseppe, G.; Stephens, D.; Feusner, J.H.; Powell, B.L.; et al. Predictors of thrombohemorrhagic early death in children and adolescents with t(15;17)-positive acute promyelocytic leukemia treated with ATRA and chemotherapy. *Ann. Hematol.* **2017**, *96*, 1449–1456. [CrossRef]
18. Orgel, E.; Genkinger, J.M.; Aggarwal, D.; Sung, L.; Nieder, M.; Ladas, E.J. Association of body mass index and survival in pediatric leukemia: A meta-analysis. *Am. J. Clin. Nutr.* **2016**, *103*, 808–817. [CrossRef] [PubMed]
19. Amankwah, E.K.; Saenz, A.M.; Hale, G.A.; Brown, P.A. Association between body mass index at diagnosis and pediatric leukemia mortality and relapse: A systematic review and meta-analysis. *Leuk. Lymphoma* **2016**, *57*, 1140–1148. [CrossRef]
20. Saenz, A.M.; Stapleton, S.; Hernandez, R.G.; Hale, G.A.; Goldenberg, N.A.; Schwartz, S.; Amankwah, E.K. Body Mass Index at Pediatric Leukemia Diagnosis and the Risks of Relapse and Mortality: Findings from a Single Institution and Meta-analysis. *J. Obes.* **2018**, *2018*, 7048078. [CrossRef]
21. Hirose, E.Y.; de Molla, V.C.; Gonçalves, M.V.; Pereira, A.D.; Szor, R.S.; da Fonseca, A.R.B.M.; Fatobene, G.; Serpa, M.G.; Xavier, E.M.; Tucunduva, L.; et al. The impact of pretransplant malnutrition on allogeneic hematopoietic stem cell transplantation outcomes. *Clin. Nutr. ESPEN* **2019**, *33*, 213–219. [CrossRef]
22. Ren, G.; Cai, W.; Wang, L.; Huang, J.; Yi, S.; Lu, L.; Wang, J. Impact of body mass index at different transplantation stages on postoperative outcomes in patients with hematological malignancies: A meta-analysis. *Bone Marrow Transplant.* **2018**, *53*, 708–721. [CrossRef]
23. Ghafoor, T. Prognostic factors in pediatric Hodgkin lymphoma: Experience from a developing country. *Leuk. Lymphoma* **2020**, *61*, 344–350. [CrossRef]
24. González, H.R.; Mejía, S.A.; Ortiz, J.O.C.; Gutiérrez, A.P.O.; López, J.E.B.; Quintana, J.E.F. Malnutrition in paediatric patients with leukaemia and lymphoma: A retrospective cohort study. *Ecancermedicalscience* **2021**, *15*, 1327. [CrossRef] [PubMed]
25. Bs, J.M.S.; Cyrus, J.; Horvai, A.; Hazard, F.K.G.; Neuhaus, J.; Matthay, K.K.; Goldsby, R.; Marina, N.; DuBois, S.G. Predictors of acute chemotherapy-associated toxicity in patients with Ewing sarcoma. *Pediatr. Blood Cancer* **2012**, *59*, 611–616. [CrossRef]
26. Goldstein, G.; Shemesh, E.; Frenkel, T.; Jacobson, J.M.; Toren, A. Abnormal body mass index at diagnosis in patients with Ewing sarcoma is associated with inferior tumor necrosis. *Pediatr. Blood Cancer* **2015**, *62*, 1892–1896. [CrossRef] [PubMed]
27. Brown, T.R.; Vijarnsorn, C.; Potts, J.; Milner, R.; Sandor, G.G.; Fryer, C. Anthracycline induced cardiac toxicity in pediatric Ewing sarcoma: A longitudinal study. *Pediatr. Blood Cancer* **2013**, *60*, 842–848. [CrossRef] [PubMed]
28. Hingorani, P.; Seidel, K.; Krailo, M.; Mascarenhas, L.; Meyers, P.; Marina, N.; Conrad, E.U.; Hawkins, D.S. Body mass index (BMI) at diagnosis is associated with surgical wound complications in patients with localized osteosarcoma: A report from the Children's Oncology Group. *Pediatr. Blood Cancer* **2011**, *57*, 939–942. [CrossRef] [PubMed]
29. Altaf, S.; Enders, F.; Jeavons, E.; Krailo, M.; Barkauskas, D.A.; Meyers, P.; Arndt, C. High-BMI at diagnosis is associated with inferior survival in patients with osteosarcoma: A report from the Children's Oncology Group. *Pediatr. Blood Cancer* **2013**, *60*, 2042–2046. [CrossRef]
30. Rodeberg, D.A.; Stoner, J.A.; Garcia-Henriquez, N.; Randall, R.L.; Spunt, S.L.; Arndt, C.A.; Kao, S.; Paidas, C.N.; Million, L.; Hawkins, D.S. Tumor volume and patient weight as predictors of outcome in children with intermediate risk rhabdomyosarcoma: A report from Children's Oncology Group. *Cancer* **2011**, *117*, 2541–2550. [CrossRef]
31. Burke, M.E.; Lyden, E.R.; Meza, J.L.; Ladas, E.J.; Dasgupta, R.; Wiegner, E.A.; Arndt, C.A. Does body mass index at diagnosis or weight change during therapy predict toxicity or survival in intermediate risk rhabdomyosarcoma? A report from the Children's Oncology Group soft tissue sarcoma committee. *Pediatr. Blood Cancer* **2013**, *60*, 748–753. [CrossRef]
32. Fernandez, C.V.; Anderson, J.; Breslow, N.E.; Dome, J.S.; Grundy, P.; Perlman, E.; Green, D.M.; The National Wilms Tumor Study Group/Children's Oncology Group. Anthropomorphic measurements and event-free survival in patients with favorable histology Wilms tumor: A report from the Children's Oncology Group. *Pediatr. Blood Cancer* **2009**, *52*, 254–258. [CrossRef]
33. Small, A.G.; Thwe, L.M.; Byrne, J.A.; Lau, L.; Chan, A.; Craig, E.M.; Cowell, C.T.; Garnett, S.P. Neuroblastoma, Body Mass Index, and Survival: A retrospective analysis. *Medicine* **2015**, *94*, e713. [CrossRef] [PubMed]
34. Yariş, N.; Akyüz, C.; Coşkun, T.; Kutluk, T.; Büyükpamukçu, M. Nutritional status of children with cancer and its effects on survival. *Turk. J. Pediatr.* **2002**, *44*, 35–39. [PubMed]
35. Tenardi, R.D.; Frühwald, M.C.; Jürgens, H.; Hertroijs, D.; Bauer, J. Nutritional status of children and young adults with Ewing sarcoma or osteosarcoma at diagnosis and during multimodality therapy. *Pediatr. Blood Cancer* **2012**, *59*, 621–626. [CrossRef] [PubMed]
36. Romano, A.; Triarico, S.; Rinninella, E.; Natale, L.; Brizi, M.G.; Cintoni, M.; Raoul, P.; Maurizi, P.; Attinà, G.; Mastrangelo, S.; et al. Clinical Impact of Nutritional Status and Sarcopenia in Pediatric Patients with Bone and Soft Tissue Sarcomas: A Pilot Retrospective Study (SarcoPed). *Nutrients* **2022**, *14*, 383. [CrossRef] [PubMed]
37. Kadenczki, O.; Nagy, A.; Kiss, C. Prevalence of Undernutrition and Effect of Body Weight Loss on Survival among Pediatric Cancer Patients in Northeastern Hungary. *Int. J. Environ. Res. Public Health* **2021**, *18*, 1478. [CrossRef] [PubMed]
38. Loeffen, E.A.H.; Brinksma, A.; Miedema, K.G.E.; de Bock, G.H.; Tissing, W.J.E. Clinical implications of malnutrition in childhood cancer patients—infections and mortality. *Support. Care Cancer* **2015**, *23*, 143–150. [CrossRef]

39. Triarico, S.; Rinninella, E.; Cintoni, M.; Capozza, A.M.; Mastrangelo, S.; Mele, M.C.; Ruggiero, A. Impact of malnutrition on survival and infections among pediatric patients with cancer: A retrospective study. *Eur. Rev. Med. Pharmacol. Sci.* **2019**, *23*, 1165–1175.
40. De Araujo, O.L.; Da Trindade, K.M.; Trompieri, N.M.; Fontenele, J.B.; Felix, F.H.C. Analysis of survival and prognostic factors of pediatric patients with brain tumor. *J. Pediatr.* **2011**, *87*, 425–432. [CrossRef]
41. Lee, J.W.; Cho, B. Prognostic factors and treatment of pediatric acute lymphoblastic leukemia. *Korean J. Pediatr.* **2017**, *60*, 129–137. [CrossRef]
42. Okui, T. Socioeconomic Predictors of Trends in Cancer Mortality among Municipalities in Japan, 2010–2019. *Asian Pac. J. Cancer Prev.* **2021**, *22*, 499–508. [CrossRef]
43. Porojnicu, A.C.; Dahlback, A.; Moan, J. Sun Exposure and Cancer Survival in Norway: Changes in the Risk of Death with Season of Diagnosis and Latitude. In *Sunlight, Vitamin D and Skin Cancer*; Springer: New York, NY, USA, 2008; pp. 43–54. [CrossRef]
44. Barr, R.D.; Stevens, M. The influence of nutrition on clinical outcomes in children with cancer. *Pediatr. Blood Cancer* **2020**, *67*, e28117. [CrossRef] [PubMed]
45. Viani, K.; Trehan, A.; Manzoli, B.; Schoeman, J. Assessment of nutritional status in children with cancer: A narrative review. *Pediatr. Blood Cancer* **2020**, *67*, e28211. [CrossRef] [PubMed]
46. Bauer, J.; Jürgens, H.; Frühwald, M.C. Important Aspects of Nutrition in Children with Cancer. *Adv. Nutr. Int. Rev. J.* **2011**, *2*, 67–77. [CrossRef]
47. Fanzani, A.; Conraads, V.M.; Penna, F.; Martinet, W. Molecular and cellular mechanisms of skeletal muscle atrophy: An update. *J. Cachex-Sarcopenia Muscle* **2012**, *3*, 163–179. [CrossRef]
48. Prado, C.M.; Antoun, S.; Sawyer, M.B.; Baracos, E.V. Two faces of drug therapy in cancer: Drug-related lean tissue loss and its adverse consequences to survival and toxicity. *Curr. Opin. Clin. Nutr. Metab. Care* **2011**, *14*, 250–254. [CrossRef]
49. Tah, P.C.; Shanita, S.N.; Poh, B.K. Nutritional status among pediatric cancer patients: A comparison between hematological malignancies and solid tumors. *J. Spéc. Pediatr. Nurs.* **2012**, *17*, 301–311. [CrossRef]
50. Hopkins, J.; Sawyer, M.B. A review of body composition and pharmacokinetics in oncology. *Expert Rev. Clin. Pharmacol.* **2017**, *10*, 947–956. [CrossRef]
51. Hoed, M.A.H.D.; Pluijm, S.M.F.; De Groot-Kruseman, H.A.; Winkel, M.L.T.; Fiocco, M.; Akker, E.V.D.; Hoogerbrugge, P.; Berg, H.V.D.; Leeuw, J.; Bruin, M.; et al. The negative impact of being underweight and weight loss on survival of children with acute lymphoblastic leukemia. *Haematologica* **2015**, *100*, 62–69. [CrossRef]
52. Horowitz, N.S.; Wright, A.A. Impact of obesity on chemotherapy management and outcomes in women with gynecologic malignancies. *Gynecol. Oncol.* **2015**, *138*, 201–206. [CrossRef]
53. Silvestris, N.; Argentiero, A.; Natalicchio, A.; D'Oronzo, S.; Beretta, G.; Acquati, S.; Adinolfi, V.; Di Bartolo, P.; Danesi, R.; Faggiano, A.; et al. Antineoplastic dosing in overweight and obese cancer patients: An Associazione Italiana Oncologia Medica (AIOM)/Associazione Medici Diabetologi (AMD)/Società Italiana Endocrinologia (SIE)/Società Italiana Farmacologia (SIF) multidisciplinary consensus position paper. *ESMO Open* **2021**, *6*, 100153. [CrossRef]
54. Quail, D.F.; Dannenberg, A.J. The obese adipose tissue microenvironment in cancer development and progression. *Nat. Rev. Endocrinol.* **2019**, *15*, 139–154. [CrossRef] [PubMed]
55. LeWitt, M.S.; Dent, M.S.; Hall, K. The Insulin-Like Growth Factor System in Obesity, Insulin Resistance and Type 2 Diabetes Mellitus. *J. Clin. Med.* **2014**, *3*, 1561–1574. [CrossRef] [PubMed]
56. Al-Mansoori, L.; Al-Jaber, H.; Prince, M.S.; Elrayess, M.A. Role of Inflammatory Cytokines, Growth Factors and Adipokines in Adipogenesis and Insulin Resistance. *Inflammation* **2022**, *45*, 31–44. [CrossRef] [PubMed]
57. Stone, T.W.; McPherson, M.; Gail Darlington, L. Obesity and Cancer: Existing and New Hypotheses for a Causal Connection. *EBioMedicine* **2018**, *30*, 14–28. [CrossRef]
58. Manna, P.; Jain, S.K. Obesity, Oxidative Stress, Adipose Tissue Dysfunction, and the Associated Health Risks: Causes and Therapeutic Strategies. *Metab. Syndr. Relat. Disord.* **2015**, *13*, 423–444. [CrossRef]
59. Casabonne, D.; Benavente, Y.; Costas, L.; Robles, C.; Gonzalez-Barca, E.; Banda, E.; Alonso, E.; Aymerich, M.; Campo, E.; Marcos-Gragera, R.; et al. Insulin-like growth factor levels and chronic lymphocytic leukaemia: Results from the MCC -Spain and EpiLymph-Spain studies. *Br. J. Haematol.* **2019**, *185*, 608–612. [CrossRef]
60. Orgel, E.; Sea, J.L.; Mittelman, S.D. Mechanisms by Which Obesity Impacts Survival from Acute Lymphoblastic Leukemia. *J. Natl. Cancer Inst. Monogr.* **2019**, *2019*, 152–156. [CrossRef]
61. Fabozzi, F.; Trovato, C.M.; Diamanti, A.; Mastronuzzi, A.; Zecca, M.; Tripodi, S.I.; Masetti, R.; Leardini, D.; Muratore, E.; Barat, V.; et al. Management of Nutritional Needs in Pediatric Oncology: A Consensus Statement. *Cancers* **2022**, *14*, 3378. [CrossRef]
62. Schwingshackl, L.; Schwedhelm, C.; Galbete, C.; Hoffmann, G. Adherence to Mediterranean Diet and Risk of Cancer: An Updated Systematic Review and Meta-Analysis. *Nutrients* **2017**, *9*, 1063. [CrossRef]
63. Totadri, S.; Trehan, A.; Mahajan, D.; Viani, K.; Barr, R.; Ladas, E.J. Validation of an algorithmic nutritional approach in children undergoing chemotherapy for cancer. *Pediatr. Blood Cancer* **2019**, *66*, e27980. [CrossRef]
64. Elbarbary, N.S.; Ismail, E.A.R.; Farahat, R.K.; El-Hamamsy, M. ω-3 fatty acids as an adjuvant therapy ameliorates methotrexate-induced hepatotoxicity in children and adolescents with acute lymphoblastic leukemia: A randomized placebo-controlled study. *Nutrition* **2016**, *32*, 41–47. [CrossRef] [PubMed]

65. Hagag, A.; AbdElaal, A.; Elfaragy, M.; Hassan, S.; Elzamarany, E. Therapeutic Value of Black Seed Oil in Methotrexate Hepatotoxicity in Egyptian Children with Acute Lymphoblastic Leukemia. *Infect. Disord. Drug Targets* **2015**, *15*, 64–71. [CrossRef] [PubMed]
66. Ward, E.; Smith, M.; Henderson, M.; Reid, U.; Lewis, I.; Kinsey, S.; Allgar, V.; Bowers, D.; Picton, S.V. The effect of high-dose enteral glutamine on the incidence and severity of mucositis in paediatric oncology patients. *Eur. J. Clin. Nutr.* **2009**, *63*, 134–140. [CrossRef] [PubMed]
67. Zhou, W.; Mukherjee, P.; Kiebish, A.M.; Markis, W.T.; Mantis, J.G.; Seyfried, T.N. The calorically restricted ketogenic diet, an effective alternative therapy for malignant brain cancer. *Nutr. Metab.* **2007**, *4*, 5. [CrossRef]
68. Touyz, L.M.; Cohen, J.; Neville, K.A.; Wakefield, C.E.; Garnett, S.P.; Mallitt, K.-A.; Grech, A.M.; Cohn, R.J. Changes in body mass index in long-term survivors of childhood acute lymphoblastic leukemia treated without cranial radiation and with reduced glucocorticoid therapy. *Pediatr. Blood Cancer* **2017**, *64*, e26344. [CrossRef]
69. Fleming, C.A.; Cohen, J.; Murphy, A.; Wakefield, C.E.; Cohn, R.J.; Naumann, F.L. Parent feeding interactions and practices during childhood cancer treatment. A qualitative investigation. *Appetite* **2015**, *89*, 219–225. [CrossRef]
70. Zhang, F.F.; Liu, S.; Chung, M.; Kelly, M.J. Growth patterns during and after treatment in patients with pediatric ALL: A meta-analysis. *Pediatr. Blood Cancer* **2015**, *62*, 1452–1460. [CrossRef]
71. Chaput, C.; Beaulieu-Gagnon, S.; Bélanger, V.; Drouin, S.; Bertout, L.; Lafrance, L.; Olivier, C.; Robitaille, M.; Laverdière, C.; Sinnett, D.; et al. Research- and Practice-Based Nutrition Education and Cooking Workshops in Pediatric Oncology: Protocol for Implementation and Development of Curriculum. *JMIR Res. Protoc.* **2018**, *7*, e2. [CrossRef]
72. Beaulieu-Gagnon, S.; Bélanger, V.; Meloche, C.; Curnier, D.; Sultan, S.; Laverdière, C.; Sinnett, D.; Marcil, V. Nutrition education and cooking workshops for families of children with cancer: A feasibility study. *BMC Nutr.* **2019**, *5*, 52. [CrossRef]
73. Bélanger, V.; Delorme, J.; Napartuk, M.; Bouchard, I.; Meloche, C.; Curnier, D.; Sultan, S.; Laverdière, C.; Sinnett, D.; Marcil, V. Early Nutritional Intervention to Promote Healthy Eating Habits in Pediatric Oncology: A Feasibility Study. *Nutrients* **2022**, *14*, 1024. [CrossRef]
74. Li, R.; Raber, M.; Chandra, J.; Tee, S.-H.; Balter, K. Developing a Healthy Web-Based Cookbook for Pediatric Cancer Patients and Survivors: Rationale and Methods. *JMIR Res. Protoc.* **2015**, *4*, e37. [CrossRef] [PubMed]
75. Wartenberg, L.; Raber, M.; Chandra, J. Unique features of a web-based nutrition website for childhood cancer populations: Availability, features, and content. (Preprint). *J. Med. Internet Res.* **2021**, *23*, e24515. [CrossRef]
76. Touyz, L.M.; Cohen, J.; Garnett, S.P.; Grech, A.M.; Gohil, P.; Cohn, R.J.; Wakefield, C.E. Acceptability and feasibility of a parent-targeted dietary intervention in young survivors of childhood cancer: "Reboot". *Pediatr. Blood Cancer* **2020**, *67*, e28353. [CrossRef] [PubMed]
77. Chargi, N.; Bashiri, F.; Wendrich, A.W.; Smid, E.J.; de Jong, P.A.; Huitema, A.D.R.; Devriese, L.A.; de Bree, R. Image-based analysis of skeletal muscle mass predicts cisplatin dose-limiting toxicity in patients with locally advanced head and neck cancer. *Eur. Arch. Oto-Rhino-Laryngol.* **2022**, *279*, 3685–3694. [CrossRef] [PubMed]
78. Hilmi, M.; Jouinot, A.; Burns, R.; Pigneur, F.; Mounier, R.; Gondin, J.; Neuzillet, C.; Goldwasser, F. Body composition and sarcopenia: The next-generation of personalized oncology and pharmacology? *Pharmacol. Ther.* **2019**, *196*, 135–159. [CrossRef] [PubMed]
79. Celik, E.; Suzan, V.; Samanci, N.S.; Suzan, A.A.; Karadag, M.; Sahin, S.; Aslan, M.S.; Yavuzer, H.; Demirci, N.S.; Doventas, A.; et al. Sarcopenia assessment by new EWGSOP2 criteria for predicting chemotherapy dose-limiting toxicity in patients with gastrointestinal tract tumors. *Eur. Geriatr. Med.* **2022**, *13*, 267–274. [CrossRef]
80. Wang, Y.; Wang, Y.; Ai, L.; Zhang, H.; Li, G.; Wang, Z.; Jiang, X.; Yan, G.; Liu, Y.; Wang, C.; et al. Linear Skeletal Muscle Index and Muscle Attenuation May Be New Prognostic Factors in Colorectal Carcinoma Treated by Radical Resection. *Front. Oncol.* **2022**, *12*, 839899. [CrossRef]
81. Division of Nutrition PA and ONC for CDP and HP. Obesity Is a Common, Serious, and Costly Disease. 2022. Available online: https://www.cdc.gov/obesity/data/adult.html (accessed on 1 January 2020).

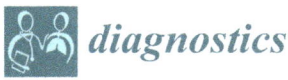

Review

Prognostic Factors for Cardiotoxicity among Children with Cancer: Definition, Causes, and Diagnosis with Omics Technologies

Kondylia Antoniadi [1,*], Nikolaos Thomaidis [2], Petros Nihoyannopoulos [3], Konstantinos Toutouzas [3], Evangelos Gikas [2], Charikleia Kelaidi [1] and Sophia Polychronopoulou [1]

[1] Department of Pediatric Hematology-Oncology (T.A.O.), "Aghia Sophia" Children's Hospital, Goudi, 11527 Athens, Greece
[2] Department of Chemistry, National and Kapodistrian University of Athens, 15772 Athens, Greece
[3] First Department of Cardiology, University of Athens, Hippokration Hospital, 11527 Athens, Greece
* Correspondence: condilia.and@gmail.com; Tel.: +30-210-745-2018 or +30-697-460-1968

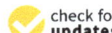

Citation: Antoniadi, K.; Thomaidis, N.; Nihoyannopoulos, P.; Toutouzas, K.; Gikas, E.; Kelaidi, C.; Polychronopoulou, S. Prognostic Factors for Cardiotoxicity among Children with Cancer: Definition, Causes, and Diagnosis with Omics Technologies. *Diagnostics* 2023, 13, 1864. https://doi.org/10.3390/diagnostics13111864

Academic Editor: Michael Henein

Received: 20 April 2023
Revised: 3 May 2023
Accepted: 23 May 2023
Published: 26 May 2023

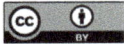

Copyright: © 2023 by the authors. Licensee MDPI, Basel, Switzerland. This article is an open access article distributed under the terms and conditions of the Creative Commons Attribution (CC BY) license (https://creativecommons.org/licenses/by/4.0/).

Abstract: Improvements in the treatment of childhood cancer have considerably enhanced survival rates over the last decades to over 80% as of today. However, this great achievement has been accompanied by the occurrence of several early and long-term treatment-related complications major of which is cardiotoxicity. This article reviews the contemporary definition of cardiotoxicity, older and newer chemotherapeutic agents that are mainly involved in cardiotoxicity, routine process diagnoses, and methods using omics technology for early and preventive diagnosis. Chemotherapeutic agents and radiation therapies have been implicated as a cause of cardiotoxicity. In response, the area of cardio-oncology has developed into a crucial element of oncologic patient care, committed to the early diagnosis and treatment of adverse cardiac events. However, routine diagnosis and the monitoring of cardiotoxicity rely on electrocardiography and echocardiography. For the early detection of cardiotoxicity, in recent years, major studies have been conducted using biomarkers such as troponin, N-terminal pro b-natriuretic peptide, etc. Despite the refinements in diagnostics, severe limitations still exist due to the increase in the above-mentioned biomarkers only after significant cardiac damage has occurred. Lately, the research has expanded by introducing new technologies and finding new markers using the omics approach. These new markers could be used not only for early detection but also for the early prevention of cardiotoxicity. Omics science, which includes genomics, transcriptomics, proteomics, and metabolomics, offers new opportunities for biomarker discovery in cardiotoxicity and may provide an understanding of the mechanisms of cardiotoxicity beyond traditional technologies.

Keywords: cardiotoxicity; childhood cancer; chemotherapeutics agents; biomarkers; omics technology

1. Introduction

With the induction of new chemotherapeutic agents over the years, the 5-year survival rate for childhood malignancies exceeds 80%. Caring for these patients includes not only early survival but also later outcomes. Chronic health conditions and health-related quality of life are noted among these, as many long-term treatment-related complications have resulted in increased morbidity and mortality rates. Cardiotoxicity represents the most serious non-hematological toxicity of chemotherapeutic drugs. It is noted that childhood cancer survivors have an 8× higher risk of mortality due to cardiovascular disease and a 6× increased risk of congestive heart failure. Most importantly, early cardiotoxicity may affect the design of chemotherapy and the omission of radiotherapy, resulting in incomplete cancer treatment, and consequently, inferior outcomes. The study of cardiotoxicity among the pediatric population is, as expected, of particular importance due to their long life expectancy [1–6].

2. Cardiotoxicity

Definition

The term cardiotoxicity was first described in 1946 as the damage to the heart caused by local anesthetics, mercurial diuretics, and digitalis. Later, in the 1970s, the term broadened to encompass cardiac complications related to anthracyclines (doxorubicin and daunorubicin), combination therapies such as doxorubicin and radiation, and drugs such as 5-fluorouracil. Presently, there is increased research interest, both basic and clinical, in detecting and managing cardiotoxicity as early as possible.

The definition of cardiotoxicity has great significance for a patient's management. According to the International Cardio-Oncology Society (IC-OS), the cardiovascular complications of chemotherapy can be separated into the following clinical entities and/or categories: (i) cardiac dysfunction: cardiomyopathy/heart failure (HF), (ii) vascular toxicity, (iii) myocarditis, (iv) arterial hypertension, and (v) arrhythmias and QT prolongation [7,8].

The most preponderant diagnosis of cardiotoxicity is based on the changes found in the left ventricular (LV) systolic function measured by the left ventricular ejection fraction (LVEF). Different organizations have defined cardiotoxicity in several ways using different threshold changes in the LVEF [8]. The need to harmonize all these definitions has been met by the International Cardio-Oncology Society (IC-OS) and is supported by the 2022 ESC Guidelines [7,8].

Cardiotoxicity can be categorized according to the time of presentation as acute, early onset, or late onset. Cardiotoxicity can be reversible if addressed while in the early stages [9]. Acute (<1%) toxicity can occur either after administrating a single dose or after a course of chemotherapeutic agents, as long as the onset of clinical manifestations is within the first two weeks following the end of the administration. If presented within the first year of treatment, it is characterized as early onset (1–18%). Late or chronic onset is manifested years or even decades following the treatment [9]. The percentage of late-onset cardiotoxicity varies in the literature mainly due to the different definitions used, the detection methods for cardiotoxicity, the population monitored, and the study design. It seems that over 50% of pediatric cancer survivors showed a subclinical decline in myocardial function and over 16% showed symptoms of clinical HF, especially those who had been exposed to anthracyclines [9].

Abnormalities in ventricular repolarization and electrocardiographic QT-interval alterations, supraventricular and ventricular arrhythmias, acute coronary syndromes, and pericarditis and/or myocarditis-like syndromes are hallmarks of acute or early onset cardiotoxicity [9]. In contrast, asymptomatic systolic and/or diastolic LVD, which can result in dilated cardiomyopathy, is the most typical indicator of chronic cardiotoxicity [9,10]. Clinical and sub-clinical cardiovascular damage, coronary artery disease, and cerebrovascular events are other conditions linked to treatment-related complications. Survivors had an almost six-fold higher risk of heart failure, a five-fold higher risk of myocardial infarction, a six-fold higher risk of pericardial disease, and an almost five-fold higher risk of valvular abnormalities compared to their siblings [11–13].

3. Chemotherapeutic Drugs

3.1. Anthracyclines

Anthracyclines, primarily doxorubicin but also daunomycin, epirubicin, and idarubicin, are some of the most commonly used agents for both hematologic and solid tumors. The basic structure of anthracyclines is that of a tetracyclic molecule with an anthraquinone backbone connected to a sugar moiety by a glycosidic linkage (Figure 1).

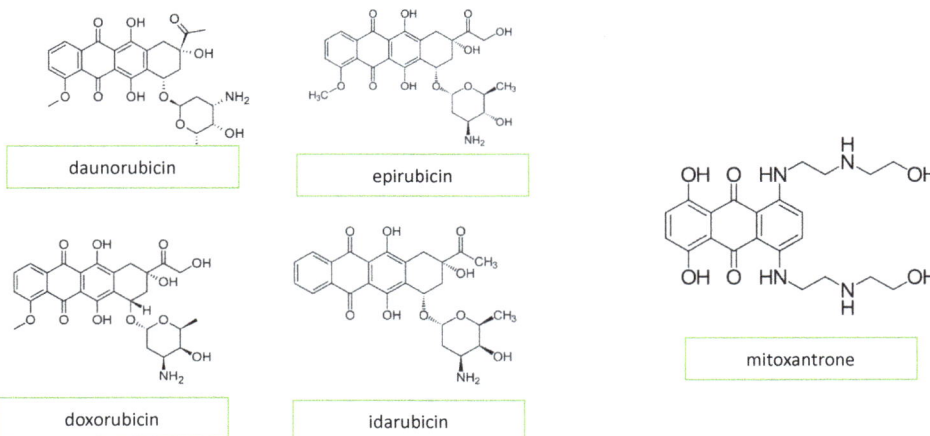

Figure 1. Chemical structure of anthracyclines and mitoxantrone.

Acute cardiotoxicity due to anthracyclines may present as hypotension, tachycardia, arrhythmia, transient depression of left ventricular function, myocarditis, pericarditis, or acute coronary syndrome. Late-onset cardiotoxicity caused by a high cumulative dose of anthracyclines mainly includes signs and symptoms of cardiomyopathy and chronic heart failure [9].

Mitoxantrone is a an anthracenedione (1,4-dihydroxy-9,10-anthraquinon, Figure 1) or anthracycline analog and has similar anthracycline mechanisms of action. Mitoxantrone might cause a wide variety of heart conditions, such as disturbances of cardiac rhythm, chronic heart failure, and persistent diastolic dysfunction in the absence of an impairment of the left ventricular ejection fraction [10].

The prevalent concept of how anthracycline action may cause heart damage involves the production of oxygen radicals, which in turn damage the DNA, proteins, and lipids, leading to cellular dysfunction and myocyte death [14–16].

Cardiolipins are abundantly found on the inner mitochondrial cell membrane. By having an increased affinity for anthracyclines, they in turn allow for their increased cell entry. Upon cell entry by passive diffusion, they can reach much higher intracellular concentrations compared to extracellular compartments. Within the cell, they form complexes by binding to iron, thus producing free radicals and reactive oxygen species, which in turn cause cell damage and death. By peroxidizing lipids of the cell membrane, those elements may also damage the cell membrane. As cardiomyocytes contain an abundance of mitochondria, they are more susceptible to anthracycline damage because of the depletion of glutathione peroxidase (an antioxidant) [15].

Other mechanisms of cardiotoxicity include alterations to gene expression and nitric oxide synthase activity, which lead to reduced creatine kinase activity and function in the mitochondria, and ultimately, cell death [15]. After exposure to anthracyclines, many of these subcellular sequelae continue to develop for weeks, shedding light on the mechanisms of chronic cardiomyopathy [14].

Another identified mechanism of doxorubicin-mediated cardiotoxicity is changes to the topoisomerase-II (Top2). Topoisomerase II (TOP2) is a molecule that anthracyclines bind to and inhibit, preventing the growth of tumors. DNA's phosphate backbone is broken, twisted, and then resealed by topoisomerases, allowing the double helix's tension to be changed during transcription and replication. Anthracyclines intercalate into DNA, forming complexes with TOP2 that halt the enzyme's activity and trigger a DNA damage reaction that results in cell death [14,15,17] (Figure 2).

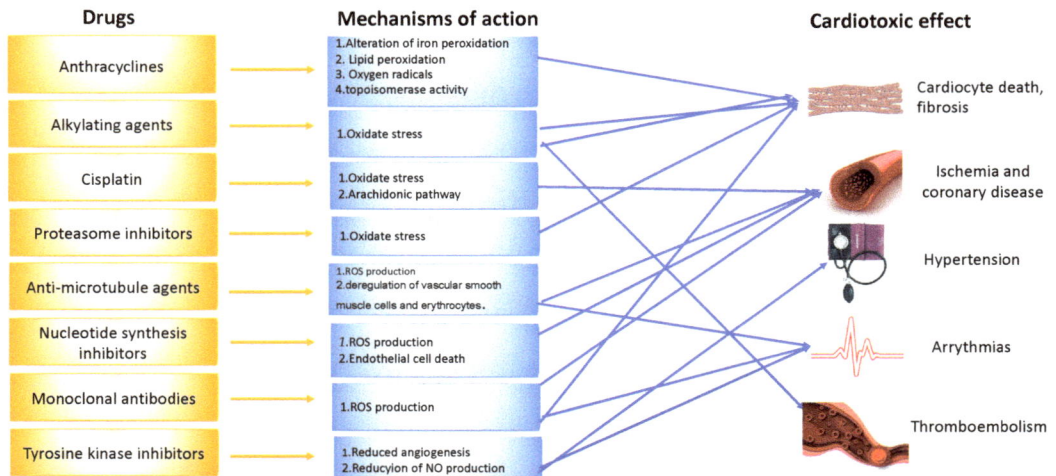

Figure 2. Mechanisms of drug-induced cardiotoxicity.

The mechanisms of mitoxantrone-associated cardiotoxicity remain to be completely understood. The formation of reactive oxygen species in myocardial cells is thought to lead to tissue damage through interactions with cellular iron metabolism [10].

3.2. Nucleotide Synthesis Inhibitors

The clinical presentation of methotrexate and fluorouracil (5-FU)-induced cardiotoxicity includes myocardial ischemia, cardiogenic shock, heart failure, and cardiomyopathy [10]. Coronary spasm is the most frequently reported mechanism of 5-FU-induced cardiotoxicity (Figure 2) [10]. The data derived from animal models indicate that these chemotherapeutic agents induce oxidative stress and the subsequent apoptosis of cardiomyocytes and endothelial cells [10,17].

3.3. Alkylating Agents

Adjuvant DNA-alkylating agents, such as cyclophosphamide (CP) and ifosfamide (IFO), suspend DNA synthesis in cancer cells. These two agents are similar in structure (Figure 3) and engender a similar pattern of cardiotoxic effects, causing acute heart failure, hemorrhagic myopericarditis, and arrhythmia [10,18]. CP- and IFO-induced acute cardiotoxicity is attributed mainly to a rise in free oxygen radicals and a lower antioxidant defense mechanism in the myocardium (Figure 2). A recent study by Sayed-Ahmed MM et al. demonstrated that CP- and IFO-induced cardiotoxicity is due to the inhibition of long-chain fatty acid oxidation via the repression of carnitine palmitoyl transferase I and fatty acid binding protein [19].

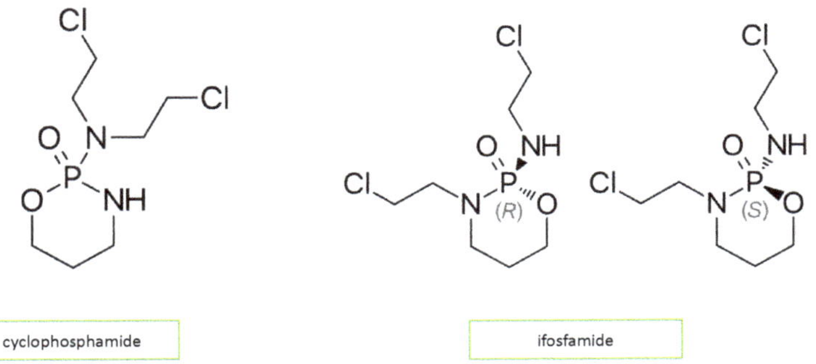

Figure 3. Chemical structure of alkylating agents.

3.4. Tyrosine Kinase Inhibitors

Dasatinib, imatinib, lapatinib, sorafenib, nilotinib, and sunitinib are examples of small molecule tyrosine kinase inhibitors (TKIs) that suppress cancer cell proliferation and induce apoptosis of cancer cells. Imatinib, dasatinib, and nilotinib are the three FDA-approved TKIs for use as first-line chronic myeloid leukemia therapy in pediatrics. In addition, sorafenib is used in young adults. The pathophysiological mechanism of TKI-induced cardiotoxicity is mitochondrial impairment and cardiomyocyte apoptosis (Figure 2) [10,18,20]. Each of the above drugs is associated with a different type of cardiotoxicity. For example, dasatinib is more often associated with pleural effusion and less with hypertension, HF, pericardial effusion, and pulmonary hypertension. Nilotinib is associated with peripheral artery disease, hypertension, and prolonged QTc. In contrast, imatinib is related to less cardiotoxicity than the other TKIs [7].

3.5. Anti-Microtubule Agents

Anti-microtubule agents, including docetaxel, paclitaxel, and vinca alkaloids, prevent the polymerization or depolymerization of microtubules [17]. The clinical features of cardiotoxicity induced by anti-microtubule agents are mostly ischemia and arrhythmia. Among all anti-microtubule agents in clinical use, paclitaxel induces the release of histamine, which in turn activates specific cardiac receptors, raising the myocardium's oxygen need, and leading to coronary vasoconstriction (Figure 2). In addition, Zhang et al. reported that the frequency of spontaneous calcium concentration in cardiomyocytes was significantly increased after paclitaxel treatment. This finding could be of great significance, as fluctuations in blood calcium levels are linked to arrhythmogenesis [10,21].

3.6. Cisplatin

Cisplatin is an efficacious chemotherapeutic drug with a strong antitumor effect against a wide range of neoplasms (Figure 4). However, the drug's acute and cumulative cardiotoxicity, including electrocardiograph (ECG) abnormalities, angina and acute myocardial infarction, hypertension and hypotension, arrhythmias, myocarditis, cardiomyopathy, and congestive heart failure, is a significant factor that restricts cisplatin treatment. Cisplatin cardiotoxicity can be caused by reactive oxygen species generation, which leads to the creation of oxidative stress and endothelial capillary damage (vascular damage) or has a direct toxic effect on cardiac myocytes (Figure 2) [10]. The prolonged cardiovascular toxicity of cisplatin, lasting up to many years, has been explained by both direct diffuse endothelial damage and an increase in risk factors for cardiovascular disease. These effects include coronary artery disease, systolic or diastolic left ventricular dysfunction, and severe congestive cardiomyopathy [10].

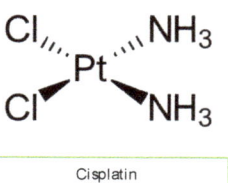

Cisplatin

Figure 4. Chemical structure of cisplatin.

3.7. Monoclonal Antibodies

Monoclonal antibodies, including bevacizumab (Avastin) and trastuzumab, not used in children, inhibit angiogenesis. Bevacizumab blocks vascular endothelial growth factor (VEGF), while trastuzumab inhibits human epidermal growth factor receptor 2 (HER2) in cancer cells (Figure 5). Bevacizumab causes mostly hypertension, congestive heart failure, and thromboembolic events of the artery and vein through the mechanism of oxidate stress induced by cardiomyocyte apoptosis. Monoclonal antibodies are not widely used in children with malignancy, so we do not discuss them further [10,18,20].

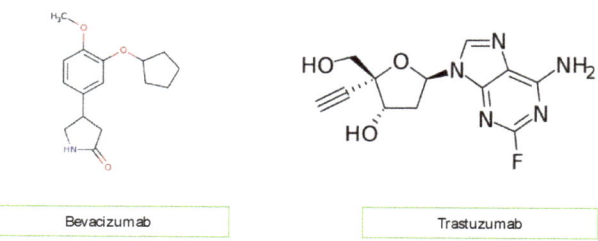

Bevacizumab   Trastuzumab

Figure 5. Chemical structure of monoclonal antibodies.

3.8. Proteasome Inhibitors

A new therapeutic option for the treatment of acute lymphoblastic leukemia (ALL) includes proteasome inhibitors (Figure 6) [18,20]. Bortezomib and carfilzomib are two newly prescribed drugs with the potential to cause cardiac dysfunction [22]. Compared to carfilzomib (up to 25%), bortezomib has a lower incidence of heart failure (up to 4%). The pathogenesis of proteasome inhibitor cardiotoxicity is not currently well understood. Exposure to proteasome inhibitors in a prenatal mouse model has shown that they can induce oxidative stress, leading to myocardial dysfunction. Carfilzomib is also known to induce renal toxicity and microangiopathy as a consequence of endothelial dysfunction. Combining these studies reveals a complicated mechanism of cardiotoxicity linked to proteasome inhibitors, including alterations to the heart's muscle and vasculature, which may be more severe with carfilzomib than bortezomib due to the irreversible nature of the proteasome inhibition of carfilzomib [23,24].

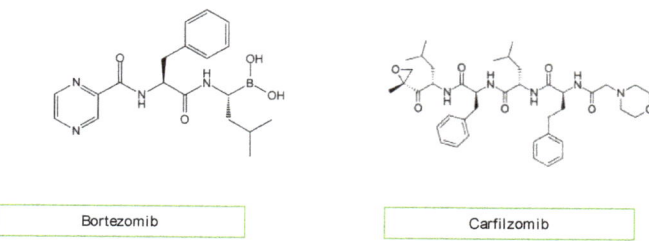

Bortezomib   Carfilzomib

Figure 6. Chemical structure of proteasome inhibitors.

4. Risk Factors

A multivariable number of factors contribute to the onset of cardiotoxicity with regard to the patient and/or the administered therapy (Figure 7). Several types of chemotherapeutic drugs may cause cardiotoxicity, as referred to above. These drugs act on cancer cells through a variety of mechanisms and promote cardiotoxicity with distinctive clinical symptoms and underlying mechanisms (Table 1) [7,10,16].

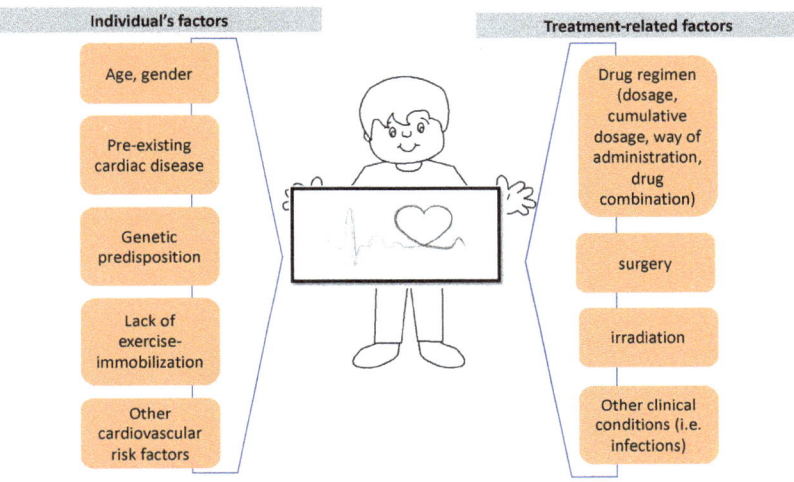

Figure 7. Multivariable factors leading to cardiotoxicity.

Table 1. Chemotherapeutic drugs and cardiovascular toxicity. (Adjusted by Rochette et al., Trends Pharmacol Sci. 2015 Jun;36(6):326–48 [25]).

Medicine/ Cardiotoxicity	Incidence (%)	Arrhythmia	Myocardial Ischemia	Vascular Toxicity	Heart Failure	QT Prolongation	Arterial Hypertension
Anthracyclines							
Doxorubicin	3–26	xxx	x	NE	xxx	NE	x
Doxorubicin Liposomal	2	x	xx	NE	x	NE	x
Epirubicin	0.9–3.3	x	x	NE	x	NE	x
Daunorubicin		xx	x	NE	x	NE	x
Idarubicin	5–18	xxx	x	NE	xx	NE	x
Antibiotics							
Mitoxantrone	0.2–30	xxx	xx	NE	xx	NE	xx
Mitomycin-c	10	xx	xx	NE	xx	xx	NE
Monoclonal antibodies							
Trastuzumab	1.7–8	xx	x	xx	xxx	NE	xx
Bevacizumab	1.6–4	xx	xx	xxx	xx	NE	xx
Pertuzumab	0.7–1.2	x	x	x	xx	NE	x
Dinutuximab beta		NE	xx	NE	xx	NE	xx
Rituximab		x	xx	xxx	x	NE	xx

Table 1. Cont.

Medicine/ Cardiotoxicity	Incidence (%)	Arrhythmia	Myocardial Ischemia	Vascular Toxicity	Heart Failure	QT Prolongation	Arterial Hypertension
Tyrosine kinase inhibitors							
Dasatinib	2–4	xxx	xx	xx	xx	xx	xx
Nilotinib	1	xx	NE	x	xx	xx	xxx
Vermurafenib		xx	xx	xx	x	NE	xx
Sorafenib	2–28	x	xx	xx	xx	NE	xx
Sunitinib	2.7–15	x	xx	xx	xxx	x	xxx
Erlotinib	7–11	NE	xx	xx	NE	NE	NE
Lapatinib	0.2–1.5	NE	xx	x	NE	xxx	NE
Pazopanib	7–11	NE	xx	xx	x	NE	xxx
Imatinib	0.2–2.7	NE	xxx	xx	xx	NE	NE
Proteasome inhibitors							
Bortezomib	2–5	x	x	x	x	NE	x
Carfilzomib	11–25	xx	xx	NE	x	NE	x
Antimetabolites							
5-fluorouracil	2–20	xxx	xxx	NE	x	NE	NE
Capecitabine		xxx	xxx	xx	NE	NE	NE
Clofarabine	27					NE	
Alkylating agents							
Cyclophosphamide	7–28	NE	NE	x	NE	NE	NE
Ifosfamide	0.5–17	NE	NE	x	xx	NE	NE
Cisplatin	rare	NE	NE	xx	NE	NE	NE
Antimicrotubule agents							
Paclitaxel	<1	xx	x	NE	x	NE	x
Docetaxel	2.3–13	xx	xx	NE	x	NE	xx
Alkaloids of vinca							
Vincristine	25	xx	x	NE	NE	xx	x
Vinblastine		NE	x	NE	NE	NE	x
Vindesin		NE	NE	NE	NE	NE	NE
Vinorelbin		NE	x	NE	NE	NE	NE

xxx: means >10%, xx: means 1–10%, x: means <1%, NE: not established.

The overall dose and mode of administration of each chemotherapeutic agent play an aggravating role in causing cardiac damage. For example, anthracycline-induced cardiotoxicity is known to be both cumulative and dose-related, indicating that each administered dose induces sequential or additional damage [18,26]. The cumulative total anthracycline dose is the most important risk factor for cardiac dysfunction [27]. In retrospective research, Von Hoff et al. [28] observed that when a patient receives a combined doxorubicin dose of 400, 550, and 700 mg/m^2, the incidence of cardiotoxicity is 3, 7, and 18%, respectively, with dose-limiting toxicity. Another study in adolescents found that even at dosages of 180–240 mg/m^2, 30% of the participants experienced subclinical episodes 13 years after therapy [29]. These results imply that there is no anthracycline dose that is considered safe. Reduced cardiac function has been correlated with dosages as low as 100 mg/m^2 [30–32].

In addition, female gender, age (under <5 years old), the patient's clinical condition (extent of disease, infection), genetic background, pre-existing cardiac disease, and the combinations of cardiotoxic drugs play an important role in causing cardiac damage [33] (Table 2). The pediatric population is more homogeneous as a study population since there are no confounding cardiovascular risk factors (diabetes, smoking, arterial hypertension) [7,14,34].

Table 2. Risk factors.

Risk Factors Related to Children	Risk Factors Related to Therapy
• Female sex • Age < 5 years • Genetic background • Pre-existing cardiac disease • Cardiovascular risk factors (diabetes, obesity, hyperlipidemia, hypertension)	• Anthracycline > 250 mg/m^2 equivalent doxorubicin • Cumulative dose • Irradiation • Combination of cardiotoxic drugs

The risk of developing cardiotoxicity is also increased by concurrent radiation exposure to the chest. In addition to the myocardium, radiation therapy has the potential for damaging the pericardium, heart vessels, and conductive tissue [18].

The carriers of certain genetic mutations are also more susceptible to cardiotoxicity [9,18]. Our understanding of genetic susceptibility to anthracycline-related cardiotoxicity has been influenced by a sizable body of research, as we describe below.

5. Diagnosis

As part of the baseline risk assessment, a thorough clinical history and physical examination are advised. Many patients with cardiac dysfunction could be asymptomatic, so both during and post-chemotherapy, cardiac monitoring is necessary. Consideration of the classic cardiovascular disease risk factors already mentioned is recommended, and children should be monitored for clinical signs and potential indicators of cardiotoxicity. The above-mentioned factors should be noted alongside the baseline electrocardiography, cardiac serum biomarkers, and cardiac imaging tests to complete baseline evaluation.

Imaging

Diagnostic approaches for chemotherapy-induced cardiotoxicity include electrocardiography and echocardiography, which are used as methods of monitoring cardiac function before, during, and after treatment.

Electrocardiography (ECG) can be used to identify any early signs of cardiac toxicity, such as resting tachycardia, ST-T wave abnormalities, conduction disturbances, QT interval prolongation, or arrhythmias. However, these ECG findings could be induced by several factors unrelated to cardiotoxic treatment. These ECG abnormalities may be reversed and are not always related to the development of chronic cardiomyopathy [7,27,34].

Two-dimensional echocardiography (2D) is the most used imaging technique to monitor cardiac function. It is non-invasive, cheap, readily available, and does not expose the patient to further radiation. However, standard echocardiographic parameters such as LVEF may lack sensitivity for the detection of systolic dysfunction [34].

Considering the poor sensitivity of 2D LVEF measurement, the use of global systolic longitudinal myocardial strain (GLS) analysis has become an area of interest [34,35]. A pathogenic percentage reduction of GLS greater than 15% from baseline is regarded as a sign of early LV dysfunction. When possible, it is preferable to use these sophisticated echocardiographic measures as the foundation for clinical decisions.

Other methods for the monitoring of these patients are cardiac magnetic resonance imaging (CMR), nuclear cardiac imaging (MUGA), and myocardial perfusion imaging (MPI). There are two techniques for MPI: single-photon emission computed tomography (SPECT) and positron emission tomography (PET). All these methods take considerably longer than follow-up echocardiography and might not be as accessible in all pediatric facilities [34].

6. Biomarkers

Several biomarkers have been assessed for their efficacy in the early prediction of patients' risk of cardiotoxicity and the identification of cardiac dysfunction. The World Health Organization defines biomarkers as any element, structure, or process that can be detected in the body (or its byproducts) and which affects or forecasts the development or course of a disease.

According to the literature, troponin and natriuretic peptide are the most studied biomarkers for the detection of both early cardiotoxicity and its later follow-up. Lipshultz et al. showed that the elevation of cardiac troponin T and N-terminal pro-brain natriuretic peptide (NT-pro-BNP) in children with acute lymphoblastic leukemia was associated with a notably reduced left ventricular (LV) mass, abnormal LV end-diastolic posterior wall thickness, and abnormal LV thickness-to-dimension ratios, all of which suggested LV remodeling, respectively, 4 years later [36]. However, further research has not pointed out an association between acute or chronic troponin release and left ventricular dysfunction, but in contrast, an association has been found with NT-pro-BNP in childhood cancer survivors [37–39].

We should be especially careful in evaluating troponin and natriuretic peptide values in children <1 year of age due to their normally elevated values at these ages [40].

Other biomarkers investigated include inflammation markers, such as C-reactive protein (CRP) and growth/differentiation factor 15 (GDF-15) [38], oxidative stress markers such as myeloperoxidase, vascular remodeling markers such as placental growth factor and soluble Fms-like tyrosine kinase receptor 3, and fibrosis markers (galectin 3) [36,41–49]. Moreover, these conventional biomarkers usually show significant changes only after heart damage occurs.

To determine the proper use of these biomarkers in clinical practice, new prospective and multicenter studies with large populations, well-standardized dosing methodologies, well-defined time of sampling, and cardiologic end points are required.

7. Omics

In the last decades, new research and clinical studies have attempted to identify possible biomarkers of early cardiac damage by chemotherapeutic agents using omics technology. Omics science offers new opportunities for biomarker discovery in cardiotoxicity and may provide an understanding of cardiotoxicity beyond traditional technologies. Omics technology includes genomics, transcriptomics, proteomics, and metabolomics.

7.1. Genomics

A cumulative anthracycline dose and other related risk factors seem to not be exclusive risk factors responsible for significant individual variation in the incidence and severity of heart failure in pediatric cancer survivors. Several studies have revealed how important host genetic polymorphisms could lead to a differential risk of cardiotoxicity among cancer survivors with otherwise identical clinical and treatment-related risk factors by using genome-wide association or candidate gene approaches [50–53]. This explains why some patients experience cardiotoxicity while other patients can tolerate high doses of chemotherapy without heart damage.

Genomic polymorphisms are small changes in a specific part of the DNA chain. One or more polymorphisms can determine a range of patient characteristics, such as their ability to metabolize and eliminate genotoxic substances. Cancer treatment-related cardiovascular toxicity risk may be influenced by genetic variation. Significant efforts using targeted and whole genome correlation studies have been made to reveal the pharmacogenomic causes of this predisposition [50,54–60].

At least 45 SNPs located in 34 genes have been associated with anthracycline-induced cardiotoxicity [61–64]. Many of these associations require further investigation through replication and/or functional and mechanistic studies to make sure we confirm and better understand the roles of these associated variants in anthracycline-related cardiotoxicity (ACT) [9].

Polymorphisms in solute carrier transporter (SLC) genes are associated with ACT. One of the functions of the SLC family is acting as drug transporters for anthracyclines, thus providing biological support for these genetic associations. Research on childhood cancer survivors has discovered correlations between ACT risk and protective variants in SLC, such as SLC28A3, SLC22A17, and SCL22A7. These findings have been successfully replicated [65–70]. In addition, different studies have reported protective variants in SLC10A2 and SLC22A1 [66]. SLC22A6 was first mentioned in the context of ACT by Sagi et al. in patients treated for childhood ALL [68].

Retinoic acid receptor gamma (RARG) has been involved in cardiac development and remodeling through the repression of Top2b [71]. A recent genome-wide association study, by Aminkeng et al. [51], uncovered a non-synonymous variant rs2229774 in *RARG*, which was significantly associated with ACT in survivors of childhood cancer. Specifically, rs2229774-carriers had a significantly increased risk of developing ACT as compared to non-carriers [51].

Studies have also revealed an elevated risk brought on by a variation in the UGT1A6 gene, a member of the glucuronosyl transferase family. Through the glucuronidation path, UGT1A6 plays a significant role in the detoxification of drugs, including the metabolites of anthracyclines [51,65,69].

Polymorphisms in adenosine triphosphate-binding cassette transporter (ABC) genes are related to cardiotoxicity in childhood patient cancers treated with anthracyclines. The ABC genes seem to play a role as efflux transporters of drugs, including anthracyclines, so may have important effects on the myocardium. Eight variants in five genes (ABCB1, ABCB4, ABCC1, ABCC2, and ABCC5) have been associated with cardiotoxicity, especially with reduced ejection fraction [54–56,68,72].

Other studies have investigated polymorphisms in carbonyl reductase genes, which have been associated with dose-dependent increases in cardiomyopathy risk. Carbonyl reductase (CBR) will reduce anthracyclines to cardiotoxic alcohol metabolites. As Blanco et al. showed, among childhood cancer survivors, homozygosity for the G allele in CBR3 leads to increased cardiomyopathy risk associated with low- to moderate-dose anthracyclines. Patients homozygous with the CBR3 V244M G allele have no safe cut-off minimum dose [57,58].

A recent study showed a gene–environment interaction between a single-nucleotide polymorphism on the CELF4 gene and a higher dose of anthracyclines [59]. CUGBP Elav-like family member 4 CELF4) protein is responsible for pre-mRNA alternative splicing of TNNT2, the gene that encodes for cardiac troponin T.

Aminkeng et al. [69] gathered evidence-based clinical practice recommendations for pharmacogenomic testing and emphasized that the RARG genes rs2229774, UGT1A6 * 4 rs1786378, and SLC28A3 rs7853758 have the potential to further discriminate patients at higher and lower risk of ACT. A pharmacogenetic test for these genetic variations in RARG, SLC28A3, and UGT1A6 has been released at the British Columbia Children's Hospital since the publication of these guidelines. Based on genetic and clinical risk variables, tested patients were divided into several risk groups, and therapy adjustments were chosen in accordance with this risk. Early evidence indicates that the British Columbia Children's Hospital's pharmacogenetic testing was effective in lowering the incidence of ACT in children, which should inspire additional clinics to utilize this pharmacogenetic test.

These findings might help develop prediction models that can spot patients who will be particularly susceptible to ACT and who will need their therapy modified or closer monitoring. Further independent research may make it possible to identify people before treatment with a genetic predisposition to cardiovascular toxicity and for whom more thorough screening, or perhaps preventive measures, should be implemented. Replication analyses, however, have occasionally failed to support the initial findings. Numerous factors, including the variability of cohorts, ambiguities in the definition of ACT, variations in the procedures, and the type or dosage of the chemotherapeutic drugs used may have contributed to this. To increase the diagnostic and prognostic role in predicting ACT, more research is required.

7.2. Transcriptomics

Another interesting area is the integration of microRNAs in the early detection of cardiotoxicity. Recently, the potential use of circulating microRNAs (miRNAs) has been studied as a possible specific biomarker and therapeutic target of cardiac disease [73–79].

MicroRNAs are small endogenous non-coding RNAs of 21–24 nucleotides, acting as post-transcriptional gene regulators by inhibiting and/or degrading target messenger RNAs (mRNAs). Bioinformatics data suggest that each miRNA molecule can control hundreds of gene targets, thus indicating the potential effect of miRNAs on virtually any genetic pathway. MiRNAs play a significant role in different biological processes, including proliferation, differentiation, development, and cell death. Furthermore, several miRNAs are involved in regulating heart development from the embryonic to the adult stage, and their dysregulation leads to various heart diseases, such as arrhythmias, essential hypertension, heart failure, cardiomyopathy, cardiac hypertrophy, and atherosclerosis [80,81].

The cardiotoxic effect of chemotherapeutic agents may lead to specific miRNAs with changed expressions. These can be used to investigate the toxicity of potential drug candidates on cardiomyocytes and cell lines originating from the heart in a preclinical in vitro setting. The potential use of circulating miRNAs in plasma as indicators of drug-induced cardiotoxicity has undergone much research during the last several years [80].

Nearly 30 circulating miRNAs have had their levels altered, both increased and decreased, and these changes have been linked to HF and associated pathologies. MiRNAs, including miR-1, miR-133, miR-208a/b, miR-499, miR-29, and miR-34, which are substantially expressed in the myocardium compared to other tissues, are the ones that are primarily being researched [73]. In addition, a variety of harmful substances alter the miRNA profile in both plasma and cardiac tissue. Even at low toxin concentrations, where other tissue damage biomarkers are not discernible, alterations in miRNAs can be measured [80]. Most studies use data from experimental animals, while those utilizing clinical patient samples are limited.

MiR-1 is a skeletal muscle-specific miRNA that has an important role in cardiac development, function, and disease. Abnormal miR-1 levels are associated with acute myocardial infarction, heart failure, arrhythmias, ventricular dysfunction, cardiac hypertrophy, and myocyte hyperplasia [82]. MiR-499 and miR-208 are associated with acute myocardial infarction and HF [82]. Circulating levels of miR-133a have been associated with an increased risk of cardiovascular diseases. Increased levels of miR-133a have been detected in patients with acute myocardial infarction earlier than cardiac troponin T increase [83]. MiR-133 includes two miRNAs, named miR-133a and miR-133b, that are highly expressed in the human heart and seem to be involved in heart development and myocyte differentiation.

The analysis of circulating miRNAs in breast cancer patients receiving doxorubicin (DOX) identified miR-1 as a potential candidate for the early detection of DOX-induced cardiotoxicity [84]. Leger et al. investigated other possible markers of cardiotoxicity in children and young adults treated with anthracycline chemotherapy (AC). Candidate plasma profiling of 24 miRNAs was performed in 33 children before and after a cycle of AC or non-cardiotoxicity chemotherapy. MiR-1, miR-29b, and miR-499 were reported to be upregulated in pediatric patients following the acute initiation of AC [85,86]. Monitoring the plasma levels of miR-208a and miR-208b showed an elevation in patients with myocardial damage and were even detected earlier than cardiac troponins [87]. This is in concordance with the findings of other studies [73,74,87,88]. Table 3 provides a summary of the major miRNAs linked to drug-induced cardiotoxicity.

Table 3. Summary of major miRNAs link to drug-induced cardiotoxicity in people.

MiRNA	Drug	Modulation	Species	System	References
miR-1	Doxorubicin	Increase	Female patients	Plasma	Riguad et al., Oncotarget 2017 [84]
miR-1, miR-29b, miR-499	Anthracyclines	Increase	Children and young adult	Plasma	Leger et al., J Am Heart Assoc. 2017 [85]
miR1254	Bevacizumub	Increase	Humans	Plasma	Zhao et al., Tumour Biol. 2014 [89]
miR29 miR499	Doxorubicin	Increase	Children	Plasma	Oatmen et al., Am J Physiol Heart Circ Physiol, 2018 [73]
miR208	Doxorubicin	Nothing	Female patients	Plasma	Carvalho et al., J Appl Toxicol 2015 [74]

In addition to anthracyclines, other cytotoxic agents have shown cardiotoxic effects, and biomarkers of their pathomechanism have been searched for, including miRNAs. Patients with bevacizumab-induced cardiotoxicity, when compared to controls, were found to have increased levels of five miRNAs. In the validation experiments, two of these (miR-1254 and miR-579) showed valuable specificity. MiR-1254 exhibited the strongest correlation with the clinical diagnosis of bevacizumab-induced cardiotoxicity [89].

With regard to a number of features of drug-induced cardiotoxicity, miRNAs appear to be a promising agent. A potentially successful method for preventing severe problems is the identification of patients with subclinical cardiotoxicity through the detection of cardio-specific miRNAs circulating in plasma that are not present under normal circumstances [80]. Many other research studies should focus on how the miRNA profile changes when interacting with drugs with proven cardiotoxicity.

7.3. Proteomics

The proteomic data available to date on chemotherapy-induced cardiac toxicity are limited, mainly involving anthracyclines, and related to experimental animal studies [90].

Proteomics is the study of proteins, which are essential components of organisms and have a variety of functions. The proteome consists of all the proteins expressed by a cell, tissue, or organism. Proteomics could give us important information for a number of biological problems.

Ohyama et al. identified cellular processes in mouse heart tissue from control rats and rats affected by different adriamycin and docetaxel dosing protocols using a toxicoproteomic approach. They identified nine different proteins that were expressed in the control and two treatment groups, and which were involved in energy production pathways, such as glycolysis, the Krebs cycle, and the mitochondrial electron transport chain [91].

Kumar et al. in 2011 used a rat model of doxorubicin-induced cardiotoxicity to show the differential regulation of several key proteins, including proteins that are stress-responsive (ATP synthase, enolase alpha, alpha B-crystallin, translocation protein 1, and stress-induced phosphoprotein 1), and apoptotic/cell damage markers (p38 alpha, lipocortin, voltage-dependent anion-selective channel protein 2, creatine kinase, and MTUS1) [86].

More recently, Desai et al. pinpointed possible biomarkers of early cardiotoxicity in the plasma of male B6C3F1 mice that received a weekly intravenous dose of 3 mg/kg doxorubicin (DOX) or saline (SAL) for 2, 3, 4, 6, or 8 weeks (corresponding to cumulative doses of 6, 9, 12, 18, or 24 mg/kg DOX). They suggested the neurogenic locus notch homolog protein 1 (NOTCH1) and von Willebrand factor (vWF) as early biomarkers of

DOX cardiotoxicity to address the clinically significant question of identifying cancer patients at risk for cardiotoxicity [92].

Finally, Yarana et al., using a mouse model of DOX-induced cardiac injury, quantified serum extracellular vehicles (EVs), assayed proteomes, counted the oxidized protein levels in serum EVs generated following DOX treatment, and examined the alteration of EV content. The release of EVs containing brain/heart glycogen phosphorylase (PYGB) before the increase in cardiac troponin in the blood following DOX therapy suggests that PYGB is an early indicator of cardiac damage, according to the proteomic profiling of DOX_EVs [93].

To find out if these pathways could result in the discovery of early markers of cardiotoxicity, more research in this area is required.

7.4. Metabolomics

Metabolomics is an upcoming new science with the potential to further increase our knowledge of cancer biology and the search for prognostic biomarkers. Up to now, most studies have either used metabolomic data from experimental animals or the cellular level, while those utilizing clinical patient samples have been extremely limited (Figure 8).

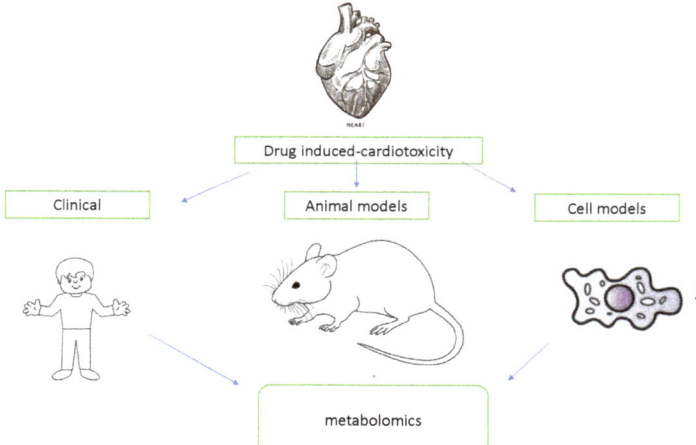

Figure 8. Diagram expressing the different research models of cardiotoxicity (clinical, animal, cellular) using metabolomic data.

Metabolism is more directly related to the phenotype and physiology of a biological system. Metabolomics is the study of all cellular metabolites (hydrocarbons, amino acids, sugars, fatty acids, organic acids, steroids, and peptides). It encompasses all levels of cellular regulation, that is, the regulation that occurs at the level of transcription, translation, and post-translational modifications, and hence, it can closely reflect the phenotype of an organism at a specific time. The human metabolome is thought to be composed of about 3000 endogenous metabolites at current estimates (the Human Metabolome Project). However, the exact size of the human metabolome is still debatable. It is also believed that nutritional compounds, xenobiotics, and microbial metabolites must be considered when defining the human metabolome [94]. Therefore, metabolome analysis can be a useful tool used to find diagnostic markers that will help us examine unknown pathological conditions effectively.

Different analytical techniques can be used in the measurement of metabolites. Such methods are nuclear magnetic resonance (NMR) spectrometry, molecular mass spectrometry (MS), gas chromatography (GC), high-performance liquid chromatography (LC), and tricarboxylic acid (TCA). The most common and higher-throughput technologies are nuclear magnetic resonance (NMR) spectrometry and molecular mass spectrometry (MS).

Mass spectrometry is an analytical platform for metabolomic analysis. It is a highly sensitive, reproductive, and versatile method, as it identifies molecules and their fragments by measuring their masses. This information is obtained by measuring the mass-to-charge ratio (m/z) of ions that are produced by inducing the loss or gain of a charge from a neutral species. The sample, which comprises a complicated mixture of metabolites, can be introduced to the mass spectrometer either directly or preceded by a separation approach (using liquid chromatography or gas chromatography) [95].

NMR spectroscopy utilizes the magnetic properties of nuclei to determine the number and type of chemical entities in a molecule. Proton NMR spectroscopy can detect soluble proton-containing molecules with a molecular weight of approximately 20 kD or less. The NMR spectra serve as the raw material for pattern recognition analyses, which simplifies the complex multivariate data into two or three dimensions that can be readily understood and evaluated. Both NMR and liquid chromatography–mass spectrometry (LC-MS) systems can be integrated into in vivo tissues or biological fluids, such as serum, plasma, urine, etc., obtained from humans. The advantages of NMR are that it requires relatively little sample preparation, it is non-destructive, and it can provide useful information regarding the exact structure of metabolites. However, NMR sensitivity is related to the magnet's strength, while available instrumentation can unambiguously detect only the most abundant metabolites in plasma. On the other hand, the most important advantage of mass spectrometry coupled with upfront chromatography is its far greater sensitivity than NMR MS-based systems, which have been used to resolve compounds in the nanomole to the picomole and even the femtomole range, whereas the identification of compounds by 1H-NMR requires concentrations of 1 nanomole or higher [96,97].

The main methodologies that are used for metabolomic analysis are untargeted and targeted metabolomics. Untargeted metabolomics allow for measuring a wider variety of metabolites present in an extracted sample without prior knowledge of the metabolome. The main advantage is that this provides an unbiased way to examine the relationships among interconnected metabolites from multiple pathways. In contrast, targeted metabolomic analyses measure the concentrations of a predefined set of metabolites and provide higher sensitivity and selectivity than untargeted metabolomics.

An overview of the main metabolomics associated with drug-induced cardiotoxicity detected in plasma/stem cells/hearts in mice and people is given in Table 4. The role of carnitine in the detection of cardiotoxicity was confirmed by a successive study in which Armenian et al. compared a metabolomics analysis in 150 symptom-free childhood cancer survivors who received anthracycline treatment. Thirty-five participants were found to have cardiac dysfunction without symptoms. So, they compared two groups (participants with cardiac dysfunction and those with normal systolic function) and discovered 15 metabolites differentially expressed among the patients. After adjusting for multiple comparisons, individuals with cardiotoxicity had significantly lower plasma carnitine levels in comparison to those with normal cardiac function [98].

Table 4. Metabolomics associated with drug-induced cardiotoxicity.

Metabolite	Plasma	Stem Cell	Heart	Mice	People	XRT	Medicine	Dose	Biomarker	References
Proline	↓//↑		↑	Yes	No		Cyclophosphamide	200 mg/kg		Li et al., J Proteome Res, 2015 [99]
LPC 20:3	↓			Yes	No		Cyclophosphamide	200 mg/kg		Li et al., J Proteome Res, 2015 [99]
Linoleic acid	↓			Yes	No		Cyclophosphamide	200 mg/kg		Li et al., J Proteome Res, 2015 [99]

Table 4. Cont.

Metabolite	Plasma	Stem Cell	Heart	Mice	People	XRT	Medicine	Dose	Biomarker	References
L-carnitine	↑//↑			Yes	No		Cyclophosphamide/ doxo/isoprotenerol/ 5-fluorouracil	200 mg/kg// 20 mg/kg// 5 mg/kg// 125 mg/kg		Li et al., J Proteome Res, 2015 [99]
19-hydroxycorticosterone	↑//↓			Yes	No		Cyclophosphamide/ doxo/isoprotenerol/ 5-fluorouracil	200 mg/kg// 20 mg/kg// 5 mg/kg// 125 mg/kg		Li et al., J Proteome Res, 2015 [99]
Phytophingosine	↓			Yes	No		Cyclophosphamide	200 mg/kg		Li et al., J Proteome Res, 2015 [99]
Cholid acid	↓			Yes	No		Cyclophosphamide	200 mg/kg		Li et al., J Proteome Res, 2015 [99]
LPC 14:0	↓//↓			Yes	No		Cyclophosphamide/ doxo/isoprotenerol/ 5-fluorouracil	200 mg/kg// 20 mg/kg// 5 mg/kg// 125 mg/kg		Li et al., J Proteome Res, 2015 [99]
LPC 18:3	↓			Yes	No		Cyclophosphamide	200 mg/kg		Li et al., J Proteome Res, 2015 [99]
LPC 16:1	↓			Yes	No		Cyclophosphamide	200 mg/kg		Li et al., J Proteome Res, 2015 [99]
LPE 18:2	↓			Yes	No		Cyclophosphamide	200 mg/kg		Li et al., J Proteome Res, 2015 [99]
LPC 22:5	↓			Yes	No		Cyclophosphamide	200 mg/kg		Li et al., J Proteome Res, 2015 [99]
LPC 22:6	↓			Yes	No		Cyclophosphamide	200 mg/kg		Li et al., J Proteome Res, 2015 [99]
LPC 22:4	↓			Yes	No		Cyclophosphamide	200 mg/kg		Li et al., J Proteome Res, 2015 [99]
LPC 20:2	↓//↓			Yes	No		Cyclophosphamide/ doxo/isoprotenerol/ 5-fluorouracil	200 mg/kg// 20 mg/kg// 5 mg/kg// 125 mg/kg		Li et al., J Proteome Res, 2015 [99]
PLE 20:3	↓			Yes	No		Cyclophosphamide	200 mg/kg		Li et al., J Proteome Res, 2015 [99]
Pyruvate			↑				Doxorubicin	20 mg/kg	Troponin T LDH	Andreadou et al., NMR Biomed, 2009 [100] /Chaudhari et al., Amino Acids 2017 [101]
Acetate		↑	↑	Yes			Doxorubicin	20 mg/kg	Troponin T LDH	Andreadou et al., NMR Biomed, 2009 [100] /Chaudhari et al., Amino Acids 2017 [101]

Table 4. Cont.

Metabolite	Plasma	Stem Cell	Heart	Mice	People	XRT	Medicine	Dose	Biomarker	References
Formate		↑					Doxorubicin	20 mg/kg	Troponin T LDH	Andreadou et al., NMR Biomed, 2009 [100] /Chaudhari et al., Amino Acids 2017 [101]
Succinate		↑	↑	Yes			Doxorubicin	20 mg/kg	Troponin T LDH	Andreadou et al., NMR Biomed, 2009 [100] /Chaudhari et al., Amino Acids 2017 [101]
Lactate	↑//↑		↓	Yes			Doxorubicin	20 mg/kg	Troponin T	Andreadou et al., NMR Biomed, 2009 [100]
Alanine	↑//↑		↑//↑	Yes			Doxorubicin	20 mg/kg	Troponin T	Andreadou et al., NMR Biomed, 2009 [100]
Glutamine	↑		↓	Yes			Doxorubicin	20 mg/kg	Troponin T	Andreadou et al., NMR Biomed, 2009 [100]
Glutamate	↑		no	Yes		↑	Doxorubicin	20 mg/kg	Troponin T	Andreadou et al., NMR Biomed, 2009 [100]
Creatine			no	Yes			Doxorubicin	20 mg/kg	Troponin T	Andreadou et al., NMR Biomed, 2009 [100]
Taurine			no	Yes		↓	Doxorubicin	20 mg/kg	Troponin T	Andreadou et al., NMR Biomed, 2009 [100]
Valine	↑		↓	Yes		↑	Doxorubicin	20 mg/kg	Troponin T	Andreadou et al., NMR Biomed, 2009 [100]
Leuline	↑		↓	Yes			Doxorubicin	20 mg/kg	Troponin T	Andreadou et al., NMR Biomed, 2009 [100]
Isoleukine	↑		↓	Yes		↑	Doxorubicin	20 mg/kg	Troponin T	Andreadou et al., NMR Biomed, 2009 [100]
Carnitine	↓//↑		↓	Yes	Yes		Anthracyclines/ doxorubicin		Troponin T	Armenian et al., Cancer Epidemiol Biomarkers Prev. 2014 [98]

Table 4. Cont.

Metabolite	Plasma	Stem Cell	Heart	Mice	People	XRT	Medicine	Dose	Biomarker	References
Threitol	↓				Yes		Anthracyclines			Armenian et al., Cancer Epidemiol Biomarkers Prev. 2014 [98]
Mannose	↓				Yes		Anthracyclines			Armenian et al., Cancer Epidemiol Biomarkers Prev. 2014 [98]
Pyroglutamine	↓				Yes		Anthracyclines			Armenian et al., Cancer Epidemiol Biomarkers Prev. 2014 [98]
N-acetylalanine	↓				Yes		Anthracyclines			Armenian et al., Cancer Epidemiol Biomarkers Prev. 2014 [98]
Creatine	↓				Yes		Anthracyclines			Armenian et al., Cancer Epidemiol Biomarkers Prev. 2014 [98]
Eicosenoate	↓				Yes		Anthracyclines			Armenian et al., Cancer Epidemiol Biomarkers Prev. 2014 [98]
Stearidonate	↓				Yes		Anthracyclines			Armenian et al., Cancer Epidemiol Biomarkers Prev. 2014 [98]
Arachidonate	↓				Yes		Anthracyclines			Armenian et al., Cancer Epidemiol Biomarkers Prev. 2014 [98]
Dihomo-linoleate	↓				Yes		Anthracyclines			Armenian et al., Cancer Epidemiol Biomarkers Prev. 2014 [98]
L-stearoylglcerophoinositol	↓				Yes		Anthracyclines			Armenian et al., Cancer Epidemiol Biomarkers Prev. 2014 [98]
Dehydroisoandrosterone sulfate	↓				Yes		Anthracyclines			Armenian et al., Cancer Epidemiol Biomarkers Prev. 2014 [98]
Pregnen-dio; disulfate	↓				Yes		Anthracyclines			Armenian et al., Cancer Epidemiol Biomarkers Prev. 2014 [98]
Pregn steroid monosulfate	↓				Yes		Anthracyclines			Armenian et al., Cancer Epidemiol Biomarkers Prev. 2014 [98]
Arginine	↑			↑	Yes		Doxorubicin			Schnackenberg et al., Appl. Toxicol. 2016 [102]
Asparagine	↑			↑	Yes		Doxorubicin		Troponin T	Schnackenberg et al., Appl. Toxicol. 2016 [102]

Table 4. *Cont.*

Metabolite	Plasma	Stem Cell	Heart	Mice	People	XRT	Medicine	Dose	Biomarker	References
Citrulline	↑		↑	Yes			Doxorubicin		Troponin T	Schnackenberg et al., Appl. Toxicol. 2016 [102]
Glycine	↑		↑	Yes		↑	Doxorubicin		Troponin T	Schnackenberg et al., Appl. Toxicol. 2016 [102]
Histidine	↑		↑	Yes			Doxorubicin		Troponin T	Schnackenberg et al., Appl. Toxicol. 2016 [102]
Lysine	↑		↑	Yes			Doxorubicin		Troponin T	Schnackenberg et al., Appl. Toxicol. 2016 [102]
Methionine	↑		↑	Yes			Doxorubicin		Troponin T	Schnackenberg et al., Appl. Toxicol. 2016 [102]
Ornithine	↑		↑	Yes			Doxorubicin		Troponin T	Schnackenberg et al., Appl. Toxicol. 2016 [102]
Phenylalanine	↑		↑	Yes			Doxorubicin		Troponin T	Schnackenberg et al., Appl. Toxicol. 2016 [102]
Serine	↑		↑	Yes			Doxorubicin		Troponin T	Schnackenberg et al., Appl. Toxicol. 2016 [102]
Threonine	↑		↑	Yes		↑	Doxorubicin		Troponin T	Schnackenberg et al., Appl. Toxicol. 2016 [102]
Tryptophan	↑		↑	Yes			Doxorubicin		Troponin T	Schnackenberg et al., Appl. Toxicol. 2016 [102]
Tyrosine	↑		↑	Yes			Doxorubicin		Troponin T	Schnackenberg et al., Appl. Toxicol. 2016 [102]
Acetylornithine	↑		↓	Yes			Doxorubicin		Troponin T	Schnackenberg et al., Appl. Toxicol. 2016 [102]
Hydroxproline	↑		No	Yes			Doxorubicin		Troponin T	Schnackenberg et al., Appl. Toxicol. 2016 [102]
Citrate	no		No	Yes			Doxorubicin		Troponin T	Schnackenberg et al., Appl. Toxicol. 2016 [102]
Propionylcarnitine	↑		No	Yes			Doxorubicin		Troponin T	Schnackenberg et al., Appl. Toxicol. 2016 [102]
Serotonine	no		↑	Yes			Doxorubicin		Troponin T	Schnackenberg et al., Appl. Toxicol. 2016 [102]
Putrescine	no		↑	Yes			Doxorubicin		Troponin T	Schnackenberg et al., Appl. Toxicol. 2016 [102]
Malate	↑		↑	Yes			Doxorubicin			Tan et al., PLoS ONE 2011 [103]
Fructose			↑	Yes			Doxorubicin			Tan et al., PLoS ONE 2011 [103]

Table 4. Cont.

Metabolite	Plasma	Stem Cell	Heart	Mice	People	XRT	Medicine	Dose	Biomarker	References
Glycose			↑	Yes			Doxorubicin			Tan et al., PLoS ONE 2011 [103]
Cholesterol			↑	Yes			Doxorubicin			Tan et al., PLoS ONE 2011 [103]
Alanine			↑	Yes			Doxorubicin			Tan et al., PLoS ONE 2011 [103]
Glutamine				Yes		↓	Doxorubicin			Tan et al., PLoS ONE 2011 [103]
Docosahexaenoic acid			↓	Yes			Sunitinib			Jensen et al., Metabolites. 2017 [104]
Arachidonic acid/eicosapetaenoic acid			↓	Yes			Sunitinib			Jensen et al., Metabolites. 2017 [104]
6-hydroxynicotinic acid			↓	Yes			Sunitinib			Jensen et al., Metabolites. 2017 [104]
O-phosphocolamine			↓	Yes			Sunitinib			Jensen et al., Metabolites. 2017 [104]
Ethanolamine	↑			Yes			Sunitinib			Jensen et al., Metabolites. 2017 [104]
Xenobiotics										

More recently, Li et al. [99] identified 39 biomarkers for detecting cardiotoxicity earlier than biochemical analysis and histopathological assessment. They used rats to create cardiotoxicity models in which the toxicity was caused by doxorubicin, isoproterenol, and 5-fluorouracil. The metabolomics analysis of plasma was performed using ultraperformance liquid chromatography quadrupole time-of-flight mass spectrometry. They used a support vector machine (SVM) to deploy a predictive model to confirm more exclusive biomarkers with more significant l-carnitine, 19-hydroxydeoxycorticosterone, lysophosphatidylcholine (LPC) (14:0), and LPC (20:2) [99].

Similarly, Schnackenberg et al. attempted to discover molecular markers of early-stage cardiotoxicity induced by doxorubicin in mice before the onset of cardiac damage. They discovered 18 metabolites significantly altered in the plasma, and another 22 metabolites were increased in cardiac tissue after a cumulative dose of 6 mg/kg, while myocardial injury and cardiac pathology were not noticed until after cumulative doses of 18 and 24 mg/kg, respectively [102]. Metabolomics analyses of plasma and heart tissue showed significant variations in the levels of many amino acids (including arginine and citrulline), biogenic amines, acylcarnitines (carnitine), and tricarboxylic acid cycle (TCA)-related metabolites (e.g., lactate, succinate).

Tan et al. conducted a study using gas chromatography–mass spectrometry to describe the metabolic profile of doxorubicin-induced cardiomyopathy in mice. They identified 24 metabolites, which were implicated in glycolysis, the citrate cycle, and the metabolism of some amino acids and lipids, and which were selected as possible biomarkers for the detection of cardiotoxicity [103].

Andreadou et al. used nuclear magnetic resonance (NMR) spectrometry to describe the metabolic profile of acute doxorubicin cardiotoxicity in rats and to evaluate the metabolic alterations conferred by co-treatment with oleuropein [90]. The mice were divided into six groups: the first group included the control group, the second group received DOX, and the other four groups of mice received doxorubicin with oleuropein in different doses and days, regarding the latter. Mice hearts were excised 72 h after doxorubicin administration and the H-NMR spectra of aqueous myocardium extracts were monitored. The results of the analysis showed an increase in the levels of acetate and succinate in the DOX group compared to the controls, while the amino acid levels were lower. The conclusion of the article was that acetate and succinate constituted novel biomarkers for the early detection of cardiotoxicity [100,105].

Geng et al. in their study, used gas chromatography—mass spectrometry analysis of the main targeted tissues (serum, heart, liver, brain, and kidney) to systemically evaluate the toxicity of DOX. Multivariate analyses revealed 21 metabolites in the serum, including cholesterol, D-glucose, D-lactic acid, glycine, L-alanine, L-glutamic acid, L-isoleucine, L-leucine, L-proline, L-serine, L-tryptophan, L-tyrosine, L-valine, N-methylphenylethanolamine, oleamide, palmitic acid, pyroglutamic acid, stearic acid, and urea, were changed in the serum in the DOX group [106].

Tantawy et al. identified a lower plasma abundance of pyruvate and a higher abundance of lactate in patients with carfilzomib-related cardiovascular adverse events. (CVAEs). They emphasized the significance of the pyruvate oxidation pathway associated with mitochondrial dysfunction. In order to better understand the mechanisms of carfilzomib-associated CVAEs, further investigation and validation are needed in a larger independent cohort [107].

Yin et al. proposed 15 different metabolites that play important roles in cyclophosphamide-induced cardiotoxicity. In their study, rat plasma samples were collected and analyzed one, three, and five days after cyclophosphamide administration using ultra-performance liquid chromatography quadrupole time-of-flight mass spectrometry (UPLC-QqTOF HRMS). Of the biomarkers studied, the proline, linoleic acid, and glycerophospholipids changed significantly in the three periods, and the changes were associated with an increasing time of occurrence of cardiotoxicity from cyclophosphamide [108].

The study of Jensen et al. [104] showed significant decreases in docosahexaenoic acid, arachidonic acid/eicosatetraenoic acid, o-phosphocolamine, and 6-hydroxynicotinic acid after sunitinib treatment with non-targeted metabolomics analysis of mice hearts [31]. The same author also showed alterations in the taurine/hypotaurine metabolism in the hearts and skeletal muscles of mice after sorafenib treatment [109].

Except for the analysis of plasma and heart tissue, NMR spectroscopy-based metabolomics may detect low-molecular-weight metabolites in urine and cell culture media. For example, Chaudhari et al. [101] showed a reduction in the utilization of pyruvate and acetate and an accumulation of formate in contrast to a control culture medium of human induced pluripotent stem cell-derived cardiomyocytes exposed to doxorubicin. In contrast, Wang et al. [59] showed in their study that tryptophan and phenylalanine metabolism in urine was also an important process in the systemic toxicity of doxorubicin. In addition, Park et al. identified 19 urinary metabolites in rats treated with doxorubicin [110].

This technology is still under development, but it seems obvious that metabolomics holds the potential to revolutionize our ability to profile samples in order to understand biological processes and find useful disease diagnostic biomarkers.

8. Conclusions

Cardiovascular toxicity continues to be a major cause of drug failure during preclinical and clinical treatment models and contributes to drug withdrawal after approval. Numerous medications that have been used frequently in adult clinical practice for a long time have demonstrated potentially harmful effects on the hearts of pediatric patients. The cardiotoxicity of these medications persists as a significant issue, having a negative impact on patients' quality of life as well as their overall survival. Several strategies for the early detection of cardiotoxicity have been developed to reduce the number of patients with cardiac mortality and morbidity. Of importance, the biomarkers identified by the "omics" approach are considered new potential markers, especially in the scenario of diagnosis and the risk stratification of acute coronary syndromes induced by chemotherapeutic drugs, and they may prove helpful in the early detection of anticancer cardiotoxicity.

Funding: This research received no external funding.

Informed Consent Statement: Not applicable.

Data Availability Statement: The article is a review, and no original data were generated.

Conflicts of Interest: The authors declare no conflict of interest.

Abbreviations

ABC	Adenosine triphosphate-binding cassette transporter
ABCC2	ATP-binding cassette subfamily C member 2
ACT	Anthracycline-related cardiotoxicity
ALL	Acute lymphoblastic leukemia
BNP	B-type natriuretic peptide
CBR	Carbonyl reductase
CELF4	CUGBP Elav-like family member 4
CHF	Congestive heart failure
CP	Cyclophosphamide
CMR	Cardiac magnetic resonance imaging
CRP	C-reactive protein
CVAEs	Cardiovascular adverse events
DOX	Doxorubicin
ECG	Electrocardiography
EVs	Extracellular vesicles
GC	Gas chromatography
GDF-15	Growth/differentiation factor 15
GLS	Global systolic longitudinal myocardial strain
HER2	Human epidermal growth factor receptor 2
HF	Heart failure
IFO	Ifosfamide
LC	Liquid chromatography high-performance
LC-MS	Liquid chromatography–mass spectrometry
LPC	Lysophosphatidylcholine
LV	Left ventricular
LVD	Left ventricular dysfunction
LVEF	Left ventricular ejection fraction
miRNAs	MicroRNAs
mRNAs	Messenger RNAs
MPI	Myocardial perfusion imaging
MS	Molecular mass spectrometry
MUGA	Nuclear cardiac imaging
NMR	Nuclear magnetic resonance spectrometry
NOTCH1	Neurogenic locus notch homolog protein 1
NT-proBNP	N-terminal pro b-natriuretic peptide
PET	Positron emission tomography
PYGB	Glycogen phosphorylase
RARG	Retinoic acid receptor gamma
SAL	Saline
SLC	Solute carrier transporters
SNP	Single-nucleotide polymorphism
SPECT	Single-photon emission computed tomography
SVM	Vector machine
TKI	Tyrosine kinase inhibitors
TCA	Tricarboxylic acid
TnT	Troponin T
TOP2	Topoisomerase II
Top2β	Topoisomerase-II β
UGT1A6	Glucuronosyltransferase family

UPLC-QqTOF HRMS		Ultra-performance liquid chromatography quadrupole time-of-flight mass spectrometry
VEGF		Vascular endothelial growth factor
vWF		Von Willebrand factor
2D		Two-dimensional echocardiography
5-FU		Fluorouracil

References

1. Pritchard-Jones, K.; Bergeron, C.; de Camargo, B.; van den Heuvel-Eibrink, M.M.; Acha, T.; Godzinski, J.; Oldenburger, F.; Boccon-Gibod, L.; Leuschner, I.; Vujanic, G.; et al. Omission of doxorubicin from the treatment of stage II-III, intermediate-risk Wilms' tumour (SIOP WT 2001): An open-label, non-inferiority, randomised controlled trial. *Lancet* **2015**, *386*, 1156–1164. [CrossRef]
2. Ampatzidou, M.; Kelaidi, C.; Dworzak, M.N.; Polychronopoulou, S. Adolescents and young adults with acute lymphoblastic and acute myeloid leukemia. *MEMO-Mag. Eur. Med. Oncol.* **2018**, *11*, 47–53.
3. Ampatzidou, M.; Panagiotou, J.P.; Paterakis, G.; Papadakis, V.; Papadimitriou, S.I.; Parcharidou, A.; Papargyri, S.; Rigatou, E.; Avgerinou, G.; Tsitsikas, K.; et al. Childhood acute lymphoblastic leukemia: 12 years of experience, using a Berlin-Frankfurt-Münster approach, in a Greek center. *Leuk. Lymphoma* **2015**, *56*, 251–255. [CrossRef] [PubMed]
4. Polychronopoulou, S.; Baka, M.; Servitzoglou, M.; Papadakis, V.; Pourtsidis, A.; Avgerinou, G.; Abatzidou, M.; Kosmidis, H. Treatment and clinical results in childhood AML in Greece. *MEM-Mag. Eur. Med. Oncol.* **2014**, *7*, 50–55. [CrossRef]
5. Georgakis, M.K.; Karalexi, M.A.; Agius, D.; Antunes, L.; Bastos, J.; Coza, D.; Demetriou, A.; Dimitrova, N.; Eser, S.; Florea, M.; et al. Incidence and time trends of childhood lymphomas: Findings from 14 Southern and Eastern European cancer registries and the Surveillance, Epidemiology and End Results, USA. *Cancer Causes Control* **2016**, *27*, 1381–1394. [CrossRef]
6. Petridou, E.T.; Dimitrova, N.; Eser, S.; Kachanov, D.; Karakilinc, H.; Varfolomeeva, S.; Belechri, M.; Baka, M.; Moschovi, M.; Polychronopoulou, S.; et al. Childhood leukemia and lymphoma: Time trends and factors affecting survival in five Southern and Eastern European Cancer Registries. *Cancer Causes Control* **2013**, *24*, 1111–1118. [CrossRef]
7. Lyon, A.R.; López-Fernández, T.; Couch, L.S.; Asteggiano, R.; Aznar, M.C.; Bergler-Klein, J.; Boriani, G.; Cardinale, D.; Cordoba, R.; Cosyns, B.; et al. 2022 ESC Guidelines on cardio-oncology developed in collaboration with the European Hematology Association (EHA), the European Society for Therapeutic Radiology and Oncology (ESTRO) and the International Cardio-Oncology Society (IC-OS). *Eur. Heart J.* **2022**, *43*, 4229–4361.
8. Herrmann, J.; Lenihan, D.; Armenian, S.; Barac, A.; Blaes, A.; Cardinale, D.; Carver, J.; Dent, S.; Ky, B.; Lyon, A.R.; et al. Defining cardiovascular toxicities of cancer therapies: An International Cardio-Oncology Society (IC-OS) consensus statement. *Eur. Heart J.* **2022**, *43*, 280–299. [CrossRef]
9. Chow, E.J.; Leger, K.J.; Bhatt, N.S.; Mulrooney, D.A.; Ross, C.J.; Aggarwal, S.; Bansal, N.; Ehrhardt, M.J.; Armenian, S.H.; Scott, J.M.; et al. Paediatric cardio-oncology: Epidemiology, screening, prevention, and treatment. *Cardiovasc. Res.* **2019**, *115*, 922–934. [CrossRef]
10. Morelli, M.B.; Bongiovanni, C.; Da Pra, S.; Miano, C.; Sacchi, F.; Lauriola, M.; D'Uva, G. Cardiotoxicity of Anticancer Drugs: Molecular Mechanisms and Strategies for Cardioprotection. *Front. Cardiovasc. Med.* **2022**, *9*, 847012, PMCID:PMC9051244. [CrossRef] [PubMed]
11. Lipshultz, S.E.; Lipshultz, E.R.; Chow, E.J.; Doody, D.R.; Armenian, S.H.; Asselin, B.L.; Baker, K.S.; Bhatia, S.; Constine, L.S.; Freyer, D.R.; et al. Cardiometabolic Risk in Childhood Cancer Survivors: A Report from the Children's Oncology Group. *Cancer Epidemiol. Biomark. Prev.* **2022**, *31*, 536–542. [CrossRef] [PubMed]
12. Ward, E.; DeSantis, C.; Robbins, A.; Kohler, B.; Jemal, A. Childhood and adolescent cancer statistics, 2014. *CA Cancer J. Clin.* **2014**, *64*, 83–103. [CrossRef] [PubMed]
13. Mulrooney, D.A.; Yeazel, M.W.; Kawashima, T.; Mertens, A.C.; Mitby, P.; Stovall, M.; Donaldson, S.S.; Green, D.M.; Sklar, C.A.; Robison, L.L.; et al. Cardiac outcomes in a cohort of adult survivors of childhood and adolescent cancer: Retrospective analysis of the Childhood Cancer Survivor Study cohort. *BMJ* **2009**, *339*, b4606. [CrossRef] [PubMed]
14. Bansal, N.; Amdani, S.; Lipshultz, E.R.; Lipshultz, S.E. Chemotherapy-induced cardiotoxicity in children. *Expert Opin. Drug Metab. Toxicol.* **2017**, *13*, 817–832. [CrossRef]
15. Minotti, G.; Menna, P.; Salvatorelli, E.; Cairo, G.; Gianni, L. Anthracyclines: Molecular advances and pharmacologic developments in antitumor activity and cardiotoxicity. *Pharmacol. Rev.* **2004**, *56*, 185–229. [CrossRef]
16. Sawyer, D.B.; Peng, X.; Chen, B.; Pentassuglia, L.; Lim, C.C. Mechanisms of anthracycline cardiac injury: Can we identify strategies for cardioprotection? *Prog. Cardiovasc. Dis.* **2010**, *53*, 105–113. [CrossRef]
17. Simbre, V.C.; Duffy, S.A.; Dadlani, G.H.; Miller, T.L.; Lipshultz, S.E. Cardiotoxicity of cancer chemotherapy: Implications for children. *Paediatr. Drugs* **2005**, *7*, 187–202. [CrossRef]
18. Herrmann, J.; Lerman, A.; Sandhu, N.P.; Villarraga, H.R.; Mulvagh, S.L.; Kohli, M. Evaluation and management of patients with heart disease and cancer: Cardio-oncology. *Mayo Clin. Proc.* **2014**, *89*, 1287–1306. [CrossRef]
19. Sayed-Ahmed, M.M.; Aldelemy, M.L.; Al-Shabanah, O.A.; Hafez, M.M.; Al-Hosaini, K.A.; Al-Harbi, N.O.; Al-Sharary, S.D.; Al-Harbi, M.M. Inhibition of gene expression of carnitine palmitoyltransferase I and heart fatty acid binding protein in cyclophosphamide and ifosfamide-induced acute cardiotoxic rat models. *Cardiovasc. Toxicol.* **2014**, *14*, 232–242. [CrossRef]

20. Rhea, I.B.; Oliveira, G.H. Cardiotoxicity of Novel Targeted Chemotherapeutic Agents. *Curr. Treat. Options Cardiovasc. Med.* **2018**, *20*, 53. [CrossRef]
21. Zhang, K.; Heidrich, F.M.; DeGray, B.; Boehmerle, W.; Ehrlich, B.E. Paclitaxel accelerates spontaneous calcium oscillations in cardiomyocytes by interacting with NCS-1 and the InsP3R. *J. Mol. Cell. Cardiol.* **2010**, *49*, 829–835. [CrossRef] [PubMed]
22. Takahashi, K.; Inukai, T.; Imamura, T.; Yano, M.; Tomoyasu, C.; Lucas, D.M.; Nemoto, A.; Sato, H.; Huang, M.; Abe, M.; et al. Anti-leukemic activity of bortezomib and carfilzomib on B-cell precursor ALL cell lines. *PLoS ONE* **2017**, *12*, e0188680. [CrossRef] [PubMed]
23. Shah, C.; Bishnoi, R.; Jain, A.; Bejjanki, H.; Xiong, S.; Wang, Y.; Zou, F.; Moreb, J.S. Cardiotoxicity associated with carfilzomib: Systematic review and meta-analysis. *Leuk. Lymphoma* **2018**, *59*, 2557–2569. [CrossRef] [PubMed]
24. Waxman, A.J.; Clasen, S.; Hwang, W.; Garfall, A.; Vogl, D.T.; Carver, J.; O'Quinn, R.; Cohen, A.D.; Stadtmauer, E.A.; Ky, B.; et al. Carfilzomib-Associated Cardiovascular Adverse Events: A Systematic Review and Meta-analysis. *JAMA Oncol.* **2018**, *4*, e174519. [CrossRef] [PubMed]
25. Rochette, L.; Guenancia, C.; Gudjoncik, A.; Hachet, O.; Zeller, M.; Cottin, Y.; Vergely, C. Anthracyclines/trastuzumab: New aspects of cardiotoxicity and molecular mechanisms. *Trends Pharmacol. Sci.* **2015**, *36*, 326–348. [CrossRef] [PubMed]
26. Lipshultz, S.E.; Karnik, R.; Sambatakos, P.; Franco, V.I.; Ross, S.W.; Miller, T.L. Anthracycline-related cardiotoxicity in childhood cancer survivors. *Curr. Opin. Cardiol.* **2014**, *29*, 103–112. [CrossRef]
27. Manrique, C.R.; Park, M.; Tiwari, N.; Plana, J.C.; Garcia, M.J. Diagnostic strategies for early recognition of cancer therapeutics-related cardiac dysfunction. *Clin. Med. Insights Cardiol.* **2017**, *11*, 1179546817697983. [CrossRef]
28. Von Hoff, D.D.; Layard, M.W.; Basa, P.; Davis, H.L., Jr.; Von Hoff, A.L.; Rozencweig, M.; Muggia, F.M. Risk factors for doxorubicin-induced congestive heart failure. *Ann. Intern. Med.* **1979**, *91*, 710–717. [CrossRef]
29. Vandecruys, E.; Mondelaers, V.; De Wolf, D.; Benoit, Y.; Suys, B. Late cardiotoxicity after low dose of anthracycline therapy for acute lymphoblastic leukemia in childhood. *J. Cancer Surviv.* **2012**, *6*, 95–101. [CrossRef]
30. Nysom, K.; Holm, K.; Lipsitz, S.R.; Mone, S.M.; Co-lan, S.D.; Orav, E.J.; Sallan, S.E.; Olsen, J.H.; Hertz, H.; Jacobsen, J.R.; et al. Relationship between cumulative anthracycline dose and late cardiotoxicity in childhood acute lymphoblastic leukemia. *J. Clin. Oncol.* **1998**, *16*, 545–550. [CrossRef]
31. Lipshultz, S.E.; Adams, M.J. Cardiotoxicity after childhood cancer: Beginning with the end in mind. *J. Clin. Oncol.* **2010**, *28*, 1276–1281. [CrossRef] [PubMed]
32. Van der Pal, H.J.; van Dalen, E.C.; Hauptmann, M.; Kok, W.E.; Caron, H.N.; van den Bos, C.; Ol-Denburger, F.; Koning, C.C.; van Leeuwen, F.E.; Kremer, L.C. Cardiac function in 5-year survivors of childhood cancer: A long-term follow-up study. *Arch. Intern. Med.* **2010**, *170*, 1247–1255. [CrossRef] [PubMed]
33. Brickler, M.; Raskin, A.; Ryan, T.D. Current State of Pediatric Cardio-Oncology: A Review. *Children* **2022**, *9*, 127. [CrossRef] [PubMed]
34. Loar, R.W.; Noel, C.V.; Tunuguntla, H.; Colquitt, J.L.; Pignatelli, R.H. State of the art review: Chemotherapy-induced cardiotoxicity in children. *Congenit. Heart Dis.* **2018**, *13*, 5–15. [CrossRef]
35. Mornoş, C.; Manolis, A.J.; Cozma, D.; Kouremenos, N.; Zacharopoulou, I.; Ionac, A. The value of left ventricular global longitudinal strain assessed by three-dimensional strain imaging in the early detection of anthracyclinemediated cardiotoxicity. *Hellenic. J. Cardiol.* **2014**, *55*, 235–244.
36. Lipshultz, S.E.; Miller, T.L.; Scully, R.E.; Lipsitz, S.R.; Rifai, N.; Silverman, L.B.; Colan, S.D.; Neuberg, D.S.; Dahlberg, S.E.; Henkel, J.M.; et al. Changes in cardiac biomarkers during doxorubicin treatment of pediatric patients with high-risk acute lymphoblastic leukemia: Associations with long-term echocardiographic outcomes. *J. Clin. Oncol.* **2012**, *30*, 1042–1049. [CrossRef]
37. Dixon, S.B.; Howell, C.R.; Lu, L.; Plana, J.C.; Joshi, V.M.; Luepker, R.V.; Durand, J.B.; Ky, B.; Lenihan, D.J.; Jefferies, J.L.; et al. Cardiac biomarkers and association with subsequent cardiomyopathy and mortality among adult survivors of childhood cancer: A report from the St. Jude Lifetime Cohort. *Cancer* **2021**, *127*, 458–466. [CrossRef]
38. Sherief, L.M.; Kamal, A.G.; Khalek, E.A.; Kamal, N.M.; Soliman, A.A.; Esh, A.M. Biomarkers and early detection of late onset anthracycline-induced cardiotoxicity in children. *Hematology* **2012**, *17*, 151–156. [CrossRef]
39. Armenian, S.H.; Gelehrter, S.K.; Vase, T.; Venkatramani, R.; Landier, W.; Wilson, K.D.; Herrera, C.; Reichman, L.; Menteer, J.D.; Mascarenhas, L.; et al. Screening for cardiac dysfunction in anthracycline-exposed childhood cancer survivors. *Clin. Cancer Res.* **2014**, *20*, 6314–6323. [CrossRef]
40. Lam, E.; Higgins, V.; Zhang, L.; Chan, M.K.; Bohn, M.K.; Trajcevski, K.; Liu, P.; Adeli, K.; Nathan, P.C. Normative Values of High-Sensitivity Cardiac Troponin T and N-Terminal pro-B-Type Natriuretic Peptide in Children and Adolescents: A Study from the CALIPER Cohort. *J. Appl. Lab. Med.* **2021**, *6*, 344–353. [CrossRef]
41. Joolharzadeh, P.; Rodriguez, M.; Zaghlol, R.; Pedersen, L.N.; Jimenez, J.; Bergom, C.; Mitchell, J.D. Recent Advances in Serum Biomarkers for Risk Stratification and Patient Management in Cardio-Oncology. *Curr. Cardiol. Rep.* **2023**, *25*, 133–146. [CrossRef] [PubMed]
42. Christensona, E.S.; Jamesa, T.; Agrawala, V.; ParkbaJohns, B.H. Use of biomarkers for the assessment of chemotherapy-induced cardiac toxicity. *Curr. Heart Fail. Rep.* **2015**, *12*, 255–262. [CrossRef] [PubMed]
43. Cardinale, D.; Biasillo, G.; Salvatici, M.; Sandri, M.T.; Cipolla, C.M. Using biomarkers to predict and to prevent cardiotoxicity of cancer therapy. *Expert Rev. Mol. Diagn.* **2017**, *17*, 245–256. [CrossRef] [PubMed]

44. Horacek, J.M.; Jebavy, L.; Vasatova, M.; Pudil, R.; Tichy, M.; Jakl, M.; Maly, J. Glycogen phosphorylase BB as a potential marker of cardiac toxicity in patients treated with anthracyclines for acute leukemia. *Bratisl. Lek. Listy.* **2013**, *114*, 708–710. [CrossRef] [PubMed]
45. Horacek, J.M.; Vasatova, M.; Tichy, M.; Pudil, R.; Jebavy, L.; Maly, J. The use of cardiac biomarkers in detection of cardiotoxicity associated with conventional and high-dose chemotherapy for acute leukemia. *Exp. Oncol.* **2010**, *32*, 97–99.
46. Horacek, J.M.; Tichy, M.; Jebavy, L.; Pudil, R.; Ulrychova, M. Maly Use of multiple biomarkers for evaluation of anthracycline-induced cardiotoxicity in patients with acute myeloid leukemia. *J. Exp. Oncol.* **2008**, *30*, 157–159.
47. Horacek, J.M.; Vasatova, M.; Pudil, R.; Tichy, M.; Zak, P.; Jakl, M.; Jebavy, L.; Maly, J. Biomarkers for the early detection of anthracycline-induced cardiotoxicity: Current status. *Biomed. Pap. Med. Fac. Univ. Palacky Olomouc. Czech. Repub.* **2014**, *158*, 511–517. [CrossRef]
48. Cao, L.; Zhu, W.; Wagar, E.A.; Meng, Q.H. Biomarkers for monitoring chemotherapy-induced cardiotoxicity. *Crit. Rev. Clin. Lab. Sci.* **2017**, *54*, 87–101. [CrossRef]
49. Arslan, D.; Cihan, T.; Kose, D.; Vatansev, H.; Cimen, D.; Koksal, Y.; Oran, B.; Akyurek, F. Growth-differentiation factor-15 and tissue doppler imaging in detection of asymptomatic anthracycline cardiomyopathy in childhood cancer survivors. *Clin. Biochem.* **2013**, *46*, 1239–1243. [CrossRef]
50. Armenian, S.; Bhatia, S. Predicting and Preventing Anthracycline-Related Cardiotoxicity. *Am. Soc. Clin. Oncol. Educ. Book* **2018**, *38*, 3–12. [CrossRef]
51. Aminkeng, F.; Bhavsar, A.P.; Visscher, H.; Rassekh, S.R.; Li, Y.; Lee, J.W.; Brunham, L.R.; Caron, H.N.; van Dalen, E.C.; Kremer, L.C.; et al. Canadian Pharmacogenomics Network for Drug Safety Consortium. A coding variant in RARG confers susceptibility to anthracycline-induced cardiotoxicity in childhood cancer. *Nat. Genet.* **2015**, *47*, 1079–1084. [CrossRef] [PubMed]
52. Madonna, R. Early diagnosis and prediction of anticancer drug-induced cardiotoxicity: From cardiac imaging to "Omics" technologies. *Rev. Espanol. Cardiol.* **2017**, *70*, 576–582. [CrossRef]
53. Linschoten, M.; Teske, A.J.; Cramer, M.J.; van der Wall, E.; Asselbergs, F.W. Chemotherapy-Related Cardiac Dysfunction: A Systematic Review of Genetic Variants Modulating Individual Risk. *Circ. Genom. Precis. Med.* **2018**, *11*, e001753. [CrossRef] [PubMed]
54. Semsei, A.F.; Erdelyi, D.J.; Ungvari, I.; Csagoly, E.; Hegyi, M.Z.; Kiszel, P.S.; Lautner-Csorba, O.; Szabolcs, J.; Masat, P.; Fekete, G.; et al. ABCC1 polymorphisms in anthracycline- induced cardiotoxicity in childhood acute lymphoblastic leukaemia. *Cell Biol. Int.* **2012**, *36*, 79–86. [CrossRef]
55. Wojnowski, L.; Kulle, B.; Schirmer, M.; Schlüter, G.; Schmidt, A.; Rosenberger, A.; Vonhof, S.; Bickeböller, H.; Toliat, M.R.; Suk, E.K.; et al. NAD(P)H oxidase and multidrug resistance protein genetic polymorphisms are associated with doxorubicin-induced cardiotoxicity. *Circulation* **2005**, *112*, 3754–3762. [CrossRef] [PubMed]
56. Vulsteke, C.; Pfeil, A.M.; Maggen, C.; Schwenkglenks, M.; Pettengell, R.; Szucs, T.D.; Lambrechts, D.; Dieudonné, A.-S.; Hatse, S.; Neven, P.; et al. Clinical and genetic risk factors for epirubicin-induced cardiac toxicity in early breast cancer patients. *Breast Cancer Res. Treat.* **2015**, *152*, 67–76. [CrossRef]
57. Blanco, J.G.; Leisenring, W.M.; Gonzalez-Covarrubias, V.M.; Kawashima, T.I.; Davies, S.M.; Relling, M.V.; Robison, L.L.; Sklar, C.A.; Stovall, M.; Bhatia, S. Genetic polymorphisms in the carbonyl reductase 3 gene CBR3 and the NAD(P)H: Quinone oxidoreductase 1 gene NQO1 in patients who developed anthracycline-related congestive heart failure after childhood cancer. *Cancer* **2008**, *112*, 2789–2795. [CrossRef]
58. Blanco, J.G.; Sun, C.L.; Landier, W.; Chen, L.; Esparza-Duran, D.; Leisenring, W.; Mays, A.; Friedman, D.L.; Ginsberg, J.P.; Hudson, M.M.; et al. Anthracycline-related cardiomyopathy after childhood cancer: Role of polymorphisms in carbonyl reductase genes—A report from the Children's Oncology Group. *J. Clin. Oncol.* **2012**, *30*, 1415–1421. [CrossRef]
59. Wang, X.; Sun, C.-L.; Quiñones-Lombraña, A.; Singh, P.; Landier, W.; Hageman, L.; Mather, M.; Rotter, J.I.; Taylor, K.D.; Chen, Y.-D.I.; et al. CELF4 variant and anthracycline-related cardiomyopathy: A Children's Oncology Group genome-wide association study. *J. Clin. Oncol.* **2016**, *34*, 863–870. [CrossRef]
60. Vos, H.I.; Coenen, M.J.; Guchelaar, H.J.; Te Loo, D.M. The role of pharmacogenetics in the treatment of osteosarcoma. *Drug Discov. Today* **2016**, *21*, 1775–1786. [CrossRef]
61. Leong, S.L.; Chaiyakunapruk, N.; Lee, S.W. Candidate Gene Association Studies of Anthracycline-induced Cardiotoxicity: A Systematic Review and Meta-analysis. *Sci. Rep.* **2017**, *7*, 39. [CrossRef] [PubMed]
62. McOwan, T.N.; Craig, L.A.; Tripdayonis, A.; Karavendzas, K.; Cheung, M.M.; Porrello, E.R.; Conyers, R.; Elliott, D.A. Evaluating anthracycline cardiotoxicity associated single nucleotide polymorphisms in a paediatric cohort with early onset cardiomyopathy. *Cardiooncology* **2020**, *6*, 5. [CrossRef] [PubMed]
63. Petrykey, K.; Andelfinger, G.U.; Laverdière, C.; Sinnett, D.; Krajinovic, M. Genetic factors in anthracycline-induced cardiotoxicity in patients treated for pediatric cancer. *Expert Opin. Drug Metab. Toxicol.* **2020**, *16*, 865–883. [CrossRef] [PubMed]
64. Lipshultz, S.E.; Lipsitz, S.R.; Kutok, J.L.; Miller, T.L.; Colan, S.D.; Neuberg, D.S.; Stevenson, K.E.; Fleming, M.D.; Sallan, S.E.; Franco, V.I.; et al. Impact of hemochromatosis gene mutations on cardiac status in doxorubicin-treated survivors of childhood high-risk leukemia. *Cancer* **2013**, *119*, 3555–3562. [CrossRef]
65. Visscher, H.; Ross, C.J.D.; Rassekh, S.R.; Sandor, G.S.S.; Caron, H.N.; van Dalen, E.C.; Kremer, L.C.; van der Pal, H.J.; Rogers, P.C.; Rieder, M.J.; et al. Validation of Variants in SLC28A3 and UGT1A6 as Genetic Markers Predictive of Anthracycline-Induced Cardiotoxicity in Children. *Pediatr. Blood Cancer* **2013**, *60*, 1375–1381. [CrossRef]

66. Visscher, H.; Ross, C.J.D.; Rassekh, S.R.; Sandor, G.S.S.; Caron, H.N.; van Dalen, E.C.; Kremer, L.C.; van der Pal, H.J.; Rogers, P.C.; Rieder, M.J.; et al. Genetic variants in *SLC22A17* and *SLC22A7* are associated with anthracycline- induced cardiotoxicity in children. *Pharmacogenomics* 2015, *16*, 1065–1076. [CrossRef]
67. Visscher, H.; Ross, C.J.D.; Rassekh, S.R.; Barhdadi, A.; Dube, M.-P.; Al-Saloos, H.; Sandor, S.; Caron, H.N.; van Dalen, E.C.; Kremer, L.C.; et al. Pharmacogenomic Prediction of Anthracycline-Induced Cardiotoxicity in Children. *J. Clin. Oncol.* 2012, *30*, 1422–1428. [CrossRef]
68. Sági, J.C.; Egyed, B.; Kelemen, A.; Kutszegi, N.; Hegyi, M.; Gézsi, A.; Herlitschke, M.A.; Rzepiel, A.; Fodor, L.E.; Ottóffy, G.; et al. Possible roles of genetic variations in chemotherapy related cardiotoxicity in pediatric acute lymphoblastic leukemia and osteosarcoma. *BMC Cancer* 2018, *18*, 704. [CrossRef]
69. Aminkeng, F.; Ross, C.J.D.; Rassekh, S.R.; Hwang, S.; Rieder, M.J.; Bhavsar, A.P.; Smith, A.; Sanatani, S.; Gelmon, K.A.; Bernstein, D.; et al. Recommendations for genetic testing to reduce the incidence of anthracycline-induced cardiotoxicity. *Br. J. Clin. Pharmacol.* 2016, *82*, 683–695. [CrossRef]
70. Marcoux, S.; Drouin, S.; Laverdière, C.; Alos, N.; Andelfinger, G.U.; Bertout, L.; Curnier, D.; Friedrich, M.G.; Kritikou, E.A.; Lefebvre, G.; et al. The PETALE study: Late adverse effects and biomarkers in childhood acute lymphoblastic leukemia survivors. *Pediatr. Blood Cancer* 2017, *64*. [CrossRef]
71. Kashyap, V.; Laursen, K.B.; Brenet, F.; Viale, A.J.; Scandura, J.M.; Gudas, L.J. RARgamma is essential for retinoic acid induced chromatin remodeling and transcriptional activation in embryonic stem cells. *J. Cell. Sci.* 2013, *126*, 999–1008. [PubMed]
72. Krajinovic, M.; Elbared, J.; Drouin, S.; Bertout, L.; Rezgui, A.; Ansari, M.; Raboisson, M.-J.; Lipshultz, S.E.; Silverman, L.B.; Sallan, S.E.; et al. Polymorphisms of ABCC5 and NOS3 genes influence doxorubicin cardiotoxicity in survivors of childhood acute lymphoblastic leukemia. *Pharm. J.* 2015, *16*, 530–535.
73. Oatmen, K.E.; Toro-Salazar, O.H.; Hauser, K.; Zellars, K.N.; Mason, K.C.; Hor, K.; Gillan, E.; Zeiss, C.J.; Gatti, D.M.; Spinale, F.G. Identification of a Novel microRNA Profile in Pediatric Patients with Cancer Treated with Anthracycline Chemotherapy. *Am. J. Physiol. Heart Circ. Physiol.* 2018, *315*, H1443–H1452. [CrossRef] [PubMed]
74. Oliveira-Carvalho, V.; Ferreira, L.R.P.; Bocchi, E.A. Circulating mir-208a fails as a biomarker of doxorubicin-induced cardiotoxicity in breast cancer patients. *J. Appl. Toxicol.* 2015, *35*, 1071–1072. [CrossRef] [PubMed]
75. Oikonomou, E.; Siasos, G.; Tousoulis, D.; Kokkou, E.; Genimata, V.; Zisimos, K.; Latsios, G.; Stefanadis, C. Diagnostic, and therapeutic potentials of microRNAs in heart failure. *Curr. Top. Med. Chem.* 2013, *13*, 1548–1558. [CrossRef] [PubMed]
76. Papageorgiou, N.; Tousoulis, D.; Androulakis, E.; Siasos, G.; Briasoulis, A.; Vogiatzi, G.; Kampoli, A.M.; Tsiamis, E.; Tentolouris, C.; Stefanadis, C. The role of microRNAs in cardiovascular disease. *Curr. Med. Chem.* 2012, *19*, 2605–2610. [CrossRef]
77. Ruggeri, C.; Gioffre, S.; Achilli, F.; Colombo, G.I.; D'Alessandra, Y. Role of microRNAs in doxorubicin-induced cardiotoxicity: An overview of preclinical models and cancer patients. *Heart Fail. Rev.* 2018, *23*, 109–122. [CrossRef]
78. Holmgren, G.; Synnergren, J.; Andersson, C.X.; Lindahl, A.; Sartipy, P. MicroRNAs as potential biomarkers for doxorubicininduced cardiotoxicity. *Toxicol. Vitr.* 2016, *34*, 26–34. [CrossRef]
79. Ludwig, N.; Leidinger, P.; Becker, K.; Backes, C.; Fehlmann, T.; Pallasch, C.; Rheinheimer, S.; Meder, B.; Stähler, C.; Meese, E.; et al. Distribution of miRNA expression across human tissues. *Nucleic Acids Res.* 2016, *44*, 3865–3877. [CrossRef]
80. Skála, M.; Hanousková, B.; Skálová, L.; Matoušková, P. MicroRNAs in the diagnosis and prevention of drug-induced Cardiotoxicity. *Arch. Toxicol.* 2019, *93*, 1–9. [CrossRef]
81. Zhou, S.-S.; Jin, J.-P.; Wang, J.-Q.; Zhang, Z.-G.; Freedman, J.H.; Zheng, Y.; Cai, L. miRNAS in cardiovascular diseases: Potential biomarkers, therapeutic targets and challenges. *Acta Pharmacol. Sin.* 2018, *39*, 1073–1084. [CrossRef]
82. Pellegrini, L.; Sileno, S.; D'Agostino, M.; Foglio, E.; Florio, M.C.; Guzzanti, V.; Russo, M.A.; Limana, F.; Magenta, A. MicroRNAs in Cancer Treatment-Induced Cardiotoxicity. *Cancers* 2020, *12*, 704. [CrossRef] [PubMed]
83. Kuwabara, Y.; Ono, K.; Horie, T.; Nishi, H.; Nagao, K.; Kinoshita, M.; Watanabe, S.; Baba, O.; Kojima, Y.; Shizuta, S.; et al. Increased MicroRNA-1 and MicroRNA-133a levels in serum of patients with cardiovascular disease indicate myocardial damage. *Circ. Cardiovasc. Genet.* 2011, *4*, 446–454. [CrossRef] [PubMed]
84. Rigaud, V.O.C.; Ferreira, L.R.P.; Ayub-Ferreira, S.M.; Ávila, M.S.; Brandão, S.M.G.; Cruz, F.D.; Santos, M.H.H.; Cruz, C.B.B.V.; Alves, M.S.L.; Issa, V.S.; et al. Circulating miR-1 as a potential biomarker of doxorubicin-induced cardiotoxicity in breast cancer patients. *Oncotarget* 2017, *8*, 6994–7002. [CrossRef] [PubMed]
85. Leger, K.J.; Leonard, D.; Nielson, D.; de Lemos, J.A.; Mammen, P.P.; Winick, N.J. Circulating microRNAs: Potential Markers of Cardiotoxicity in Children and Young Adults Treated with Anthracycline Chemotherapy. *J. Am. Heart Assoc.* 2017, *6*, e004653. [CrossRef]
86. Kumar, S.N.; Konorev, E.A.; Aggarwal, D.; Kalyanaraman, B. Analysis of Proteome Changes in Doxorubicin-Treated Adult Rat Cardiomyocyte. *J. Proteom.* 2011, *74*, 683–697. [CrossRef] [PubMed]
87. Creemers, E.E.; Tijsen, A.J.; Pinto, Y.M. Circulating microRNAs: Novel biomarkers and extracellular communicators in cardiovascular disease? *Circ. Res.* 2012, *110*, 483–495. [CrossRef]
88. Todorova, V.K.; Makhoul, I.; Wei, J.N.; Klimberg, V.S. Circulating miRNA profiles of doxorubicin-induced cardiotoxicity in breast cancer patients. *Ann. Clin. Lab. Sci.* 2017, *47*, 115–119.
89. Zhao, Z.Y.; He, J.; Zhang, J.; Liu, M.; Yang, S.; Li, N.; Li, X. Dysregulated miR1254 and miR579 for cardiotoxicity in patients treated with bevacizumab in colorectal cancer. *Tumor. Biol.* 2014, *35*, 5227–5235. [CrossRef]

90. Petricoin, E.F.; Rajapaske, V.; Herman, E.H.; Arekani, A.M.; Ross, S.; Johann, D.; Knapton, A.; Zhang, J.; Hitt, B.A.; Conrads, T.P.; et al. Toxicoproteomics: Serum Proteomic Pattern Diagnostics for Early Detection of Drug Induced Cardiac Toxicities and Cardioprotection. *Toxicol. Pathol.* **2004**, *32* (Suppl. S1), 122–130. [CrossRef]
91. Ohyama, K.; Tomonari, M.; Ichibangase, T.; To, H.; Kishikawa, N.; Nakashima, K.; Imai, K.; Kuroda, N. A Toxicoproteomic Study on Cardioprotective Effects of Pre-Administration of Docetaxel in a Mouse Model of Adriamycin-Induced Cardiotoxicity. *Biochem. Pharmacol.* **2010**, *80*, 540–547. [CrossRef]
92. Desai, V.G.; Lee, T.; Moland, C.L.; Vijay, V.; Han, T.; Lewis, S.M.; Herman, E.H.; Fuscoe, J.C. Candidate Early Predictive Plasma Protein Markers of Doxorubicin-Induced Chronic Cardiotoxicity in B6C3F 1 Mice. *Toxicol. Appl. Pharmacol.* **2019**, *363*, 164–173. [CrossRef] [PubMed]
93. Yarana, C.; Carroll, D.; Chen, J.; Chaiswing, L.; Zhao, Y.; Noel, T.; Alstott, M.; Bae, Y.; Dressler, E.V.; Moscow, J.A.; et al. Extracellular Vesicles Released by Cardiomyocytes in a Doxorubicin-Induced Cardiac Injury Mouse Model Contain Protein Biomarkers of Early Cardiac Injury. *Clin. Cancer Res.* **2018**, *24*, 1644–1653. [CrossRef] [PubMed]
94. Claudino, W.M.; Goncalves, P.H.; di Leo, A.; Philip, P.A.; Sarkar, F.H. Metabolomics in cancer: A bench-to-bedside intersection. *Crit. Rev. Oncol. Hematol.* **2012**, *84*, 1–7. [CrossRef] [PubMed]
95. Johnson, C.H.; Ivanisevic, J.; Siuzdak, G. Metabolomics: Beyond biomarkers and towards mechanisms. *Nat. Rev. Mol. Cell. Biol.* **2016**, *17*, 451–459. [CrossRef]
96. Lewis, G.D.; Asnani, A.; Gerszten, R.E. Application of metabolomics to cardiovascular biomarker and pathway discovery. *J. Am. Coll. Cardiol.* **2008**, *52*, 117–123. [CrossRef]
97. Deidda, M.; Mercurio, V.; Cuomo, A.; Noto, A.; Mercuro, G.; Cadeddu Dessalvi, C. Metabolomic Perspectives in Antiblastic Cardiotoxicity and Cardioprotection. *Int. J. Mol. Sci.* **2019**, *20*, 4928. [CrossRef]
98. Armenian, S.H.; Gelehrter, S.K.; Vase, T.; Venkatramani, R.; Landier, W.; Wilson, K.D.; Herrera, C.; Reichman, L.; Menteer, J.-D.; Mascarenhas, L. Carnitine and cardiac dysfunction in childhood cancer survivors treated with anthracyclines. *Cancer Epidemiol. Biomark. Prev.* **2014**, *23*, 1109–1114. [CrossRef]
99. Li, Y.; Ju, L.; Hou, Z.; Deng, H.; Zhang, Z.; Wang, L.; Yang, Z.; Yin, J.; Zhang, Y. Screening, Verification, and Optimization of Biomarkers for Early Prediction of Cardiotoxicity Based on Metabolomics. *J. Proteome Res.* **2015**, *14*, 2437–2445. [CrossRef] [PubMed]
100. Andreadou, I.; Papaefthimiou, M.; Constantinou, M.; Sigala, F.; Skaltsounis, A.L.; Tsantili-Kakoulidou, A.; Iliodromitis, E.K.; Kremastinos, D.T.; Mikros, E. Metabolomic identification of novel biomarkers in doxorubicin cardiotoxicity and protective eggect of the natural antioxidant oleuropein. *NMR Biomed.* **2009**, *22*, 585–592.
101. Chaudhari, U.; Ellis, J.K.; Wagh, V.; Nemade, H.; Hescheler, J.; Keun, H.C.; Sachinidis, A. Metabolite signatures of doxorubicin induced toxicity in human induced pluripotent stem cell-derived cardiomyocytes. *Amino Acids* **2017**, *49*, 1955–1963. [CrossRef] [PubMed]
102. Schnackenberg, L.K.; Pence, L.; Vijay, V.; Moland, C.L.; George, N.; Cao, Z.; Yu, L.R.; Fuscoe, J.C.; Beger, R.D.; Desai, V.G.J. Early metabolomics changes in heart and plasma during chronic doxorubicin treatment in B6C3F1mice. *Appl. Toxicol.* **2016**, *36*, 1486–1495. [CrossRef]
103. Tan, G.; Lou, Z.; Liao, W.; Zhu, Z.; Dong, X.; Zhang, W.; Chai, W.L. Potential Biomarkers in Mouse Myocardium of Doxorubicin-Induced Cardiomyopathy: A Metabonomic Method and Its Application. *PLoS ONE* **2011**, *6*, e27683. [CrossRef] [PubMed]
104. Jensen, B.C.; Parry, T.L.; Huang, W.; Ilaiwy, A.; Bain, J.R.; Muehlbauer, M.J.; O'Neal, S.K.; Patterson, C.; Johnson, G.L.; Willis, M.S. Non-Targeted Metabolomics Analysis of the Effects of Tyrosine Kinase Inhibitors Sunitinib and Erlotinib on Heart, Muscle, Liver and Serum Metabolism In Vivo. *Metabolites* **2017**, *7*, E31. [CrossRef]
105. Andreadou, I.; Mikros, E.; Ioannidis, K.; Sigala, F.; Naka, K.; Kostidis, S.; Farmakis, D.; Tenta, R.; Kavantzas, N.; Bibli, S.I. Oleuropein prevents doxorubicin-induced cardiomyopathy interfering with signaling molecules and cardiomyocyte metabolism. *J. Mol. Cell. Cardiol.* **2014**, *69*, 4–16. [CrossRef]
106. Geng, C.; Cui, C.; Wang, C.; Lu, S.; Zhang, M.; Chen, D.; Jiang, P. Systematic Evaluations of Doxorubicin-Induced Toxicity in Rats Based on Metabolomics. *ACS Omega* **2020**, *6*, 358–366. [CrossRef]
107. Tantawy, M.; Chekka, L.M.; Huang, Y.; Garrett, T.J.; Singh, S.; Shah, C.P.; Cornell, R.F.; Baz, R.C.; Fradley, M.G.; Waheed, N.; et al. Lactate Dehydrogenase B and Pyruvate Oxidation Pathway Associated with Carfilzomib-Related Cardiotoxicity in Multiple Myeloma Patients: Result of a Multi-Omics Integrative Analysis. *Front. Cardiovasc. Med.* **2021**, *8*, 645122. [CrossRef]
108. Yin, Y.J.; Xie, J.; Guo, X.; Ju, L.; Li, Y.; Zhang, Y. Plasma metabolic profiling analysis of cyclophosphamide-induced cardiotoxicity using metabolomics coupled with UPLC/Q-TOF-MS and ROC curve. *Technol. Biomed. Life Sci.* **2016**, *1033*, 428–435. [CrossRef]
109. Jensen, B.C.; Parry, T.L.; Huang, W.; Beak, J.Y.; Ilaiwy, A.; Bain, J.R.; Newgard, C.B.; Muehlbauer, M.J.; Patterson, C.; Johnson, G.L.; et al. Effects of the kinase inhibitor sorafenib on heart, muscle, liver and plasma metabolism in vivo using non-targeted metabolomics analysis. *Br. J. Pharmacol.* **2017**, *174*, 4797–4811. [CrossRef] [PubMed]
110. Park, B.; Sim, S.H.; Lee, K.S.; Kim, H.J.; Park, I.H. Genome-wide association study of genetic variants related to anthracycline-induced cardiotoxicity in early breast cancer. *Cancer Sci.* **2020**, *111*, 2579–2587. [CrossRef]

Disclaimer/Publisher's Note: The statements, opinions and data contained in all publications are solely those of the individual author(s) and contributor(s) and not of MDPI and/or the editor(s). MDPI and/or the editor(s) disclaim responsibility for any injury to people or property resulting from any ideas, methods, instructions or products referred to in the content.

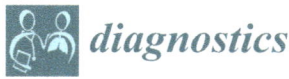

Article

Impact of Cancer Type and Treatment Protocol on Cardiac Function in Pediatric Oncology Patients: An Analysis Utilizing Speckle Tracking, Global Longitudinal Strain, and Myocardial Performance Index

Andrada Mara Ardelean [1,2,3], Ioana Cristina Olariu [1,3], Raluca Isac [1,3], Akhila Nalla [4], Ruxandra Jurac [1,3], Cristiana Stolojanu [2,3], Mircea Murariu [2,3], Roxana Manuela Fericean [2,5], Laurentiu Braescu [2,6,7], Adelina Mavrea [8,*], Catalin Dumitru [9] and Gabriela Doros [1,3]

[1] Department of Pediatrics, "Victor Babes" University of Medicine and Pharmacy, Eftimie Murgu Square 2, 300041 Timisoara, Romania; andrada.micsescu-olah@umft.ro (A.M.A.); olariu.cristina@umft.ro (I.C.O.); isac.raluca@umft.ro (R.I.); steflea.ruxandra@umft.ro (R.J.); gdoros@gmail.com (G.D.)

[2] Doctoral School, "Victor Babes" University of Medicine and Pharmacy, Eftimie Murgu Square 2, 300041 Timisoara, Romania; stolojanu.cristiana@umft.ro (C.S.); mircea.1192@yahoo.com (M.M.); manuela.fericean@umft.ro (R.M.F.); braescu.laurentiu@umft.ro (L.B.)

[3] Louis Turcanu Emergency Hospital for Children, Iosif Nemoianu Street 2, 300011 Timișoara, Romania

[4] Department of General Medicine, MNR Medical College, Sangareddy 502294, Telangana, India; akhila.nalla@gmail.com

[5] Methodological and Infectious Diseases Research Center, Department of Infectious Diseases, "Victor Babes" University of Medicine and Pharmacy, 300041 Timisoara, Romania

[6] Department of Cardiovascular Surgery, "Victor Babes" University of Medicine and Pharmacy, Eftimie Murgu Square 2, 300041 Timisoara, Romania

[7] Center for Translational Research and Systems Medicine (CERT-MEDS), "Victor Babes" University of Medicine and Pharmacy, Eftimie Murgu Square 2, 300041 Timisoara, Romania

[8] Department of Internal Medicine I, Cardiology Clinic, "Victor Babes" University of Medicine and Pharmacy Timisoara, Eftimie Murgu Square 2, 300041 Timisoara, Romania

[9] Department of Obstetrics and Gynecology, "Victor Babes" University of Medicine and Pharmacy Timisoara, 300041 Timisoara, Romania; dumitru.catalin@umft.ro

* Correspondence: mavrea.adelina@umft.ro

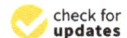

Citation: Ardelean, A.M.; Olariu, I.C.; Isac, R.; Nalla, A.; Jurac, R.; Stolojanu, C.; Murariu, M.; Fericean, R.M.; Braescu, L.; Mavrea, A.; et al. Impact of Cancer Type and Treatment Protocol on Cardiac Function in Pediatric Oncology Patients: An Analysis Utilizing Speckle Tracking, Global Longitudinal Strain, and Myocardial Performance Index. Diagnostics 2023, 13, 2830. https://doi.org/10.3390/diagnostics13172830

Academic Editors: Emmanouel Hatzipantelis and Maria Kourti

Received: 1 July 2023
Revised: 15 August 2023
Accepted: 30 August 2023
Published: 31 August 2023

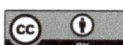

Copyright: © 2023 by the authors. Licensee MDPI, Basel, Switzerland. This article is an open access article distributed under the terms and conditions of the Creative Commons Attribution (CC BY) license (https://creativecommons.org/licenses/by/4.0/).

Abstract: Pediatric hemato-oncology patients undergoing anthracycline therapy are at risk of cardiotoxicity, with disease type and treatment intensity potentially affecting cardiac function. Novel echocardiographic measures like speckle tracking echocardiography (STE), global longitudinal strain (GLS), and the myocardial performance index (MPI) may predict early changes in cardiac function not detected by traditional methods. This study aimed to assess the impact of cancer type and treatment protocol on these parameters and their potential in predicting long-term cardiac complications. We conducted a single-center, retrospective cohort study of 99 pediatric oncology patients and 46 controls that were assessed at 3, 6, and 12 months. The median age was 10.7 ± 4.4 years for cases and 10.2 ± 3.6 years for controls. STE, GLS, and MPI were measured, and statistical analyses were performed to determine any significant correlations with cardiotoxicity. Significant variations were observed in traditional cardiac function measurements between the patient and control groups, with a lower average ejection fraction (EF) of 62.8 ± 5.7% in patients vs. 66.4 ± 6.1% in controls ($p < 0.001$), poorer GLS of −16.3 ± 5.1 in patients compared to −19.0 ± 5.4 in controls ($p = 0.004$), and higher MPI values of 0.37 ± 0.06 in patients compared to 0.55 ± 0.10 in controls, indicating worse overall cardiac function ($p < 0.001$). However, differences in cardiac function measurements by cancer histology or treatment protocol were not statistically significant. Regression analyses showed that the combination of GLS, SMOD, and MPI increased the odds of cardiac toxicity with an odds ratio of 7.30 (95% CI: 2.65–12.81, $p < 0.001$). The study underscores the predictive value of the combined GLS, SMOD, and MPI measurements in pediatric oncology patients undergoing anthracycline treatment for cardiotoxicity. Although variations across cancer types and treatment protocols were not significant, the study emphasizes the potential utility of these novel echocardiographic measures in early detection and long-term prediction of anthracycline-induced cardiotoxicity. Further studies in larger, multi-center cohorts are required for validation.

Keywords: pediatrics; oncology; chemotherapy; cardiac function tests

1. Introduction

The continued advancements in pediatric oncology have led to a steady increase in survival rates, providing a truly encouraging trend [1]. Despite this promising development, the life-saving interventions, which often include aggressive chemotherapy and radiotherapy, often cause considerable long-term morbidity [2,3]. One of the most significant and alarming late effects is cardiotoxicity [4]. It is well established that cancer treatments, particularly anthracyclines and chest irradiation, can lead to various cardiac complications such as cardiomyopathy, ischemic heart disease, pericarditis, arrythmia, and congestive heart failure [5]. Furthermore, cardiac damage can occur years or even decades after the completion of therapy, adding an extra dimension to this already complex issue [6].

Traditionally, cardiac function in pediatric oncology patients has been monitored using conventional echocardiographic methods such as ejection fraction (EF) and fractional shortening (FS) [7]. However, these measures have significant limitations, since they are influenced by several factors, including loading conditions and heart rate, and may not accurately represent true myocardial function [8]. Moreover, significant reductions in EF and FS often occur late, when irreversible myocardial damage has already occurred [9]. Therefore, there is an urgent need to improve the early detection of cardiotoxicity in this population.

The damaging effects of treatments like anthracyclines on the heart cannot be understated. Anthracyclines are known to induce cardiotoxicity, a significant side effect that can severely affect the quality of life and overall survival of cancer patients, independent of the oncological prognosis [10]. This cardiotoxicity usually starts with myocardial cell injury, progresses to reductions in left ventricular ejection fraction (LVEF), and, if undetected and untreated, can eventually lead to symptomatic heart failure [10]. Specifically, anthracycline-induced cardiotoxicity can manifest even in a subclinical phase, making early detection paramount. Traditional measures like LVEF may not suffice in capturing these early changes. Advanced echocardiographic techniques, such as 2D Speckle tracking echocardiography (STE), have shown the capability of detecting early myocardial changes, especially during chemotherapy [11,12]. Peak systolic global longitudinal strain, a parameter derived from STE, stands out as an especially consistent indicator of early myocardial damage. Thus, the use of STE, GLS, and MPI can be pivotal, not just in detecting these changes, but also in driving the implementation of cardioprotective treatments before irreversible damage ensues.

In recent years, speckle tracking echocardiography (STE), global longitudinal strain (GLS), and the myocardial performance index (MPI) have emerged as promising tools for the evaluation of myocardial function [13,14]. STE is an angle-independent imaging technique that provides a detailed assessment of myocardial deformation [15]. GLS measures the degree of deformation of the myocardium longitudinally and is considered more sensitive and specific for the early detection of myocardial damage than traditional echocardiographic methods [16]. MPI, also known as the Tei index, is a Doppler-derived index that evaluates both systolic and diastolic cardiac function [17]. These innovative techniques may enable us to detect subtle changes in cardiac function and improve patient outcomes.

However, while these novel methods show great promise, there are still many unknowns regarding their utility in pediatric oncology patients [18,19]. Previous studies have been limited by small sample sizes, heterogeneous patient populations, and lack of long-term follow-up data. Moreover, there is limited research on the potential impact of different disease types and treatment intensity on the results of these measures. In addition, it is unclear whether these measures can predict long-term cardiac outcomes. Early detection of cardiotoxicity is crucial, but it is equally important to understand the implications of these findings. If changes in cardiac function were identified at an early stage, it would be possible to intervene and alter the course of the disease. However, to do this effectively, there is a need to understand how these early changes are associated with long-term outcomes.

Therefore, the hypotheses of the present study are that disease type and treatment intensity have a significant impact on cardiac function as measured by speckle tracking, global longitudinal strain, and the myocardial performance index in pediatric oncology patients. It is assumed that these novel echocardiographic measures can detect early changes in cardiac function that traditional methods cannot. Moreover, these early changes might predict long-term cardiac outcomes in this population. Accordingly, the objectives of this study are to evaluate the impact of cancer type and treatment protocol on cardiac function in pediatric oncology patients; to compare the sensitivity of STE, GLS, and MPI with that of traditional echocardiographic methods for detecting early cardiac dysfunction; and to explore the potential of these measures to predict long-term cardiac complications in this population.

2. Materials and Methods

2.1. Design and Ethics

This study was designed as a single-center, retrospective cohort study conducted over a four-year period from 2019 to 2022. The study protocol and ethical considerations were reviewed and approved by an institutional review board (IRB). All study procedures complied with the ethical standards of the 1964 Helsinki declaration and its later amendments. The investigators ensured that confidentiality was maintained, and data privacy was protected according to local data protection laws. The investigators clarified to the parents/guardians that participation was voluntary and that they could withdraw from the study at any time without affecting the child's medical care. Before participation, written informed consent was obtained from the parents or guardians of all pediatric patients. For patients who reached the age of consent during the course of the study, assent was sought in addition to parental consent. The research team ensured that all participants and their guardians fully understood the study's objectives, procedures, potential benefits, and risks.

Studies have consistently highlighted the potential cardiotoxic effects of oncology treatments, especially in pediatric patients. While our research primarily focuses on a specific patient cohort, it is imperative to contextualize our findings within the broader scope of evidence. Several meta-analyses have aggregated results from multiple studies, providing a comprehensive understanding of cardiac effects in pediatric oncology patients across diverse treatment protocols, cancer stages, and demographics. Such meta-analyses underscore the importance of regular cardiac monitoring, especially considering the multifaceted nature of oncology treatments and the variabilities in patient response. By delving deep into the oncological characteristics of our population, such as clinical stage, total dose of cardiotoxic drug administered, and detailed echocardiogram timelines, our study aims to bridge the gaps in knowledge and offer nuanced insights into pediatric cardiac care in oncology settings.

2.2. Inclusion and Exclusion Criteria

The inclusion criteria were pediatric patients diagnosed with a new oncological pathology requiring anthracycline therapy between 2019 and 2022. Baseline measurements were taken upon the patient's first presentation at the oncology ward, before initiation of any therapeutic interventions. Patients, both neoadjuvant and metastatic, were included to provide a comprehensive view of the impact of different cancer stages on cardiac function. The study focused primarily on the diagnosis of a new oncological pathology and did not differentiate based on the specific stage of cancer. However, the clinical stage of each patient was documented and will be presented in the Results section for a more detailed understanding. The inclusion criteria comprised: (1) Pediatric patients (aged 0–18 years) diagnosed with a new oncological pathology requiring anthracycline therapy between 2019 and 2023; (2) patients with measurable cardiac function at baseline and at regular intervals during the course of treatment; (3) patients whose clinical and treatment data, including disease type, treatment protocol, and cumulative dosage of anthracyclines and other chemotherapy agents, were available and complete.

On the contrary, the exclusion criteria comprised: (1) Patients with known pre-existing cardiac pathology that could affect the cardiac function measurements; (2) patients who had already started oncological treatment before baseline measurements could be established; (3) patients with any contraindications to echocardiography, such as severe skin condition or chest deformity; (4) patients who initiated treatment at our institution but decided to continue treatment at another facility; and (5) patients with other concurrent severe medical conditions (e.g., severe infections, metabolic diseases, genetic syndromes, etc.) that could independently impact cardiac function.

The control group consisted of healthy children admitted to our hospital for minor conditions such as chest wall pain, syncope spells, minor respiratory infections, or athletes who came in for their mandatory annual check-ups and required a cardiology assessment. The cases and control groups were matched by age, gender, and body mass index. The control group included healthy children admitted to our hospital for various minor conditions. Among these, some were athletes. For the purpose of this study, "athletes" were defined as individuals who engage in regular, structured physical training for a specific sport and participate in competitive events related to that sport at least once a year. Out of all the controls, seven were athletes.

Additional factors including patient age, sex, disease, fractional shortening (FS), left-ventricular global longitudinal strain (GLS), Simpson's method of discs (SMOD) measurements, myocardial performance index (MPI), presence of cardiotoxicity, 12-lead electrocardiogram (ECG) findings, echocardiography results, biomarkers of cardiac injury, protocol intensity, surface area (m^2), total anthracycline dose, cumulative dosage of other chemotherapy agents (including cytarabine administered intravenously, subcutaneously, and intrathecally, etoposide, cyclophosphamide, vincristine, asparaginase, ifosfamide, methotrexate administered intravenously and intrathecally, mercaptopurine orally, Oncaspar intravenously, mitoxantrone intravenously), and radiation therapy received were collected and analyzed.

2.3. Materials Used and Definitions

The diagnosis of cardiac toxicity was made by identifying ultrasound alterations after chemotherapy. Cardiac function was measured using a GE VIVID E9 echocardiograph. High-quality images with ECG signals were captured in apical views (3, 4, and 2 chambers). When satisfactory images were obtained, the machine software identified the end-systolic frame and automatically traced the endocardial and epicardial borders, spanning from one end of the mitral annulus to the other. This process generated a region of interest (ROI) that encompassed the entire myocardial wall. Cardiac function measurements were taken at regular intervals post the initiation of therapy. Specifically, echocardiograms were performed every three months. Cardioxane, although not a primary chemotherapy agent under consideration, was documented if administered to any patient.

Adjustments were then made to the ROI manually, and speckle placement was corrected to select for optimal myocardial wall thickness. Speckles, which are myocardial reflectors, were tracked throughout the cardiac cycle to determine myocardial strain. Care was taken not to include the pericardium or the base of the valves to avoid a false reduction in global longitudinal strain (GLS). Decreases in GLS (less negative values, closer to 0) may indicate decreased cardiac function and potentially cardiac injury.

In addition to GLS, cardiac function was assessed using traditional methods such as M mode dimension ejection fraction (Teicholtz) and volume ejection fraction (Simpson's method of disks, SMOD), and tissue Doppler was used to measure the myocardial performance index. The normal range for SMOD is generally considered to be between 55% and 70%, while values below 55% are usually considered indicative of reduced systolic function. Normal MPI values are generally considered to be less than 0.40, and these may vary slightly depending on whether they are measured by tissue Doppler imaging or flow Doppler imaging. Values above 0.40 indicate worsening global cardiac function. Any abnormalities that arose during treatment, such as pericardial or pleural effusion, valve regurgitations or stenoses, pulmonary hypertension, diastolic dysfunction, dilated cardiomyopathy or electrocardiographic modifications, were documented and monitored.

2.4. Statistical Analysis

Statistical analysis was performed using the Statistical Package for the Social Sciences (SPSS v.26). Descriptive statistics were utilized to summarize the data. Continuous variables were expressed as the mean ± standard deviation, while categorical variables were presented as frequencies and percentages. The paired t-test was used to compare baseline and post-treatment measurements within the same group, and the independent t-test was used to compare differences between the patient and control groups, while the ANOVA test was employed to compare means of more than two groups. Multivariate logistic regression was employed to identify independent predictors of chemotherapy-induced cardiotoxicity, adjusting for potential confounders. Before performing multivariate logistic regression, a univariate analysis was conducted to determine which variables were to be included in the multivariate analysis. Additionally, to assess the effectiveness of our cardiac function measurements against established standards, a predictive analysis was carried out. This involved computing predictive values, sensitivity, and specificity of our measures in relation to the gold standard. The ANOVA test was primarily utilized to compare means of cardiac function measurements at different time points, including baseline, 3 months, 6 months, and 12 months. A p-value of less than 0.05 was considered statistically significant. All graphs and tables were created using GraphPad Prism v.9.

3. Results

3.1. Background Data of Patients

The current study incorporated a total of 145 participants, including 99 cases and 46 controls (Table 1). The average age of the case group was 10.7 ± 4.4 years, whereas the control group averaged slightly younger at 10.2 ± 3.6 years, without a significant difference. The body mass index (BMI) was comparable between the two groups, with mean BMI values of 20.5 and 21.3 for the cases and control groups, respectively, but with no significant difference. Moreover, the BMI percentile categories displayed a balanced distribution among both case and control groups, and the statistical comparison between the two groups did not yield a significant p-value (0.361). Gender distribution in both groups was also similar, with 58.6% of the case group being male compared to 63.0% in the control group. Female participants accounted for 41.4% of the case group and 37.0% of the control group, yielding a p-value of 0.610. Therefore, gender did not significantly differ between the two groups. The most common cancer histology was B-cell acute lymphocytic leukemia (B-ALL), followed by T-ALL (14.1%), and acute myeloid leukemia (AML) in 12.1% of cases, as presented in Figure 1.

Table 1. Background data of study participants.

Variables *	Cases (n = 99)	Controls (n = 46)	p-Value
Age (mean ± SD)	10.7 ± 4.4	10.2 ± 3.6	0.471
Age range	1–18	1–17	–
BMI, kg/m^2 (mean ± SD)	20.5 ± 4.6	21.3 ± 5.8	0.308
BMI percentile categories			0.361
>85%	9 (9.1%)	2 (4.3%)	
50–85%	47 (27.3%)	9 (19.6%)	
15–50%	75 (35.4%)	17 (37.0%)	
5–15%	81 (21.2%)	16 (34.8%)	
<5%	4 (7.0%)	2 (4.3%)	
Gender (n,%)			0.610
Male	58 (58.6%)	29 (63.0%)	
Female	41 (41.4%)	17 (37.0%)	

*—Mean and SD compared using Student's t-test; BMI—body mass index; SD—standard deviation.

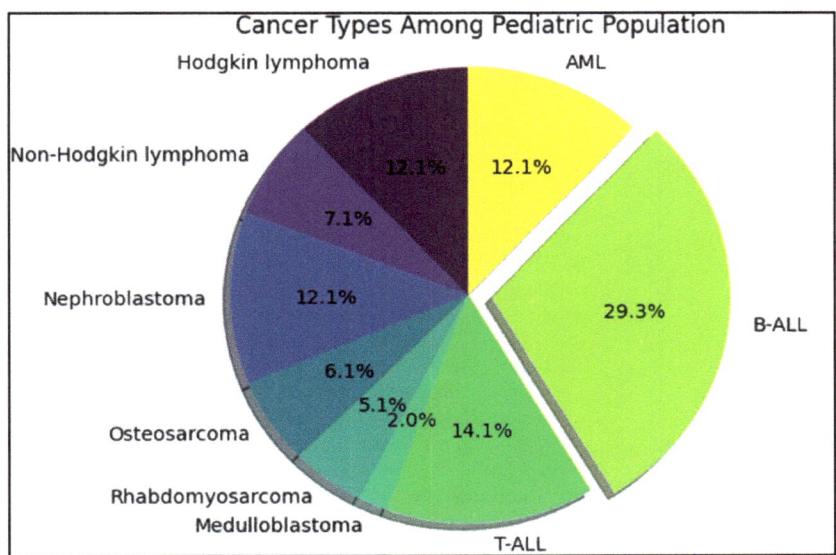

Figure 1. Prevalence of cancer histology types among the pediatric population.

3.2. Cardiac Parameters

Table 2 outlines the analysis of cardiac function measurements between pediatric oncology patients post-chemotherapy (n = 99) and healthy controls (n = 46). Ejection fraction (EF), a marker of systolic function, showed significant variation between the two cohorts. The mean EF in the cases was 62.8 ± 5.7%, which was lower than that in the controls (66.4 ± 6.1%), and this difference was statistically significant ($p < 0.001$). Additionally, EF distribution across categories revealed that a higher proportion of controls had an EF above 70% (30.4%) compared to that of cases (11.1%), also statistically significant ($p = 0.005$). A similar trend was observed in the global longitudinal strain (GLS) measurement. The cases had a mean GLS of −16.3 ± 5.1, whereas the controls had a more negative mean GLS of −19.0 ± 5.4, indicating a more substantial contraction and hence better cardiac function in the controls ($p = 0.004$).

Table 2. Cardiac function measurements between children after chemotherapy and healthy controls.

Variables *	Cases (n = 99)	Controls (n = 46)	p-Value
EF (mean ± SD,%)	62.8 ± 5.7	66.4 ± 6.1	<0.001
EF categories (initial)			0.005
50–60%	16 (16.2%)	2 (4.3%)	
60–70%	72 (72.7%)	30 (65.2%)	
>70%	11 (11.1%)	14 (30.4%)	
GLS (mean ± SD,%)	−16.3 ± 5.1	−19.0 ± 5.4	0.004
SMOD (mean ± SD,%)	55.1 ± 6.0	59.3 ± 6.7	<0.001
MPI (mean ± SD, score)	0.37 ± 0.06	0.55 ± 0.10	<0.001
ECG (%)			
Normal findings	66 (66.7%)	40 (87.0%)	0.010
Abnormal	33 (33.3%)	6 (13.0%)	
Cardiac ultrasound (%)			0.610
Normal findings	47 (47.5%)	11 (76.1%)	0.001
Abnormal	52 (52.5%)	6 (23.9%)	

*—Mean and SD compared using Student's t-test; SD—standard deviation; GLS—global longitudinal strain; SMOD—Simpson's method of discs; MPI—myocardial performance index; ECG—electrocardiogram; EF—ejection fraction.

When assessed using Simpson's method of discs (SMOD), the mean score in cases was found to be 55.1 ± 6.0, which was again significantly lower than that in controls (59.3 ± 6.7, $p < 0.001$). The myocardial performance index (MPI), a measure of both systolic and diastolic function, was higher in cases (0.37 ± 0.06) compared to that in controls (0.55 ± 0.10). A higher MPI usually represents worse cardiac performance, reflecting poorer overall cardiac function in cases ($p < 0.001$). Electrocardiogram (ECG) findings revealed a significantly higher proportion of normal findings in controls (87.0%) compared to that in cases (66.7%, $p = 0.010$). This was mirrored in the cardiac ultrasound findings, with a higher rate of normal findings among controls (76.1%) compared to that in cases (47.5%, $p = 0.001$). Conversely, the percentage of abnormal findings was higher in cases for both ECG and cardiac ultrasound.

Table 3 illustrates the comparison of cardiac function measurements stratified by cancer histology. Although there was variation among the different cancer types, none of the observed differences reached statistical significance. Global longitudinal strain (GLS) was calculated using speckle tracking echocardiography and ranged from −15.3 ± 4.6 in Hodgkin's lymphoma patients to −18.1 ± 5.1 in T-cell acute lymphoblastic leukemia (T-ALL) patients. However, these differences were not statistically significant ($p = 0.442$).

Table 3. Cardiac measurements based on cancer histology.

Variables (Mean ± SD)	Speckle (GLS, %)	Simpson (SMOD, %)	MPI Score	EF (%)
Cancer histology				
Hodgkin's lymphoma	−15.3 ± 4.6	58.4 ± 6.8	0.36 ± 0.05	62.0 ± 5.9
Non-Hodgkin's lymphoma	−16.2 ± 5.8	59.2 ± 6.6	0.41 ± 0.07	64.6 ± 5.5
Nephroblastoma	−16.0 ± 4.2	54.6 ± 5.1	0.40 ± 0.04	59.3 ± 5.1
Osteosarcoma	−15.3 ± 4.7	52.1 ± 5.3	0.44 ± 0.10	58.0 ± 5.4
Rhabdomyosarcoma	−15.9 ± 5.3	55.0 ± 6.2	0.42 ± 0.06	62.4 ± 5.8
Medulloblastoma	−17.6 ± 4.8	52.8 ± 5.6	0.48 ± 0.09	60.8 ± 5.6
T-ALL	−18.1 ± 5.1	53.3 ± 6.1	0.40 ± 0.05	61.1 ± 4.7
B-ALL	−17.3 ± 4.9	54.9 ± 5.4	0.45 ± 0.12	59.3 ± 5.5
AML	−16.4 ± 5.2	51.0 ± 6.3	0.41 ± 0.07	60.6 ± 4.9
p-value	0.442	0.150	0.306	0.084

SD—standard deviation; MPI—myocardial performance index; T-ALL—T-cell acute lymphoblastic leukemia; B-ALL—B-cell acute lymphoblastic leukemia; AML—acute myeloid leukemia; GLS—global longitudinal strain; SMOD—Simpson's method of discs; EF—ejection fraction.

Cardiac function measured by Simpson's method of discs (SMOD) ranged from 51.0 ± 6.3 in acute myeloid leukemia (AML) patients to 59.2 ± 6.6 in non-Hodgkin's lymphoma patients. Again, the differences across the various types of cancers did not attain statistical significance (p = 0.150). The myocardial performance index (MPI), a combined measure of both systolic and diastolic function, varied between 0.36 ± 0.05 in Hodgkin's lymphoma patients and 0.48 ± 0.09 in medulloblastoma patients, but these variations were not statistically significant (p = 0.306). Lastly, mean ejection fraction (EF), a measure of systolic function, varied between 58.0 ± 5.4 in osteosarcoma patients and 64.6 ± 5.5 in non-Hodgkin's lymphoma patients. Despite this range, the differences were not statistically significant (p = 0.084).

Table 4 illustrates the cardiac function measurements in relation to the different treatment protocols implemented for the various types of cancer. Despite observable differences in the measurements, none of the variations among the treatments reached statistical significance. Global longitudinal strain (GLS), calculated using speckle tracking echocardiography, varied across treatment protocols from −16.5 ± 4.6 under the EURAMOS protocol to −15.0 ± 4.8 under the RCHOP protocol. However, these variations did not achieve statistical significance (p = 0.095). Regarding the Simpson's method of discs (SMOD), values ranged from 55.0 ± 6.6 under the EURAMOS protocol to 60.1 ± 4.3 under the ICE protocol, and this range did not reach statistical significance (p = 0.317).

Table 4. Cardiac measurements based on treatment protocol.

Variables (Mean ± SD)	Speckle (GLS, %)	Simpson (SMOD, %)	MPI Score	EF (%)	Developed Cardiac Toxicity (n,%)
Treatment protocol					
AML BFM	−16.1 ± 4.3	56.2 ± 4.4	0.39 ± 0.04	58.3 ± 3.5	2 (2.0%)
ALL BFM	−15.5 ± 5.4	57.0 ± 4.3	0.44 ± 0.06	61.5 ± 4.3	12 (12.1%)
ABVD	−16.2 ± 3.5	57.9 ± 5.2	0.42 ± 0.10	59.6 ± 3.7	4 (4.0%)
ICE	−15.8 ± 6.6	60.1 ± 4.3	0.46 ± 0.12	60.4 ± 4.0	2 (2.0%)
ISPO	−16.3 ± 3.7	59.3 ± 6.4	0.43 ± 0.09	62.6 ± 3.8	2 (2.0%)
RCHOP	−15.0 ± 4.8	57.6 ± 4.5	0.40 ± 0.05	60.1 ± 4.7	2 (2.0%)
EURAMOS	−16.5 ± 4.6	55.0 ± 6.6	0.42 ± 0.10	57.6 ± 3.9	3 (3.0%)
CWS	−15.9 ± 5.4	56.8 ± 5.7	0.44 ± 0.16	59.0 ± 3.6	3 (3.0%)
p-value	0.095	0.317	0.063	0.139	0.247

SD—standard deviation; GLS—global longitudinal strain; SMOD—Simpson's method of discs; MPI—myocardial performance index; AML—acute myeloid leukemia; ALL—acute lymphoid leukemia; BFM—Berlin-Frankfurt-Münster; ABVD (for Hodgkin's lymphoma)—Adriamycin (doxorubicin), bleomycin, vinblastine, and dacarbazine; ICE—ifosfamide, carboplatin, and etoposide; ISPO (for nephroblastoma)—International Society of Pediatric Oncology; RCHOP (for non-Hodgkin's lymphoma)—rituximab, cyclophosphamide, hydroxydaunorubicin (doxorubicin), Oncovin (vincristine), and prednisone; EURAMOS—European and American Osteosarcoma Study Group; CWS (for rhabdomyosarcoma)—Cooperative Weichteilsarkom Studiengruppe; EF—ejection fraction.

The myocardial performance index (MPI), a combined measure of both systolic and diastolic function, varied between 0.39 ± 0.04 under the AML BFM protocol and 0.46 ± 0.12 under the ICE protocol, but these differences were not statistically significant (p = 0.063). Ejection fraction (EF), a measure of systolic function, ranged from 57.6 ± 3.9 under the EURAMOS protocol to 62.6 ± 3.8 under the ISPO protocol, but these differences were not statistically significant (p = 0.139). The percentage of patients who developed cardiac toxicity also varied by treatment protocol, with the highest occurrence in patients under the ALL BFM protocol (12.1%) and the lowest in multiple protocols, including AML BFM, ICE, ISPO, and RCHOP, each at 2.0%. However, the variance in incidence of cardiac toxicity among the different treatment protocols did not reach statistical significance (p = 0.247).

3.3. Risk Evaluation

Table 5 and Figure 2 show the results of the regression analysis, providing odds ratios for the associations between various cardiac function measurements and the development of cardiac toxicity. The odds ratios have been adjusted for potential confounders. Global longitudinal strain (GLS) alone had an odds ratio of 2.20, indicating that for each unit increase in GLS, the odds of cardiac toxicity were approximately doubled. However, this finding was not statistically significant (95% CI: 0.92–4.31, p = 0.106). Simpson's method of discs (SMOD) had a similar odds ratio of 2.16, indicating a slightly more than double increase in the odds of cardiac toxicity for each unit increase in the SMOD measure, but again, this finding was not statistically significant (95% CI: 0.99–5.16, p = 0.098).

Table 5. Regression analysis for factors associated with cardiac toxicity.

Adjusted Factors *	Odds Ratio	(95% CI)	p-Value
GLS	2.20	0.92–4.31	0.106
SMOD	2.16	0.99–5.16	0.098
MPI	1.24	0.81–4.03	0.221
GLS + SMOD	4.05	1.33–7.40	<0.001
GLS + MPI	2.49	1.08–7.24	0.030
SMOD + MPI	5.02	2.14–10.09	<0.001
GLS + SMOD + MPI	7.30	2.65–12.81	<0.001

*—The control group serves as reference; CI—confidence interval; GLS—global longitudinal strain; SMOD—Simpson's method of discs; MPI—myocardial performance index.

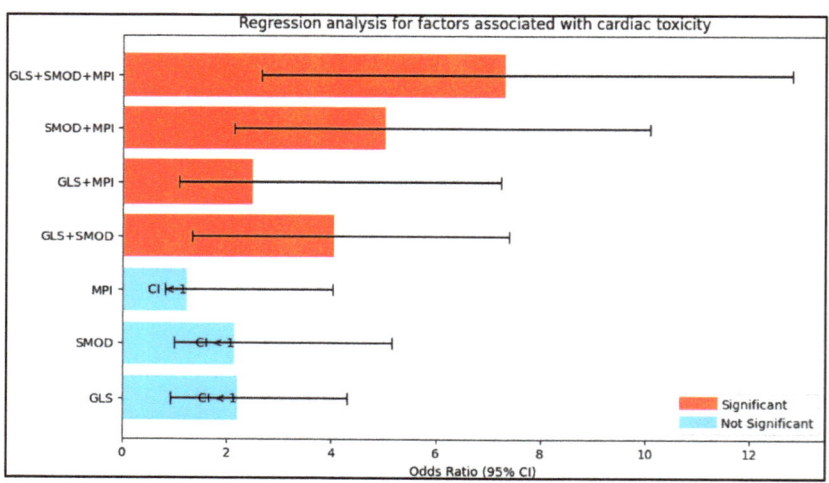

Figure 2. Risk analysis for factors associated with cardiac toxicity.

The myocardial performance index (MPI) showed a less marked association, with an odds ratio of 1.24 suggesting only a slight increase in the odds of cardiac toxicity for each unit increase in MPI. This association was also not statistically significant (95% CI: 0.81–4.03, p = 0.221). However, combinations of these measures showed stronger and statistically significant associations with cardiac toxicity. The combination of GLS and SMOD had an odds ratio of 4.05, showing a significant quadrupling in the odds of cardiac toxicity (95% CI: 1.33–7.40, p < 0.001). Similarly, the combination of GLS and MPI showed a significant increase in the odds of cardiac toxicity, with an odds ratio of 2.49 (95% CI: 1.08–7.24, p = 0.030). The combination of SMOD and MPI showed an even greater odds ratio of 5.02, indicating a more than fivefold increase in the odds of cardiac toxicity (95% CI: 2.14–10.09, p < 0.001). The combination of all three measurements—GLS, SMOD, and MPI—showed the greatest odds ratio of 7.30, indicating more than a sevenfold increase in the odds of cardiac toxicity (95% CI: 2.65–12.81, p < 0.001).

4. Discussion

4.1. Literature and Current Study Findings

The present study's findings underscored a significant impact of disease type and treatment intensity on cardiac function in pediatric oncology patients. These results were consistent with the initial hypotheses that traditional echocardiographic methods might not detect early changes in cardiac function that these novel methods can discern. Importantly, these early changes might predict long-term cardiac outcomes in this population, lending further weight to the potential utility of these novel approaches in this clinical context.

The observed differences in cardiac function parameters, such as ejection fraction (EF), global longitudinal strain (GLS), the myocardial performance index (MPI), and results from Simpson's method of discs (SMOD), underscored the potential deleterious effects of cancer and its treatment on cardiac function. These findings align with earlier studies, such as Lipshultz et al. [20], which identified a higher risk of cardiac dysfunction in childhood cancer survivors, particularly in those exposed to anthracycline therapy or chest radiation.

Importantly, our study revealed no statistically significant differences in cardiac function parameters when stratified by cancer histology, suggesting a consistent impact across various cancer types. While this seems to be in contrast to prior research such as that by Mulrooney et al. [21] and Getz et al. [22], it is crucial to consider several factors. First, the chemotherapeutic agents used in those studies were different from those in ours, with some using agents like dexrazoxane instead of doxorubicin for AML. The cardiotoxic profile of different chemotherapy agents can vary widely, potentially accounting for the disparate findings. Additionally, population characteristics, such as the age group, baseline health status, and the presence of other comorbidities, might have been different in these studies, leading to varied results. Moreover, sample size, methodology, and the instruments used to measure cardiac function can also influence findings. For instance, if Mulrooney et al. [21] had a larger sample size, they might have had more statistical power to detect subtle differences that our study could not. Similarly, variations in methodology, such as the time intervals between chemotherapy sessions and cardiac function measurements, can yield different results.

The uniform impact of treatment intensity on cardiac function across various protocols, as observed in our study, deviates from previous literature. Studies like Armenian et al. [23] have indicated differential impacts based on treatment protocols. Several reasons could account for this discrepancy. The definition and classification of treatment intensity might differ between studies. What was considered "intense" in our study could potentially be "moderate" or "mild" in another. Furthermore, the follow-up duration and intervals to check cardiac function post-treatment could vary, leading to differences in the observed impacts. Lastly, the previous studies might have included more diverse treatment protocols, or their patient population might have had different vulnerabilities to certain treatments. However, it is possible that the robustness and sensitivity of the novel echocardiographic measures used in the present study allowed for a more nuanced and sensitive detection of early cardiac dysfunction, thus capturing changes that traditional methods might have missed.

Interestingly, the regression analysis results showed a significant association between combinations of novel echocardiographic measures (GLS, SMOD, and MPI) and the development of cardiac toxicity. This finding suggests that the combined use of these novel measures might provide more accurate and early detection of cardiac dysfunction in pediatric oncology patients. This supports the contention of several previous studies, such as Thavendiranathan et al. [24] and Poterucha et al. [25], who argued for the combined use of novel echocardiographic measures to improve the prediction of chemotherapy-related cardiac dysfunction. Moreover, this combined approach may have the potential to facilitate early intervention, thus mitigating the risk of long-term cardiac complications in this vulnerable population. This aligns with recent research by Narayan et al. [26], who demonstrated that early detection and intervention can improve cardiac outcomes in pediatric oncology patients.

Our results accentuate that pediatric oncology patients post-chemotherapy demonstrated significant decrements in cardiac function when compared to healthy controls. Parameters such as EF and GLS showcased notably lower values in the cases than in controls, indicative of reduced systolic function and compromised cardiac health, respectively. These findings align with the prevailing literature suggesting potential cardiotoxic effects of certain chemotherapy agents on pediatric patients, warranting heightened surveillance and potential interventions to ameliorate these impacts [27,28]. Additionally, while variations in cardiac measurements based on cancer histology and treatment protocol were noted, these were not statistically significant. This underlines the need for more expansive studies, possibly integrating multi-center data, to discern the nuanced effects of different treatment modalities and disease types on pediatric cardiac health. As childhood cancer survivors continue to live longer due to advances in therapy, understanding these cardiac repercussions becomes paramount for tailoring long-term care and optimizing quality of life.

The findings of this study also highlight the potential predictive value of these novel echocardiographic measures in forecasting long-term cardiac outcomes in pediatric oncology patients. This echoes the findings of studies such as Cheung et al. [29] and Kang et al. [30], which identified a significant correlation between early changes in these measures and long-term cardiac outcomes. Therefore, these results underscore the significant impact of cancer and its treatment on cardiac function in pediatric oncology patients. The present study's use of novel echocardiographic measures (GLS, SMOD, and MPI) offers a valuable approach to detecting early cardiac dysfunction and potentially forecasting long-term cardiac outcomes in this population. These findings underscore the importance of ongoing research in this area to further refine these methods and to develop targeted interventions to mitigate the cardiac risks associated with pediatric oncology treatment. Lastly, there is a need for a follow-up study that looks into the time of initial detection of cardiac function abnormalities by the different echocardiographic methods, spanning a period longer than four years. This would help in drawing a more definitive comparison between traditional and novel measures in predicting anthracycline-induced cardiotoxicity.

4.2. Study Limitations

While this study provides valuable insights into the potential of speckle tracking echocardiography, global longitudinal strain, and the myocardial performance index as sensitive indicators of early anthracycline-induced cardiotoxicity, it has several limitations. Firstly, the study's single-center, retrospective design might limit the generalizability of its findings. Data from a single institution might not adequately capture the variability of clinical practices across different centers, potentially biasing the results. Furthermore, the retrospective nature of the study might introduce selection bias, with the potential for missing or incomplete data. The reliance on historical records could also lead to information bias due to inaccuracies in documentation. Secondly, the study was conducted over a four-year period, which might be insufficient to determine the long-term cardiac effects of anthracycline therapy. Late-onset cardiotoxicity can occur many years after treatment cessation; thus, the follow-up period might need to be extended to fully assess these effects.

Additionally, the study did not account for other factors that might influence cardiac function, such as patients' physical activity levels, nutritional status, or other comorbidities. The impact of these confounding variables on cardiac function should be considered in future studies. The exclusion of patients who had started treatment before baseline measurements could be established might have resulted in a selection bias, potentially excluding patients with more aggressive disease who needed immediate treatment. Furthermore, patients with severe infections or metabolic diseases were also excluded, potentially creating a cohort of patients in better overall health than the general population of pediatric oncology patients.

Lastly, while the study included a healthy control group, these controls were patients who sought medical care for minor conditions, possibly introducing a "healthy patient bias". Furthermore, matching cases and controls by age, gender, and body mass index might not have controlled for all potential confounding variables. Other factors such as socioeconomic status or genetic predispositions might also influence cardiac outcomes and were not considered in this study. Despite these limitations, the study provides valuable insights into the potential use of novel echocardiographic measures to detect early cardiac dysfunction in pediatric oncology patients. Further research, particularly multicenter, prospective studies with longer follow-up periods, is needed to validate these findings and to better understand the long-term cardiac outcomes in this population.

5. Conclusions

The study concluded that pediatric oncology patients exhibited significant differences in cardiac function post-chemotherapy compared to that of healthy controls, as evidenced by measurements including the ejection fraction (EF), global longitudinal strain (GLS), Simpson's method of discs (SMOD), and the myocardial performance index (MPI). These measurements suggested an increased prevalence of cardiac dysfunction in patients, corroborating the hypothesis that cancer type and treatment intensity significantly impacted cardiac function. Notably, early changes detected by GLS, SMOD, and MPI were associated with long-term cardiac outcomes, establishing these methods as potentially superior to traditional echocardiographic measures in identifying early cardiac dysfunction. However, the variations in cardiac function measurements among different cancer histologies and treatment protocols did not reach statistical significance. Interestingly, the combination of GLS, SMOD, and MPI demonstrated the highest association with the development of cardiac toxicity, indicating a sevenfold increase in risk. While the data indicated a promise of these novel measures, further longitudinal studies, spanning longer durations, are needed to truly validate their long-term predictive value.

Author Contributions: Conceptualization, A.M.A. and I.C.O.; methodology, A.M.A. and I.C.O.; software, R.I. and R.J.; validation, R.I. and R.J.; formal analysis, C.S. and M.M.; investigation, C.S. and M.M.; resources, R.M.F.; data curation, R.M.F.; writing—original draft preparation, A.M.A.; writing—review and editing, L.B., C.D. and A.N.; visualization, L.B., C.D., and A.N.; supervision, A.M. and G.D.; project administration, A.M. and G.D. All authors have read and agreed to the published version of the manuscript.

Funding: This research received no external funding.

Institutional Review Board Statement: The study was conducted in accordance with the Declaration of Helsinki and approved by the Institutional Review Board of the Emergency Hospital for Children "Louis Țurcanu", from Timisoara, Romania.

Informed Consent Statement: Informed consent was obtained for all subjects involved in the study.

Data Availability Statement: Data available on request.

Conflicts of Interest: The authors declare no conflict of interest.

References

1. Williams, A.M.; Liu, Q.; Bhakta, N.; Krull, K.R.; Hudson, M.M.; Robison, L.L.; Yasui, Y. Rethinking Success in Pediatric Oncology: Beyond 5-Year Survival. *J. Clin. Oncol.* **2021**, *39*, 2227–2231. [CrossRef]
2. Tan, T.C.; Scherrer-Crosbie, M. Cardiac complications of chemotherapy: Role of imaging. *Curr. Treat. Options Cardiovasc. Med.* **2014**, *16*, 296. [CrossRef] [PubMed]
3. Chen, H.H.W.; Kuo, M.T. Improving radiotherapy in cancer treatment: Promises and challenges. *Oncotarget* **2017**, *8*, 62742–62758. [CrossRef] [PubMed]
4. Angsutararux, P.; Luanpitpong, S.; Issaragrisil, S. Chemotherapy-Induced Cardiotoxicity: Overview of the Roles of Oxidative Stress. *Oxidative Med. Cell. Longev.* **2015**, *2015*, 795602. [CrossRef]
5. Herrmann, J. Adverse cardiac effects of cancer therapies: Cardiotoxicity and arrhythmia. *Nat. Rev. Cardiol.* **2020**, *17*, 474–502. [CrossRef] [PubMed]
6. Aleman, B.M.; Moser, E.C.; Nuver, J.; Suter, T.M.; Maraldo, M.V.; Specht, L.; Vrieling, C.; Darby, S.C. Cardiovascular disease after cancer therapy. *EJC Suppl.* **2014**, *12*, 18–28. [CrossRef] [PubMed]

7. Border, W.L.; Sachdeva, R.; Stratton, K.L.; Armenian, S.H.; Bhat, A.; Cox, D.E.; Leger, K.J.; Leisenring, W.M.; Meacham, L.R.; Sadak, K.T.; et al. Longitudinal Changes in Echocardiographic Parameters of Cardiac Function in Pediatric Cancer Survivors. *JACC CardioOncology* **2020**, *2*, 26–37. [CrossRef]
8. Li, C.K.; Sung, R.Y.; Kwok, K.L.; Leung, T.F.; Shing, M.M.; Chik, K.W.; Yu, C.W.; Yam, M.C.; Yuen, P.M. A longitudinal study of cardiac function in children with cancer over 40 months. *Pediatr. Hematol. Oncol.* **2000**, *17*, 77–83. [CrossRef]
9. Löffler, A.I.; Salerno, M. Cardiac MRI for the evaluation of oncologic cardiotoxicity. *J. Nucl. Cardiol.* **2018**, *25*, 2148–2158. [CrossRef]
10. Cardinale, D.; Iacopo, F.; Cipolla, C.M. Cardiotoxicity of Anthracyclines. *Front. Cardiovasc. Med.* **2020**, *7*, 26. [CrossRef]
11. Bergamini, C.; Dolci, G.; Truong, S.; Zanolla, L.; Benfari, G.; Fiorio, E.; Rossi, A.; Ribichini, F.L. Role of Speckle Tracking Echocardiography in the Evaluation of Breast Cancer Patients Undergoing Chemotherapy: Review and Meta-analysis of the Literature. *Cardiovasc. Toxicol.* **2019**, *19*, 485–492. [CrossRef] [PubMed]
12. Laufer-Perl, M.; Gilon, D.; Kapusta, L.; Iakobishvili, Z. The Role of Speckle Strain Echocardiography in the Diagnosis of Early Subclinical Cardiac Injury in Cancer Patients-Is There More Than Just Left Ventricle Global Longitudinal Strain? *J. Clin. Med.* **2021**, *10*, 154. [CrossRef]
13. Zhu, H.; Guo, Y.; Wang, X.; Yang, C.; Li, Y.; Meng, X.; Pei, Z.; Zhang, R.; Zhong, Y.; Wang, F. Myocardial Work by Speckle Tracking Echocardiography Accurately Assesses Left Ventricular Function of Coronary Artery Disease Patients. *Front. Cardiovasc. Med.* **2021**, *8*, 727389. [CrossRef] [PubMed]
14. Verbeke, J.; Calle, S.; Kamoen, V.; De Buyzere, M.; Timmermans, F. Prognostic value of myocardial work and global longitudinal strain in patients with heart failure and functional mitral regurgitation. *Int. J. Cardiovasc. Imaging* **2021**, *38*, 803–812. [CrossRef]
15. Salvo, G.D.; Pergola, V.; Fadel, B.; Bulbul, Z.A.; Caso, P. Strain Echocardiography and Myocardial Mechanics: From Basics to Clinical Applications. *J. Cardiovasc. Echogr.* **2015**, *25*, 1–8. [CrossRef]
16. Diao, K.Y.; Yang, Z.G.; Ma, M.; He, Y.; Zhao, Q.; Liu, X.; Gao, Y.; Xie, L.J.; Guo, Y.K. The Diagnostic Value of Global Longitudinal Strain (GLS) on Myocardial Infarction Size by Echocardiography: A Systematic Review and Meta-analysis. *Sci. Rep.* **2017**, *7*, 10082. [CrossRef]
17. Goroshi, M.; Chand, D. Myocardial Performance Index (Tei Index): A simple tool to identify cardiac dysfunction in patients with diabetes mellitus. *Indian Heart J.* **2016**, *68*, 83–87. [CrossRef]
18. Muntean, I.; Melinte, M.; Făgărășan, A.; Șuteu, C.C.; Togănel, R. A Novel Speckle-Tracking Echocardiography Derived Parameter That Predicts Clinical Worsening in Children with Pulmonary Arterial Hypertension. *Appl. Sci.* **2022**, *12*, 5494. [CrossRef]
19. Wilke, L.; Abellan Schneyder, F.E.; Roskopf, M.; Jenke, A.C.; Heusch, A.; Hensel, K.O. Speckle tracking stress echocardiography in children: Interobserver and intraobserver reproducibility and the impact of echocardiographic image quality. *Sci. Rep.* **2018**, *8*, 9185. [CrossRef]
20. Lipshultz, S.E.; Scully, R.E.; Lipsitz, S.R.; Sallan, S.E.; Silverman, L.B.; Miller, T.L.; Barry, E.V.; Asselin, B.L.; Athale, U.; Clavell, L.A.; et al. Assessment of dexrazoxane as a cardioprotectant in doxorubicin-treated children with high-risk acute lymphoblastic leukaemia: Long-term follow-up of a prospective, randomised, multicentre trial. *Lancet Oncol.* **2010**, *11*, 950–961. [CrossRef]
21. Mulrooney, D.A.; Yeazel, M.W.; Kawashima, T.; Mertens, A.C.; Mitby, P.; Stovall, M.; Donaldson, S.S.; Green, D.M.; Sklar, C.A.; Robison, L.L.; et al. Cardiac outcomes in a cohort of adult survivors of childhood and adolescent cancer: Retrospective analysis of the Childhood Cancer Survivor Study cohort. *BMJ* **2009**, *339*, b4606. [CrossRef]
22. Getz, K.D.; Sung, L.; Alonzo, T.A.; Leger, K.J.; Gerbing, R.B.; Pollard, J.A.; Cooper, T.; Kolb, E.A.; Gamis, A.S.; Ky, B.; et al. Effect of Dexrazoxane on Left Ventricular Systolic Function and Treatment Outcomes in Patients with Acute Myeloid Leukemia: A Report From the Children's Oncology Group. *J. Clin. Oncol.* **2020**, *38*, 2398–2406. [CrossRef] [PubMed]
23. Armenian, S.H.; Hudson, M.M.; Mulder, R.L.; Chen, M.H.; Constine, L.S.; Dwyer, M.; Nathan, P.C.; Tissing, W.J.; Shankar, S.; Sieswerda, E.; et al. Recommendations for cardiomyopathy surveillance for survivors of childhood cancer: A report from the International Late Effects of Childhood Cancer Guideline Harmonization Group. *Lancet Oncol.* **2015**, *16*, e123–e136. [CrossRef]
24. Thavendiranathan, P.; Poulin, F.; Lim, K.D.; Plana, J.C.; Woo, A.; Marwick, T.H. Use of myocardial strain imaging by echocardiography for the early detection of cardiotoxicity in patients during and after cancer chemotherapy: A systematic review. *J. Am. Coll. Cardiol.* **2014**, *63*, 2751–2768. [CrossRef]
25. Poterucha, J.T.; Kutty, S.; Lindquist, R.K.; Li, L.; Eidem, B.W. Changes in left ventricular longitudinal strain with anthracycline chemotherapy in adolescents precede subsequent decreased left ventricular ejection fraction. *J. Am. Soc. Echocardiogr.* **2012**, *25*, 733–740. [CrossRef] [PubMed]
26. Narayan, H.K.; French, B.; Khan, A.M.; Plappert, T.; Hyman, D.; Bajulaiye, A.; Domchek, S.; DeMichele, A.; Clark, A.; Matro, J.; et al. Noninvasive Measures of Ventricular-Arterial Coupling and Circumferential Strain Predict Cancer Therapeutics-Related Cardiac Dysfunction. *JACC Cardiovasc. Imaging* **2016**, *9*, 1131–1141. [CrossRef]
27. Avila, M.S.; Siqueira, S.R.R.; Ferreira, S.M.A.; Bocchi, E.A. Prevention and Treatment of Chemotherapy-Induced Cardiotoxicity. *Methodist DeBakey Cardiovasc. J.* **2019**, *15*, 267–273. [CrossRef] [PubMed]
28. Hitawala, G.; Jain, E.; Castellanos, L.; Garimella, R.; Akku, R.; Chamavaliyathil, A.K.; Irfan, H.; Jaiswal, V.; Quinonez, J.; Dakroub, M.; et al. Pediatric Chemotherapy Drugs Associated With Cardiotoxicity. *Cureus* **2021**, *13*, e19658. [CrossRef]

29. Cheung, Y.F.; Hong, W.J.; Chan, G.C.; Wong, S.J.; Ha, S.Y. Left ventricular myocardial deformation and mechanical dyssynchrony in children with normal ventricular shortening fraction after anthracycline therapy. *Heart* **2010**, *96*, 1137–1141. [CrossRef]
30. Kang, Y.; Cheng, L.; Li, L.; Chen, H.; Sun, M.; Wei, Z.; Pan, C.; Shu, X. Early detection of anthracycline-induced cardiotoxicity using two-dimensional speckle tracking echocardiography. *Cardiol. J.* **2013**, *20*, 592–599. [CrossRef]

Disclaimer/Publisher's Note: The statements, opinions and data contained in all publications are solely those of the individual author(s) and contributor(s) and not of MDPI and/or the editor(s). MDPI and/or the editor(s) disclaim responsibility for any injury to people or property resulting from any ideas, methods, instructions or products referred to in the content.

MDPI
St. Alban-Anlage 66
4052 Basel
Switzerland
www.mdpi.com

Diagnostics Editorial Office
E-mail: diagnostics@mdpi.com
www.mdpi.com/journal/diagnostics

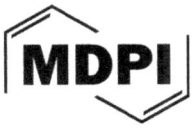

Disclaimer/Publisher's Note: The statements, opinions and data contained in all publications are solely those of the individual author(s) and contributor(s) and not of MDPI and/or the editor(s). MDPI and/or the editor(s) disclaim responsibility for any injury to people or property resulting from any ideas, methods, instructions or products referred to in the content.

www.ingramcontent.com/pod-product-compliance
Lightning Source LLC
LaVergne TN
LVHW070718100526
838202LV00013B/1120